Early Detection and Treatment
of Head & Neck Cancers

Rami El Assal
Dyani Gaudilliere
Stephen Thaddeus Connelly

Editors

Early Detection and Treatment of Head & Neck Cancers

Theoretical Background and Newly Emerging Research

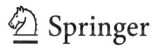 Springer

Editors
Rami El Assal
Canary Center at Stanford for Cancer Early Detection
Stanford University School of Medicine
Palo Alto, CA
USA

Dyani Gaudilliere
Division of Plastic & Reconstructive Surgery, Department of Surgery
Stanford University School of Medicine
Palo Alto, CA
USA

Stephen Thaddeus Connelly
Department of Oral and Maxillofacial Surgery
University of California, San Francisco
San Francisco, CA
USA

ISBN 978-3-030-69854-6   ISBN 978-3-030-69852-2   (eBook)
https://doi.org/10.1007/978-3-030-69852-2

This Springer imprint is published by the registered company Springer Nature Switzerland AG
The registered company address is: Gewerbestrasse 11, 6330 Cham, Switzerland

This book is dedicated to the late Professor Sam Gambhir of Stanford.

Sam was the pioneer in the foundation of cancer early detection. He dedicated his life to developing methods of early disease detection, ushering in a new era of molecular imaging and nanotechnologies to flag signals of disease in its nascent stages. Dr. Gambhir was the Virginia and D.K. Ludwig professor of cancer research and chair of radiology at Stanford University School of Medicine. He was the founding director of the Canary Center at Stanford for Cancer Early Detection, Precision Health and Integrated Diagnostics Center at Stanford, and the director of the molecular imaging program at Stanford.

The editor-in-chief, Dr. Rami El Assal, would like to express his gratitude for the selfless devotion of Dr. Gambhir, a kind and honest man. Dr. El Assal commented, "In our last meeting while I was transitioning out of Stanford, Dr. Gambhir demonstrated the care and support to me at multi-level including stating that 'if you wanted to come back to Stanford, just let me know.'"

Dr. El Assal added, "I still remember that in the 2015 Department of Radiology Retreat, Sam stated, 'I want to make an impact on human health even if it is not recognized in my lifetime.'" "And I believe he did," *Dr. El Assal said.*

Foreword

It is with great pleasure that I write this foreword for the first edition of *Early Detection and Treatment of Head and Neck Cancer* (HNC). The fields of early detection and early treatment in cancer biology are advancing rapidly as both the concept and practical applications have entered clinical practice.

The recent release of the most comprehensive genomic HNC data to date (Nature, 2015) from The Cancer Genome Atlas, a project funded by the National Institute of Health to characterize cancer genomes, is enabling scientists to refine their list of candidate biomarkers and to identify new ones for early detection of HNCs. Such an expanding body of knowledge is essential given that roughly two-thirds of HNCs present at advanced stages, and the prognosis remains poor. Therefore, new approaches are urgently needed for early HNC detection to improve treatment outcomes. For example, circulating DNA has shown great promise as a non-invasively obtained biomarker in a number of HNC cohorts. Using the known mutational signatures of HNC to identify tumor DNA in body fluids has demonstrated the potential for detecting tumors at early stages and for monitoring tumor relapse and response to treatment.

In the era of precision health and medicine, there are opportunities to select treatment plans that are most likely to succeed based on an individual's personal data. HNC can be monitored and treated more efficiently by taking multiple forms of medical data into consideration and by implementing more effective methodologies that are currently being validated, including liquid biopsy, salivary biomarkers, imaging, and treatments, including gene therapy, immunotherapy, surgery, radiotherapy, and many others.

Early detection is an evidence-based field in which we have come a long way, but it is still in its infancy. We have discovered many of the fundamental principles but still need to develop, translate, and improve detection and diagnostics as well as treatment standards to, hopefully, prevent cancer, including HNC.

Here, I would like to invite readers to enjoy the carefully and expertly prepared material by the authors of this book series (Volumes I and II), which are based on solid scientific evidence and diverse clinical experience achieved through many years of professional practice.

R. Bruce Donoff, DMD, MD
Dean of Harvard School of Dental Medicine (1991–2019)
Boston, MA, USA

Dean Emeritus R. Bruce Donoff in Few Words

Dr. R. Bruce Donoff served as dean of Harvard School of Dental Medicine (HSDM) from 1991 to 2019. He was born in New York City and attended Brooklyn College as an undergraduate. He received his DMD from HSDM in 1967 and his MD from Harvard Medical School in 1973. Dr. Donoff's professional career has centered on Harvard's Faculty of Medicine and the Massachusetts General Hospital's Department of Oral and Maxillofacial Surgery. He began as an intern in 1967, served as chairman and chief of service from 1982 through 1993, and continues to see patients today.

In addition to leading HSDM as its dean, Dr. Donoff has made major contributions in research to the specialty of oral and maxillofacial surgery with interest in oral and head and neck cancers. He has published over one hundred papers, authored textbooks, and lectured worldwide. He recently helped launch the HSDM Initiative – Integrating Oral Health and Medicine, a project of great importance to him.

Dr. Donoff served 12 years on the board of the Oral and Maxillofacial Surgery Foundation and is former president of the Friends of the National Institute of Dental and Craniofacial Research. He is editor of the *MGH Manual of Oral and Maxillofacial Surgery* and a member of the editorial board of the *Journal of Oral and Maxillofacial Surgery* and the *Massachusetts Dental Society Journal*.

Dr. Donoff has received numerous honors during his academic career, including the American Association of Oral and Maxillofacial Surgeons Research Recognition Award, the William J. Gies Foundation Award for Oral and Maxillofacial Surgery, Fellow of the American Association for the Advancement of Science, the Alpha Omega Achievement Award, and the Distinguished Alumni and Faculty Awards from HSDM. In 2014, he was a Shils-Meskin awardee for leadership in the dental profession.

Acknowledgments

A Historic Perspective

> I shall be telling this with a sigh somewhere ages and ages hence;
> Two roads diverged in a wood, and I took the road less traveled by,
> And that has made all the difference.

– The Road Not Taken by Robert Frost, 1916

I would like to acknowledge first and foremost my family:

To my mother who endured this long process with me, always offering support and for whom grace is all in her steps, heaven in her eye, in every gesture dignity and love. Everything I am or ever hope to be, I owe to my angel mother.

To my wife, Somayeh, and my son, Adam, you all are my world and reason for being. My gratitude for your understanding that my career being of service to others often entails long hours. Thank you for your patience and compassion.

To my sister, Lina, who always supported and guided me all the way, and my devoted brother-in-law, Ghiath, and my elegant nieces, Sana, Maria, Naya, and Zeina.

To my brother, Shadi, who was always there for me.

I can never forget my father, who was a blend of strength (may he rest in peace).

To my cousin, Hussein, whose friendship and support I treasure.

To my wife's family: my father- and mother-in-law; brother-in-law, Wahid; and my sisters-in-law, Susan, Samira, Sudaba, and Saeeda.

To my close friends whom I consider part of my family. They helped shape my education and supported me throughout my academic and professional journey.

Additionally, I would like to thank my friends and co-editors, Dyani and Thaddeus; without their help, this book would not have come to fruition. I am so proud of you and wish to let you know that your friendship touches me deeply. I know we will continue to work closely in the future and support one another's ideas and projects.

I would like to express my sincere gratitude to all authors who contributed to these two volumes; this project would not be possible without their contribution.

I feel a deep sense of gratitude to Emeritus Dean R. Bruce Donoff, who kindly wrote the foreword to this book series.

To all of my past teachers, mentors, and fellow students, I hope this book is worthy of the many contributions you have given me.

I am very grateful to all my colleagues and friends around the world.

Lastly, to head and neck cancer (HNC) patients, my respectful and gentle gratitude goes to you all. As a part of our commitment to service HNC patients, I recently co-founded with Thaddeus an "Early Disease Detection & Treatment Fund" to translate innovations from research labs, bringing them close to patients. We are proud to have partnered and invested with visionary entrepreneurs who are tackling head and neck cancers.

Palo Alto, CA, USA   Rami El Assal

Preface

Volume II of this book series provides an up-to-date overview of the theoretical background in the field of head and neck cancer (HNC) as well as of the emerging research that is impacting our understanding of this disease.

Volume II begins with a comprehensive review of the epidemiology, etiology, symptoms, diagnosis, and staging of HNC. Next, it covers the essentials of potentially malignant disorders of the oral cavity, an important variety of HNC.

Subsequently, Volume II covers the newly emerging research in the field of HNC. For example, the advances in genomics research during the past few decades allowed us to better understand the mutational landscape of HNC. In addition, a comprehensive understanding of the pro-inflammatory signaling pathways in HNC could lead to the identification of novel biomarkers for early detection and the development of new therapeutic strategies. Furthermore, an increasing number of studies demonstrate that circulating biomarkers, such as circulating tumor DNA (ctDNA), circulating tumor cells (CTCs), and exosomal miRNAs, can open up new avenues to comprehensively study, early detect, and precisely treat HNC. The overall goal is to shift towards precision medicine (discussed in detail in Volume I), which will bring individualized clinical benefit to patients with HNC.

We conclude this volume with the topic of chronic pain associated with HNC, including both the mechanisms of pain and the management strategies, and the emerging oral mucoadhesive drug delivery approach for HNC. All HNC surgeons, scientists, residents, and individuals, whose lives have been touched by this disease, will recognize the impact pain has upon a patient's health and his or her recovery trajectory.

The editors and the authors of the chapters herein hope that the valuable information presented will help you grow your knowledge base and improve your ability to successfully treat a wide variety of HNCs.

Palo Alto, CA, USA   Rami El Assal
Palo Alto, CA, USA   Dyani Gaudilliere
San Francisco, CA, USA   Stephen Thaddeus Connelly

Contents

Contributors

Hamzah Alkofahi Division of Plastic & Reconstructive Surgery, Department of Surgery, Stanford University School of Medicine, Stanford, CA, USA

Department of Oral and Maxillofacial Surgery, Jordanian Royal Medical Services, Irbid, Jordan

Zhong Chen Tumor Biology Section, Head and Neck Surgery Branch, National Institute on Deafness and Other Communication Disorders, National Institutes of Health, Bethesda, MD, USA

Stephen Thaddeus Connelly Department of Oral and Maxillofacial Surgery, University of California San Francisco (UCSF) School of Dentistry, San Francisco, CA, USA

San Francisco VA Health Care System, San Francisco, CA, USA

Mehdi Ebrahimi Prince Philip Dental Hospital, The University of Hong Kong, Pok Fu Lam, Hong Kong, China

Lisa M. Evangelista Department of Otolaryngology/Head & Neck Surgery, University of California at Davis Medical Center, Sacramento, CA, USA

Ayman Fouad Department of Otolaryngology, Head & Neck Surgery, Stanford University, Stanford, CA, USA

Department of Otolaryngology, Head & Neck Surgery, Tanta University, Tanta, Egypt

Jennifer R. Grandis Department of Otolaryngology – Head and Neck Surgery, University of California at San Francisco, San Francisco, CA, USA

Jun Jeon Tumor Biology Section, Head and Neck Surgery Branch, National Institute on Deafness and Other Communication Disorders, National Institutes of Health, Bethesda, MD, USA

Daniel E. Johnson Department of Otolaryngology – Head and Neck Surgery, University of California at San Francisco, San Francisco, CA, USA

Nagarjun Konduru Department of Cellular and Molecular Biology, University of Texas Health Science Center at Tyler, Tyler, TX, USA

Shilpa Kusampudi Department of Cellular and Molecular Biology, University of Texas Health Science Center at Tyler, Tyler, TX, USA

Peter Luke Santa Maria Department of Oral Rehabilitation, Prince Philip Dental Hospital, The University of Hong Kong, Pok Fu Lam, Hong Kong, USA

Solange Massa Department of Otolaryngology, Head & Neck Surgery, Stanford University, Stanford, CA, USA

Ethan L. Morgan Tumor Biology Section, Head and Neck Surgery Branch, National Institute on Deafness and Other Communication Disorders, National Institutes of Health, Bethesda, MD, USA

Taichiro Nonaka Center for Oral/Head and Neck Oncology Research, School of Dentistry, University of California, Los Angeles, Los Angeles, CA, USA

Division of Oral Biology and Medicine, School of Dentistry, University of California, Los Angeles, Los Angeles, CA, USA

Kelechi Nwachuku School of Medicine, University of California at San Francisco, San Francisco, CA, USA

M. Anthony Pogrel Department of Oral and Maxillofacial Surgery, University of California, San Francisco, San Francisco, CA, USA

Carter Van Waes Tumor Biology Section, Head and Neck Surgery Branch, National Institute on Deafness and Other Communication Disorders, National Institutes of Health, Bethesda, MD, USA

Ramya Viswanathan Tumor Biology Section, Head and Neck Surgery Branch, National Institute on Deafness and Other Communication Disorders, National Institutes of Health, Bethesda, MD, USA

David T. W. Wong Center for Oral/Head and Neck Oncology Research, School of Dentistry, University of California, Los Angeles, Los Angeles, CA, USA

Division of Oral Biology and Medicine, School of Dentistry, University of California, Los Angeles, Los Angeles, CA, USA

Justin M. Young Private Practice, San Francisco, CA, USA

Department of Oral & Maxillofacial Surgery, University of the Pacific, Arthur A. Dugoni School of Dentistry, San Francisco, CA, USA

Chapter 1
General Introduction to Head and Neck Cancer: Etiology, Symptoms, Diagnosis, Staging, Prevention, and Treatment

Shilpa Kusampudi and Nagarjun Konduru

Introduction

Head and neck cancer (HNC) is a terminology used for a group of cancers originating in the lips, oral cavity, oropharynx, salivary glands, larynx, pharynx, hypopharynx, nasopharynx, and sinuses (Fig. 1.1). These cancers most commonly affect squamous cells, accounting for about 90% of all HNC [1–4]. In the 1950s, tumors of the facial bones, as well as primary and metastatic tumors of the neck and thyroid neoplasms were also termed head and neck tumors [5]. However, presently these tumors fall under different categories of malignancies such as thyroid and parathyroid malignancies under endocrine neoplasms and lymph nodes under hematological malignancies.

Neoplasms in various regions of the body are assigned codes, with C00–C14, C30, and C32 coding for head and neck cancers (Table 1.1).

Epidemiology

HNC is the sixth most common type of cancers, based on the estimated number of new cases (Fig. 1.2). In 2018, 710,237 out of 18 million new cases of all cancers recorded worldwide were HNC.

Based on Globocan world cancer data for 2018, the global incidence of HNC is 4.9% of all cancers (Fig. 1.3). Among the various HNCs, lip and oral cavity cancers together accounted for the highest percentage of the global HNC cases (40%),

S. Kusampudi · N. Konduru (✉)
Department of Cellular and Molecular Biology, University of Texas Health Science
Center at Tyler, Tyler, TX, USA
e-mail: nagarjun.konduruvenkata@uthct.edu

© Springer Nature Switzerland AG 2021   1
R. El Assal et al. (eds.), *Early Detection and Treatment of Head & Neck
Cancers*, https://doi.org/10.1007/978-3-030-69852-2_1

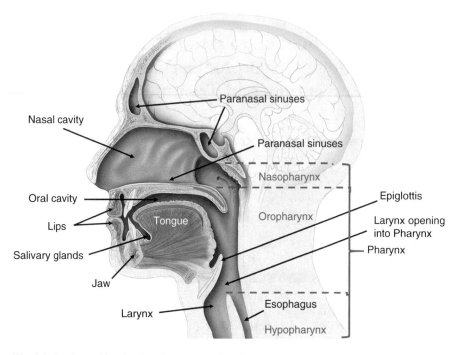

Fig. 1.1 Regions of head and neck cancer. (Edited from [6])

Table 1.1 Head and neck cancer codes

Cancer code	Cancer
C00–C06	Lip, oral cavity
C000	Malignant neoplasm of external upper lip
C001	Malignant neoplasm of external lower lip
C002	Malignant neoplasm of external lip, unspecified
C003	Malignant neoplasm of upper lip, inner aspect
C004	Malignant neoplasm of lower lip, inner aspect
C005	Malignant neoplasm of lip, unspecified, inner aspect
C006	Malignant neoplasm of commissure of lip, unspecified
C008	Malignant neoplasm of overlapping sites of lip
C009	Malignant neoplasm of lip, unspecified
C010	Malignant neoplasm of base of tongue
C020	Malignant neoplasm of dorsal surface of tongue
C021	Malignant neoplasm of border of tongue
C022	Malignant neoplasm of ventral surface of tongue
C023	Malignant neoplasm of anterior two-thirds of tongue, part unspecified
C024	Malignant neoplasm of lingual tonsil
C028	Malignant neoplasm of overlapping sites of tongue
C029	Malignant neoplasm of tongue, unspecified
C030	Malignant neoplasm of upper gum

Table 1.1 (continued)

Cancer code	Cancer
C031	Malignant neoplasm of lower gum
C039	Malignant neoplasm of gum, unspecified
C040	Malignant neoplasm of anterior floor of mouth
C041	Malignant neoplasm of lateral floor of mouth
C048	Malignant neoplasm of overlapping sites of floor of mouth
C049	Malignant neoplasm of floor of mouth, unspecified
C050	Malignant neoplasm of hard palate
C051	Malignant neoplasm of soft palate
C052	Malignant neoplasm of uvula
C058	Malignant neoplasm of overlapping sites of palate
C059	Malignant neoplasm of palate, unspecified
C060	Malignant neoplasm of cheek mucosa
C061	Malignant neoplasm of vestibule of mouth
C062	Malignant neoplasm of retromolar area
C0680	Malignant neoplasm of overlapping sites of unspecified parts of mouth
C0689	Malignant neoplasm of overlapping sites of other parts of mouth
C069	Malignant neoplasm of mouth, unspecified
C07–08	Salivary glands
C07	Malignant neoplasm of parotid gland
C080	Malignant neoplasm of submandibular gland
C081	Malignant neoplasm of sublingual gland
C089	Malignant neoplasm of major salivary gland, unspecified
C09–10	Oropharynx
C090	Malignant neoplasm of tonsillar fossa
C091	Malignant neoplasm of tonsillar pillar (anterior) (posterior)
C098	Malignant neoplasm of overlapping sites of tonsil
C099	Malignant neoplasm of tonsil, unspecified
C100	Malignant neoplasm of vallecula
C101	Malignant neoplasm of anterior surface of epiglottis
C102	Malignant neoplasm of lateral wall of oropharynx
C103	Malignant neoplasm of posterior wall of oropharynx
C104	Malignant neoplasm of branchial cleft
C108	Malignant neoplasm of overlapping sites of oropharynx
C109	Malignant neoplasm of oropharynx, unspecified
C11	Nasopharynx
C110	Malignant neoplasm of superior wall of nasopharynx
C111	Malignant neoplasm of posterior wall of nasopharynx
C112	Malignant neoplasm of lateral wall of nasopharynx
C113	Malignant neoplasm of anterior wall of nasopharynx
C118	Malignant neoplasm of overlapping sites of nasopharynx
C119	Malignant neoplasm of nasopharynx, unspecified
C12–13	Hypopharynx
C12	Malignant neoplasm of pyriform sinus

(continued)

Table 1.1 (continued)

Cancer code	Cancer
C130	Malignant neoplasm of postcricoid region
C131	Malignant neoplasm of aryepiglottic fold, hypopharyngeal aspect
C132	Malignant neoplasm of posterior wall of hypopharynx
C138	Malignant neoplasm of overlapping sites of hypopharynx
C139	Malignant neoplasm of hypopharynx, unspecified
C14	Unspecified
C140	Malignant neoplasm of pharynx, unspecified
C142	Malignant neoplasm of Waldeyer's ring
C148	Malignant neoplasm of overlapping sites of lip, oral cavity, and pharynx
C30–31	Sinus cancer
C30	Malignant neoplasm of nasal cavity
C301	Malignant neoplasm of middle ear
C310	Malignant neoplasm of maxillary sinus
C311	Malignant neoplasm of ethmoidal sinus
C312	Malignant neoplasm of frontal sinus
C313	Malignant neoplasm of sphenoid sinus
C318	Malignant neoplasm of overlapping sites of accessory sinuses
C319	Malignant neoplasm of accessory sinus, unspecified
C32	Malignant neoplasm of glottis
C321	Malignant neoplasm of supraglottis
C322	Malignant neoplasm of subglottis
C323	Malignant neoplasm of laryngeal cartilage
C328	Malignant neoplasm of overlapping sites of larynx
C329	Malignant neoplasm of larynx, unspecified

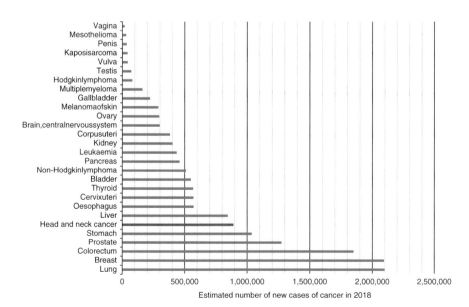

Fig. 1.2 The number of new cases of cancer estimated worldwide in 2018

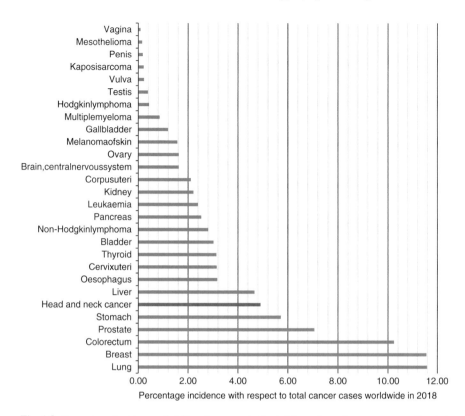

Fig. 1.3 Percentage incidence of different cancers to the total number of cancer cases estimated worldwide

followed by larynx 4 (20%), nasopharynx (15%), oropharynx (10%), hypopharynx (9%), and salivary glands (6%) (Fig. 1.4).

Based on 2018 Globocan data, the highest number of new cases of HNC was recorded in Asia, followed by Europe, North America, Latin America and the Caribbean, Africa, and Oceania. HNC in southeast Asia is actually ranked #1 among all other cancers, and in the US ranking #6. The percentage incidence of HNC to other cancers in the respective continent was highest in the Asian continent (6.3%) followed by Africa, Latin America and the Caribbean, Europe, Oceania, and North America (Fig. 1.5). In Asia, lip and oral cavity cancer accounted for the highest incidence (41%) of HNC cases, followed by nasopharynx, larynx, hypopharynx, oropharynx, and salivary glands.

As the Asian continent had the highest percentage incidence of HNC compared to other continents, the incidence of HNC was focused in various countries of Asia. Based on the year 2018 cancer statistics the top 10 countries with increased new incidences of HNC were India, China, Bangladesh, Indonesia, Pakistan, Japan, Thailand, Myanmar, Turkey, and the Philippines. In India, lip and oral cavity

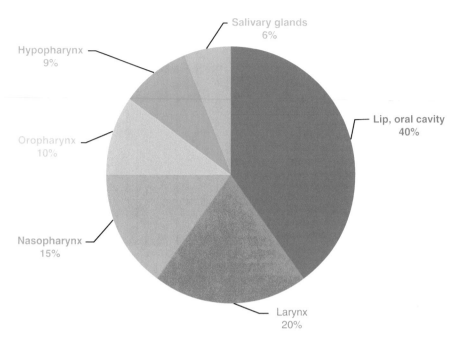

Fig. 1.4 The percentage incidence of various types of HNC (C00–14, 32) in the world

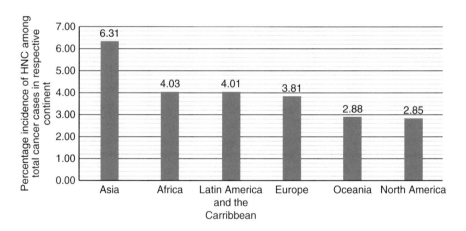

Fig. 1.5 Percentage incidence of HNC (C00–14, 32) by continent

cancers were recorded to be 58% of HNC followed by larynx (14%), hypopharynx (13%), oropharynx (9%), salivary glands (4%), and nasopharynx (2%).

The number of new incidences of HNC was highest in India and China; the reason could be their billion-plus population. However, Bangladesh is the Asian country recorded with the highest percentage (20.5%) of HNC incidence to all cancers reported in the respective country, and Armenia (1%) is recorded with the least

percentage incidence of HNC. The top 10 countries with highest percentage inci-
dence of HNC among other cancer incidences in their respective countries are
Bangladesh, India, Pakistan, Sri Lanka, Bhutan, Myanmar, Afghanistan, Nepal,
Indonesia, and Malaysia.

In Bangladesh among the various HNC, 43% incidence of the lip and oral cavity
cancer was observed, followed by hypopharynx (23%), larynx (16%), oropharynx
(12%), salivary gland (3%), and nasopharyngeal carcinoma (3%), respectively.

The percentage incidence of different types of head and neck cancer vary by
continent and are summarized in Fig. 1.6. Based on 2018 Globocan world cancer
data, HNC is among the top 10 cancers in North America with its place being in the
ninth place with 2.9% (Fig. 1.7). Among the various HNCs, lip and oral cavity

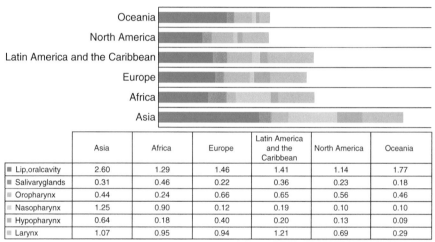

	Asia	Africa	Europe	Latin America and the Caribbean	North America	Oceania
▪ Lip,oralcavity	2.60	1.29	1.46	1.41	1.14	1.77
▪ Salivaryglands	0.31	0.46	0.22	0.36	0.23	0.18
▪ Oropharynx	0.44	0.24	0.66	0.65	0.56	0.46
▪ Nasopharynx	1.25	0.90	0.12	0.19	0.10	0.10
▪ Hypopharynx	0.64	0.18	0.40	0.20	0.13	0.09
▪ Larynx	1.07	0.95	0.94	1.21	0.69	0.29

Percentage incidence compared to all cancer incidences in respective continent

Fig. 1.6 Percentage incidence of each type of HNC (C00–14, 32) in comparison to total cancers
occurring in the respective continents

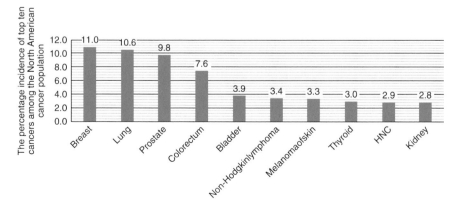

Fig. 1.7 The percentage incidence of the top 10 cancers among the North American cancer population in 2018

cancers together accounted for the highest percentage of the global HNC cases (40%), followed by larynx (24%), oropharynx (20%), salivary glands (8%), hypo-pharynx (5%), and nasopharynx (3%).

Age-adjusted statistics of HNC in the United States for the years 2013–2017 are presented in Table 1.2. The rate of cancer-related deaths increased till 1991,

Table 1.2 Head and neck cancer statistics in the United States' Surveillance, Epidemiology, and End Results (SEER 21) 2013–2017, age-adjusted [9]

	Oral cavity and pharynx cancer	Lip cancer	Tongue cancer	Laryngeal cancer
Estimated new cases in 2020	53,260		17,660	12,370
Percentage of all new cancer cases	2.9%		1.0%	0.7%
Estimated deaths in 2020	10,750		2830	3750
Percentage of all cancer deaths	1.8%		0.5%	0.6%
5-year Relative Survival (2010–2016)	66.2%	92.0%	67.1%	60.6%
Rate of new cases per 100,000 men and women per year (2013–2017)	11.4	0.6	3.5%	2.9
Rate of deaths per 100,000 men and women per year (2013–2017)	2.5	0.02	0.7%	1
Percent of men and women with lifetime risk of developing cancer	1.2%	0.1%	0.4%	0.3%
Percentage of all new cancer cases in the US	2.9%		1.0%	0.7%
Prevalence of this cancer in US in the year 2017	383,415			96,231
Frequently diagnosed among people aged between	55–64	65–74	55–64	55–64
Laryngeal cancer deaths is highest among people aged between	65–74	85+	65–74	65–74
Race and gender exhibiting increased number of new cases	Non-Hispanic male	White male	White male	Black male
Race and gender exhibiting increased number of deaths	Black male	Non-Hispanic male and White male	Non-Hispanic and white	Black male
Age-adjusted death rates on average each year over 2008–2017	Raising by 0.5%	Stable	Raising on average 1.2%	Falling by 2.3%

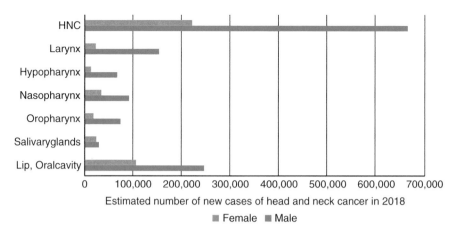

Fig. 1.8 The number of new cases of the male and female population with HNC (C00–14, 32) estimated worldwide in the year 2018

then decreased through 2017, thereby projecting 2.9 million less deaths due to cancer in comparison to the deaths estimated in case the rates persisted [8]. In 2018, North America stands in third position in the number of new incidences of head and neck cancer in the world. While this continent rank sixth in percentage incidence of HNC in comparison to total cancers by continent (Globocan 2018). American Cancer Society has projected 1,806,590 new cases of cancer and 606,520 deaths due to cancer in year 2020, in the United States [8].

Based on the Globocan 2018 data, the estimated number of new cases of HNC as well as the percentage incidence of each type of HNC was globally higher in the male population in comparison to the female population (Figs. 1.8 and 1.9). The discrepancy in the incidence of HNC in males and females is generally related to the population exposed to risk factors such as tobacco smoking or chewing, betel nut chewing, and alcohol consumption [10]. This was confirmed by a retrospective and hospital-based study conducted by Addala et al. (2012) focusing only on the histologically confirmed cases of HNC patients suggested a preponderance of cancer in males compared to females due to indulgence of males in the habits that increase risk for HNC (smoking and chewing tobacco, drinking alcohol, and using them in combination) [11]. Exposure to these risk factors for longer duration together with diet and occupation increased the incidence of HNC [11]. However, the incidence of lip, oral cavity cancers, salivary gland cancer, and nasopharyngeal carcinoma was higher in females than in males. Whereas the percentage incidence of oropharynx, hypopharynx, and larynx cancer were higher males than in females (Fig. 1.10).

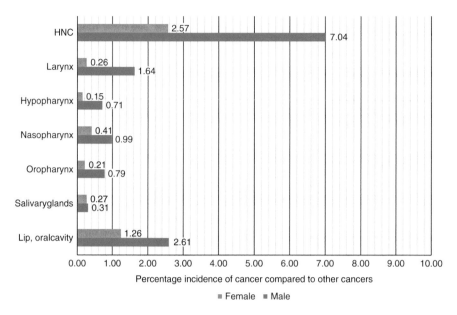

Fig. 1.9 Percentage incidence of HNC (C00–14, 32) in comparison to total cancers occurring worldwide

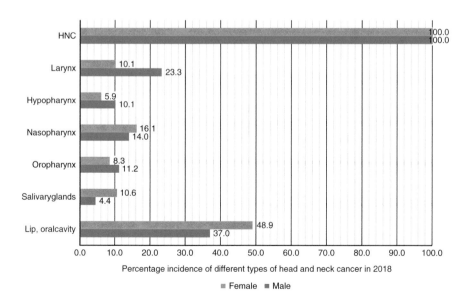

Fig. 1.10 Percentage incidence of different types of HNC (C00–14, 32) compared to total incidences of HNC in respective male and female populations

Etiology

"Exposome" is a term defined as the measure of all the internal and external exposure a person is introduced to in a lifetime and its effect on health [12]. People are exposed to various environmental and occupational sources before birth and throughout their life. Understanding the relationship between the exposomes and an individual's genetics and epigenetics impact our health. Assessment of internal exposome occurs at the level of the genes, proteins, lipids, and metabolites [12]. External exposure assessment relies on measuring environmental stressors, and these influence the occurrence of HNC. The various external agents causing HNC will be discussed in detail (Table 1.3).

Tobacco

Tobacco is used in several ways such as smoking cigarettes, cigars, pipes, chewing, and snuffing tobacco and is considered to be the prime risk factor for HNC [4, 10]. Exposure to tobacco and related products is a component of the external exposome, contributing to development of oral cavity cancer, pharyngeal cancer, oropharyngeal cancer, hypopharyngeal cancer, supraglottis cancer, and nasopharyngeal cancer.

In the Arabian peninsula, a traditional smokeless tobacco habit called "shammah" is associated with the incidence of leukoplakia in a dose-dependent manner [13]. Use of tobacco with products socially acceptable in Southeast Asia, the South Pacific Islands, and India, such as betel nuts, *paan*, *chaalia*, *gutka*, *naswar*, and areca also increase the risk for oral cavity cancer [13]. Smokeless tobacco contains carcinogenic substances such as nitrosamines and is considered to be a significant risk factor for oral cavity cancer. South Asia is known to be a hub for global smokeless tobacco use [14]. Khan et al. (2014) have reported that chewing *paan* with tobacco increases the risk of oral cavity cancer [14]. A large portion of the population of the Asia-Pacific region chews betel quid regularly [15, 16]. Areca nut alone is an age-old carcinogen and causes oral cavity cancer [17, 18].

Alcohol

Increased consumption of alcohol increases the risk of developing oral cavity, pharyngeal, and laryngeal cancer. Elwood et al. (1984) have reported increased risks with alcohol consumption in comparison to smoking [19].

Table 1.3 The various agents causing HNC

Exposomes	Subtype of the exposome	Type/site of head and neck cancer	Reference
Tobacco	Smoking cigarettes Cigars Pipes Reverse smoking Hookli Chillum Chewing tobacco Snuffing tobacco Betel nuts *Paan* *Chaalia* *Gutka* *Naswar* Areca nut Smokeless tobacco (*shammah*) Bidis/ Keeyo (a form of cheap cigarette made by sundried, uncured tobacco rolled in a dried leaf of temburni (Diospyros melanoxylon) or banana) Smokeless tobacco (nitrosamines) *Paan* with tobacco Smoking tobacco Chewing tobacco in the form of "*nass*" (a combination of betel leaf, ash, lime, cotton and sesame oil, tobacco and slaked shell)	Oral cavity cancer Cancer at the base of the tongue Cancer of the hard palate Pharyngeal cancer Oropharyngeal cancer Hypopharyngeal cancer Supraglottic cancer Nasopharyngeal carcinoma	[4, 10, 13, 14, 18, 20–30]
Alcohol	Drinking alcohol	Oral cavity cancer Pharyngeal cancer Laryngeal cancer	[18–21, 24, 31–33]
Alcohol and tobacco		Oropharynx cancer Hypopharynx cancer Salivary gland cancer Oral cancer Pharyngeal cancer	[19, 24, 31–37]

Viruses	Human papillomavirus (HPV)	Oropharyngeal cancer Oropharyngeal squamous cell carcinoma Oral cavity cancer	[18, 38–45]
	Epstein–Barr virus (EBV)	Nasopharyngeal cancer Malignant salivary gland tumors	[46, 47]
Diet	Poor nutrition Low consumption of vegetables and fruit Diet low in vitamins A, B, C, E, iron, selenium, folate, and other trace elements Low consumption of β-carotene due to reduced vegetable and fruit intake, and cholesterol rich diets	Oral cavity cancer Pharyngeal cancer Salivary gland malignancies	[13, 21, 47–51]
	Mate drinking	Oral cavity cancer	[38, 52]
	Chewing of kola nuts	Oral cavity cancer	[53, 54]
	Salted fish consumption	Nasopharyngeal carcinoma	[29, 30, 55–58]
	Canton-style salted fish	Nasopharyngeal carcinoma	[59]
	Preserved vegetables	Nasopharyngeal carcinoma	[59]
	Preserved/cured meat	Nasopharyngeal carcinoma	[59]
	Salt-preserved foods, including eggs, leafy vegetables, and roots	Nasopharyngeal carcinoma	[57, 58]
	Consumption of other preserved foods	Nasopharyngeal carcinoma	[46]
	Nitrosamine in some food items traditionally used in southern China	Nasopharyngeal carcinoma	[29, 60, 61]
	Traditional herbal medicines in the Asian population	Nasopharyngeal carcinoma	[29, 30, 62]
Oral hygiene	Polymicrobial supragingival dental plaque	Oral cavity cancer	[13, 19]
	Periodontal disease	Oral cavity cancer	[18, 63, 64]
	Wearing poorly fitting; defective complete dentures; faulty restorations; sharp teeth and ill-fitting dentures	Oral cavity cancer	[18, 38, 65, 66]

(continued)

Table 1.3 (continued)

Exposomes	Subtype of the exposome	Type/site of head and neck cancer	Reference
Diseases	Polyendocrinopathy–candidiasis–ectodermal dystrophy Diabetes mellitus Gastroesophageal reflux disease (GERD) Laryngopharyngeal reflux disease (LPRD)	Oral cavity cancer	[13]
	Diabetes	Head and neck cancer	[18, 67]
	Plummer–Vinson syndrome	Oral cavity Oropharynx cancer	[18]
Immunosuppressive agents	Kidney transplantation Azathioprine and cyclosporin	Oral cavity cancer	[18, 38, 68, 69]
	AIDS oral carcinoma	Lip Cancer	[18]
	Immunosuppression	Malignant salivary gland tumors	[47]
Oral microbiota	Fusobacterium, Dialister, Peptostreptococcus, Filifactor, Peptococcus, Catonella and Parvimonas Fusobacterium	Oral cavity cancer	[70]
Low socioeconomic status		Oral cavity cancer Oral cavity cancer Head and neck cancer	[4, 38, 71–74]
Free radicals	ROS, RNS	Oral cavity cancer	[13]
Atmospheric gases	Sulfur dioxide	Laryngeal cancer Pharyngeal cancer	[75]
	Atmospheric smoke	Laryngeal cancer Pharyngeal cancer	[75]
	Smoke	Nasopharyngeal carcinoma	[29, 30, 46]
	Acid mists	Laryngeal cancer	[75]
	Indoor air pollution by solid fuels such as oil/coal/wood	Oral cavity cancer Head and neck cancer	[38, 76, 77]

Occupational exposure			
	Agriculture/farming	Laryngeal cancer Salivary gland cancer Head and neck cancer	[75, 78–81]
	Textile industry	Laryngeal cancer Pharyngeal cancer Nasal cancer Sinonasal cancer	[75, 82, 83]
	Dyes	Laryngeal cancer Glottic cancer	[75, 84]
	Painters and varnishers (paints containing chromium-VI compounds)	Laryngeal cancer	[85]
	Craftsmen Laborers	Laryngeal cancer	[78, 79]
	Coal mining	Laryngeal cancer	[75]
	Railroad industry	Laryngeal cancer	[79]
	Lumber industry	Laryngeal cancer	[79]
	Sheet metal workers/foundry/structural metal preparers and erectors	Laryngeal cancer Nasal cancer Head and neck cancer	[79, 81, 82]
	Material-handling equipment operators	Head and neck cancer	[81]
	Welders	Head and neck cancer	[81]
	Soldering fumes (electrical works)	Oral cavity cancer Pharyngeal cancer	[86]
	Welding fumes (electrical works)	Pharyngeal cancer Laryngeal cancer	[87]
	Grinding wheel operators	Laryngeal cancer	[79]
	Automobile mechanics/automotive industries	Laryngeal cancer Salivary gland cancer	[79, 80]
	Wood workers/forestry/carpentry	Malignant salivary gland carcinoma Nasal/paranasal sinus cancer	[75, 88–90]
	Rubber industry workers	Malignant salivary gland carcinoma Head and neck cancer	[31, 80, 81, 88]
	Building/construction industries	Pharyngeal cancer Head and neck cancer Sinonasal cancer	[75, 81, 83]
	Firefighters	Head and neck cancer	[81]
	Launderers	Head and neck cancer	[81]
	Cleaners	Head and neck cancer	[81]

(continued)

Table 1.3 (continued)

Exposomes	Subtype of the exposome	Type/site of head and neck cancer	Reference
Dust	Construction dust	Laryngeal cancer	[85, 89]
	Cement dust	Laryngeal cancer Supraglottis cancer Pharyngeal cancer Head and neck squamous cell carcinomas	[75, 84, 85, 89, 91]
	Asbestos	Laryngeal cancer Pharyngeal cancer	[18, 87, 89, 91–93]
	Silica/silica dust	Salivary gland cancer	[47, 51, 80]
	Metal dust	Laryngeal cancer Head and neck squamous cell carcinomas	[82, 89]
	Wood dust	Nasal/paranasal sinus cancer Nasal cancer Laryngeal cancer Pharyngeal cancer Sinonasal cancer Nasopharyngeal carcinoma	[18, 29, 75, 82, 83, 89, 90]
	Coal dust	Hypopharyngeal Cancer	[36]
	Saw dust	Laryngeal cancer Head and neck squamous cell carcinomas	[89]
	Leather dust	Head and neck squamous cell carcinomas Nasal/paranasal sinus cancer Nasal cancer Larynx and pharynx cancer Sinonasal cancer	[18, 75, 82, 83, 89, 90]
	Chimney soot	Head and neck squamous cell carcinomas	[89]

Solvents and chemicals	Ethanol	Laryngeal cancer	[75]
	Oil	Laryngeal cancer	[75, 84]
	Grease	Supraglottis cancer	
	Kerosene as cooking fuel	Salivary gland cancer	[80]
	Perchloroethylene and trichloroethylene	Head and neck cancer	[94]
	Petroleum	Nasal/paranasal sinus cancer	[75]
	Formaldehyde	Hypopharyngeal cancer	[29, 36, 83]
		Sinonasal cancer	
		Nasopharyngeal carcinoma	
Radiation	Head X-ray examinations	Salivary gland cancer	[80]
	Ionizing radiation	Malignant salivary gland carcinoma	[88, 95, 96]
	High or prolonged doses of radiation	Salivary gland malignancies	[47, 51]
	Ultraviolet radiation	Malignant salivary gland tumors	[18, 47, 97–100]
		Lip cancer	
	Ultraviolet light treatment to the head or neck	Head and neck cancer	[31]
	Solar irradiation	Lip cancer	[13]
	Atomic bombs (high-level ionizing radiation)	Head and neck cancer	[101]
	Radiation/radioactive materials	Head and neck cancer	[31]
	Head or neck radiation treatment, radiotherapy	Head and neck cancer	[31, 102]
	Repeated medical and full mouth dental X-ray examinations	Head and neck cancer	[31]
Metal	Nickel compounds/alloys	Malignant salivary gland carcinoma	[31, 75, 83, 88, 95, 103]
		Nasal/paranasal sinus cancer	
		Head and neck cancers	
		Sinonasal cancer	
	Cd	Head and neck cancers	[103]
		Sinonasal cancer	
	Cr	Sinonasal cancer	[83]
Others	Age (<45 years)	HNC	[104, 105]
	Gender	HNC	[40]
	Black race	Salivary gland cancer	[106]
	Never-smoker and never-drinker (NSND)	HNC	[107]
	Family history	Nasopharyngeal carcinoma	[46]

Alcohol and Tobacco in Combination

The consumption of both alcohol and tobacco significantly increases the risk of developing an HNC [4, 10]. Horn-Ross et al. (1997) reported smoking and heavy alcohol consumption to be associated with increased risk of salivary gland cancer in men, but these factors were not strongly related to salivary gland cancer in women [31].

The risk of oral cavity cancer increases with the consumption of alcohol in combination with tobacco in any form such as bidi smoking and/or pan tobacco chewing [18, 108].

Viruses

Human papillomavirus (HPV) is a well-established risk factor for HNCs [39]. HPV is associated with head and neck squamous cell carcinoma and is strongly related to oropharyngeal cancer [40]. The HPV-attributable fraction of HNC varies substantially between countries. Gheit et al. (2017) conducted a study in the Indian subcontinent and reported the highest percentage of HPV DNA/RNA double positivity in the oropharynx (9.4%), followed by larynx (1.7%) and oral cavity (1.6%). Different strains of HPV are associated with the development of certain types of cancers. HPV16 was the major type associated with HNC [109]. Smith et al. (2012) reported an increased risk of cancer in the oral cavity amid HPV-positive/higher tobacco and alcohol level users in comparison to controls. However, their study also reported a higher risk of oropharynx cancer among HPV-negative/higher tobacco and alcohol level users than among HPV-positive/higher tobacco and alcohol users [39].

Epstein–Barr Virus (EBV) is commonly known to cause nasopharyngeal carcinoma. Among the several cancers caused with EBV infection, undifferentiated nasopharyngeal carcinoma has been identified to have a close association with this infection in endemic areas such as southern Chinese population [110]. A relation between EBV antigens presentation to host immune cells and nasopharyngeal carcinoma risk has been identified with a strong association between NPC risk and the HLA locus at chromosome 6p [110].

Immunosuppressive Agents

Post kidney transplantation the use of immunosuppressive agents such as azathioprine and cyclosporin increases the risk of lip cancer [68, 111]. During inflammatory bowel disorders (Crohn's disease) extended use of immunosuppressive agents such as azathioprine increase the risk of tongue cancer [38, 69].

Diet

Studies have linked poor diet quality diet to the occurrence of HNC. Low intake of fresh vegetables and fruits, and consuming a diet low in vitamins A, B, C, E, iron, selenium, folate, and other trace elements increases the risk of oral cavity cancer [13, 38, 104, 112–114]. Consumption of too much meat and processed meat products increases the risk for many HNC [18, 38, 48, 115]. Consumption of salted fish, preserved vegetables, nitrosamine in food, and traditional herbal medicines have been reported to increase the risk of nasopharyngeal carcinoma [29, 59]. Mate is a drink which is consumed very hot using a metal straw in Argentina, Uruguay, Paraguay, and southern Brazil. Mate is an infusion made of the herb Ilex paraguariensis. The herb is cultivated throughout South America. Mate drinking increases the risk of oral cavity cancer [38, 52].

Oral Hygiene

Poor dental and oral hygiene increase the risk of oral cavity cancer [19]. Poor oral hygiene and poor dentition, including faulty restorations, sharp teeth, and ill-fitting dentures, increases the incidence of oral cavity cancer [38, 66, 116]. Polymicrobial supragingival dental plaque possesses a relevant mutagenic interaction with saliva and is considered to be an independent risk factor for oral cavity cancer [13]. Divaris et al. (2010) have reported the association of periodontitis with the risk of squamous cell carcinoma of head and neck [63].

Diseases

Polyendocrinopathy–Candidiasis–Ectodermal Dystrophy An autosomal recessive disease called polyendocrinopathy–candidiasis–ectodermal dystrophy, which is common in Finland, is associated with a limited T lymphocyte defect and seems to favor the growth of *Candida albicans* and predispose individuals to chronic mucositis and oral cavity cancer [13].

Diabetes Mellitus Based on epidemiological studies, diabetes mellitus is suggested to be associated with oral squamous cell carcinomas (OSCC) involving molecular targets such as insulin receptor substrate-1 and focal adhesion kinase [13].

Gastroesophageal Reflux Disease (GERD) and Laryngopharyngeal Reflux Disease (LPRD) Gastroesophageal reflux disease (GERD) and laryngopharyngeal reflux disease (LPRD) cause reflux of stomach acid into the upper airway and throat, thereby increasing the risk of HNC [13].

Oral Microbiota

Oral microbes and their biofilms may facilitate the metabolism of ethanol to acetaldehyde (a potent carcinogen) in the oral cavity of chronic alcohol users. Acetaldehyde increases the risk for oral cavity cancer in cells among chronic users [38]. Zhao et al. (2017) have reported bacterial dysbiosis within OSCC surface lesion samples, with drastic changes in bacterial composition and bacterial gene functions in comparison to controls [70]. Their team observed that a group of periodontitis-correlated taxa, including Fusobacterium, Dialister, Peptostreptococcus, Filifactor, Peptococcus, Catonella, and Parvimonas significantly enriched in OSCC samples. Also, several Fusobacterium operational taxonomic units were involved in OSCC and were found to have good diagnostic power. Bacterial dysbiosis changes the local microenvironment driving carcinogenesis in bacterial habitats, allowing bacteria suitable for a tumor microenvironment to thrive, resulting in shifts in bacterial communities [70].

Socioeconomic Status

Increased risk of HNC has been associated with low socioeconomic status [71]. The prevalence of HNC in developing countries is reported to be higher due to the increased consumption of smoking and alcohol consumption [4] and poor diet [38]. However, lower socioeconomic status measured in terms of occupation, income, or education is a significant risk factor for oral cavity cancer independent of lifestyle behaviors [38].

Free Radicals

In carcinogenesis, free radicals such as reactive oxygen species (ROS) and reactive nitrogen species (RNS) function as initiators and promoters. The increase in ROS and RNS may have been the event that led to the consumption and reduction of salivary antioxidant systems, thus explaining the oxidative damage to DNA and proteins and, possibly, the promotion of oral cavity cancer [13].

Atmospheric Gases

In 1993, Wake correlated atmospheric sulfur dioxide or its biological products or consequences with increased risk of laryngeal and pharyngeal cancer. He also reported an increased risk of laryngeal cancer with atmospheric smoke [75].

Occupational Exposures

Although both Elwood et al. (1984) [19] and Purdue et al. (2006) [91] reported no significant association with specific occupational exposures in separate studies involving construction workers, other studies suggest that environmental or occupational inhalants increase the risk of HNC. In 1994, Pukkala et al. reported an increased risk of oral and pharyngeal cancer among electrical workers exposed to soldering fumes [86]. In 1998, Gustavsson et al. (1998) associated increased risk of pharyngeal cancer and laryngeal cancer with long-term exposure to welding fumes [87].

Occupations with possible exposure to rubber are associated with an increased risk of salivary gland cancer [80]. Horn-Ross et al. (1997) also reported an increased risk of HNC in individuals employed in the rubber industry [31].

Williams et al. (1977) reported different ratios for the rates of incidence of laryngeal cancer in in individuals with certain occupations, including ratios of 1.3, 1, 0.9, and 0.4 for operatives, craftsmen, laborers, and farmers, respectively [78]. Similarly, in 1982, Flanders and Rothman (1982) estimated the rates for the same occupations to be 1.4, 1.2, 1.6, and 0.5, respectively [79]. They also reported the increased occurrence of laryngeal cancer in workers of the railroad industry, lumber industry, sheet metal workers, grinding wheel operators, and automobile mechanics [79].

Occupations with possible exposure to automotive industries and farming have been linked to an elevated risk of salivary gland cancer [80]. Comba et al. (1992) have reported the increased risk of nasal cancer to be associated with individuals working in the wood, leather, and textile industries [82]. Paget-Bailly et al. (2013) reported that in the French population, the risk of HNC increases with the duration of employment in occupations such as cleaning, laundry, firefighting, several agricultural occupations, welding, structural metal preparation, building, rubber working, several construction occupations, and material-handling equipment operations [81].

Dust Dust is small solid particles temporarily suspended in air, ranging from 1 to 100 μm in diameter. It contains a heterogeneous group of organic (such as wood or leather dust) or inorganic (such as metal dust) exposures. Dust can induce a carcinogenic effect through chronic inflammation caused due to its inherent chemical properties, or a carrier of other carcinogenic compounds. Wood and leather dust are two forms of occupational dust that are associated with cancers of the nasal cavity and paranasal sinus. These two types of dust are classified as type 1 carcinogens by the International Agency for Cancer Research (IARC) [89]. Langevin et al. reported an increased risk of laryngeal carcinoma with sawdust and metal dust exposure, whereas leather dust exposure increased the risk of Head and Neck Squamous Cell Carcinoma (HNSCC) [89].

Construction Dust Increased risk of laryngeal carcinoma is reported for building and construction workers, as construction dust is composed of several substances, for example, asbestos, mineral fibers, sand, metal powders, tar, bitumen, and cement dust [85].

Cement Dust In 1990, Cauvin et al. reported an increased risk of supraglottic cancer associated with exposure to cement [84]. A study by Dietz et al. (2004) concluded that exposure of building and construction workers to cement dust increases the risk for laryngeal carcinoma [85]. Purdue et al. (2006) also reported an increased risk of pharyngeal cancer in workers exposed to cement dust [91].

Asbestos In 1998, Gustavsson et al. reported an association between asbestos exposure and laryngeal cancer [87]. Similar results were obtained by Purdue et al. (2006), who related asbestos exposure to an increased laryngeal cancer incidence [91]. Straif et al. (2009) have mentioned that the IARC recognized asbestos exposure as a cause of laryngeal cancer [92]. A study conducted by Menvielle et al. (2016) in France recommend avoiding exposure to asbestos-containing materials because their study also showed a significant incidence of laryngeal cancer in individuals exposed to asbestos in combination with tobacco and alcohol [93].

Silica Dust A study conducted by Zheng et al. (1996) reported a 2.5-fold increase in the risk of salivary gland cancer on exposure to silica dust [80].

Metal Dust Comba et al. (1992) have reported an increased risk for individuals working in foundries. The metal dust is associated with a higher risk of nasal cancer [82].

Wood Dust A study by Elwood (1981) suggested an occupational risk of tumors of the nasal cavity and paranasal sinuses may extend beyond furniture manufacturers to those handling wood in primary industries, including forestry and carpentry [90].

Solvent A study conducted by Cauvin et al. (1990) showed that supraglottic cancer is associated with exposure to oil and grease [84]. Zheng et al. (1996) reported an increased risk of salivary gland cancer in individuals using kerosene as cooking fuel [80]. Gustavsson et al. (1998) reported that increased exposure to polycyclic aromatic hydrocarbons (PAHs) is associated with esophageal cancer [87]. Carton et al. (2017) conducted a study on the effect of occupational exposure to solvents on HNC in women [94]. The solvents used for the study were five chlorinated solvents (i.e., carbon tetrachloride, chloroform, methylene chloride, perchloroethylene, trichloroethylene), five petroleum solvents (i.e., benzene, special petroleum product, gasoline, white spirits and other light aromatic mixtures, diesel, fuels, and kerosene), and five oxygenated solvents (i.e., alcohols, ketones and esters, ethylene glycol, diethyl ether, tetrahydrofuran). The increased risk was observed in women exposed to perchloroethylene and trichloroethylene, and the risk increased with exposure duration. Carton et al. (2017) reported no significant risk of HNSCC in occupational exposure to the other chlorinated, petroleum, or oxygenated solvents [94].

Radiation High-level ionizing radiation from the atomic bombs on Hiroshima and Nagasaki [101], radiotherapy [102], and repeated medical and dental radiograph examinations [117] increase the risk of cancer. Zheng et al. (1996) reported an association of head radiograph examinations with an increased risk of salivary gland cancer [80]. Horn-Ross et al. (1997) reported increased risk associated with a higher dose of therapeutic medical radiation treatment to the head or neck, full mouth dental radiographs, ultraviolet light treatment to the head or neck, and radiation or radioactive materials [31].

Prolonged exposure to solar irradiation is a major risk factor for cancer of the lip. Typically, lip cancers arise on the lower lip, and many patients have outdoor occupations with increased sun exposure. Lip cancer is three times more common in men than in women, which may be an effect of occupation, smoking, and sun exposure [13].

Metals Horn-Ross et al. (1997) reported an increased risk of HNC upon exposure to nickel compounds/alloys [31]. Khlifi and Hamza-Chaffai (2010) have indicated smoking to increase the total body burden of heavy metals for metals workers [103]. It is widely accepted that heavy metals such as nickel [31, 103], chromium, and cadmium are carcinogens and increase the risk of HNC in humans [103].

In 1990, Cauvin et al. reported glottic cancer to be associated with exposure to dye [84]. Painters and varnishers likely have an increased risk of developing laryngeal cancer as paints contain carcinogenic substances, such as chromium VI compounds [85].

Other Risk Factors

Age The risk of HNC is higher above the age of 40, with an average age of diagnosis of 62 years [118]. HNSCC is typically regarded as a disease of elderly people. However, increasing numbers of patients worldwide with HNSCC at a younger age (defined as <45 years old) have been reported in recent years [105].

Gender In Central and South America, the occurrence of HNC in males is around four times higher than in females [40]. Based on Globocan data for the year 2018 a similar observation was made where HNC ranks as the fifth most prevalent cancer in men, after lung, prostate, colorectal, and stomach cancers, while it is the eleventh most common cancer in women, after breast, colorectal, lung, cervical uteri, thyroid, corpus uteri, stomach, ovarian, and liver cancers and non-Hodgkin lymphoma.

Race South Asians have been reported with higher rates of oral cavity cancer than people from most other countries. In the United States, black males have an increased risk of oropharyngeal cancer than white males [38].

Never-Smoker and Never-Drinker (NSND) Dahlstrom et al. (2008) reported female NSND at extremes of age to be more likely to develop HNC and were significantly younger than ever-smoker and ever-drinker (ESED) patients [107]. NSND patients exhibited a higher proportion of oral cavity and oropharyngeal cancers than ESED patients. Regular environmental tobacco smoke exposure was reported in cases of HNC in 45% of NSND women and 41% of men. Increased risk of HNC was also observed in 24% NSND women and 36% NSND men exposed to carcinogens or toxins during their occupations. NSND patients with a history of GERD accounted for 30% incidence. More than half of the NSND patients who were serologically positive for HPV type 16 were reported to have oropharyngeal primary. It was observed that no specific single known factor is responsible for a majority of HNSCC in NSNDs [107].

Diz et al. (2017) reported regional differences in oral cavity and pharyngeal cancer in terms of incidence and mortality due to differences in lifestyle and exposure to risk factors such as smoking (e.g., the high incidence in Danish women), alcohol (e.g., in Lithuanian men) or both (e.g., in Belgium and Portugal). Other traditional factors, such as actinic radiation, are responsible for the increased incidence of lip cancer (e.g., in Spain), and oncogenic potential of HPV explains the rising trend in oropharyngeal cancer in some countries (e.g., in Denmark and Scotland) [119].

Symptoms

In the early stages of HNC, the tumor is often asymptomatic, causing the symptoms of HNC to be overlooked by the patient or the practitioner [120]. However, the most common symptoms that do occur are swelling or a sore in the mouth that is persistent. A red or white patch in the mouth or a lump or mass in the head or neck area, with or without pain, is the manifestation of HNC [121]. Additional symptoms include foul mouth odor observed even after following proper oral hygiene, persistent nasal congestion, frequent nose bleeds, and unusual nasal discharge, pain or difficulty in chewing, swallowing, or moving the jaw or tongue, jaw pain, blood in the saliva or phlegm, loosening of teeth, dentures that no longer fit, hoarseness or change in voice, difficulty breathing, double vision, numbness or weakness of a body part in the head and neck region, unexplained weight loss, fatigue, and ear pain or infection. Facial pain, mild trismus, earaches, and headaches are subtle signs of nasopharyngeal carcinoma that are generally confused with benign disorders. Pharyngeal cancers are detected mostly at an advanced stage, and have a poor prognosis due to the late emergence of symptoms [121, 122].

Diagnosis

Clinical Examination

Palpation of the tumor and regional lymph nodes in the neck are performed in addition to endoscopic examination for clinical examination of the tumor to determine the stage of the disease. HNC allows diagnosis and staging by clinical examination due to its uncomplicated endoscopic and diagnostic biopsy through a natural orifice in almost all cases [4, 123–125]. During diagnosis, the patient's history is evaluated, and physical examination is performed with complete head and neck examination and biopsy [4, 126]. However, during the physical examination, it is advised to perform bimanual palpation of the oral cavity and examination of the neck lymph nodes [4]. The examination with a mirror or fiberoptic scope is essential in diagnosing and staging lesions involving the larynx and pharynx [126]. Nasolaryngoscope usage by an otolaryngologist is essential for the diagnosis and staging of HNC. When examining neck masses, fine needle aspiration (FNA) is a useful diagnostic tool.

Imaging

Ultrasound Ultrasound can be used in combination with a FNA biopsy to evaluate tumor presence in cervical lymph nodes or to measure the depth of infiltration in oral cavity cancer [127, 128]. It has been noted that the accuracy of clinical examination in evaluating neck lymphadenopathy improves by ultrasound-guided FNA [129, 130] and is considered better than other imaging modalities for this purpose. Retropharyngeal lymph node areas cannot be assessed by ultrasonography due to their innate location, whereas aspirating small-sized lymph nodes is technically demanding. Instead, ultrasound-guided FNA may detect malignancy in lymph nodes which appear normal by CT scan and, therefore, might prove to be a valuable helper diagnostic tool for the evaluation of the neck [127, 128, 131]. However, its role in the management of patients with HNC is yet to be determined [132].

Computed Tomography (CT) Scanning *CT scanning* is used to visualize the location and size of the tumor and cervical lymph nodes and with respect to HNC, it mostly helps in the detection of cancers in paranasal sinuses and nasal cavity [133]. It usually produces multiple images, the cross-sectional images produced during a CT scan can help in reconstruction of 3-D images. It is used to measure tumor volumes or to determine the extent of the radiation fields [127, 128, 132].

The risk of developing distant metastases for the advanced stage of cancer, especially nasopharyngeal and hypopharyngeal primaries, can spread to the lungs, bone, liver, and mediastinal lymph nodes. Patients with considerable risk for distant metastasis are evaluated with a CT scan of the chest, including the upper abdomen, along with a bone scan which might be low yield [132].

CT and MRI of the neck region provide information about the lymph node involvement and invasion of adjacent structures. CT scanning is faster and more affordable than MRI, and it is used to assess neck lymphadenopathy. CT scanning has better accuracy for the evaluation of bony erosions (e.g., invasion of the mandible or base of the skull) and larynx as it has areas that may produce motion artifact on an MRI [131, 132].

Magnetic Resonance Imaging (MRI) MRI scanning provides multiplanar imaging and is often used to visualize and outline head and neck tumors and to get better soft-tissue contrast, as it can detect subtle differences in the soft tissues. Also, different scanning protocols can be used to image different structures more clearly or to study different tissue characteristics like diffusion or perfusion [127, 128]. MRI is better than CT scanning for evaluation of the nasopharynx, paranasal sinuses, salivary glands, retropharyngeal and prevertebral spaces, and oropharynx [131]. Multiplanar imaging during MRI scanning detects subtle differences in the soft tissues [132].

Positron Emission Tomography (PET) This is another method to produce functional images using diverse molecules labeled with a positron-emitter such as fludeoxyglucose (glucose labeled with fluorine-18, FDG). When injected, these labeled molecules distribute throughout the body and provide real-time biological information. PET tracer such as FDG can be used to detect metabolically active tumor cells by studying glucose uptake in different tissues. PET scanning has the advantage of using a variety of molecules as PET tracer, depending on the process to be investigated [134]. The tracers other than FDG used in radiation oncology include thymidine labeled with carbon-11 to measure proliferation, FMISO ([^{18}F] Fluoromisonidazole) and Cu-ATSM for hypoxia imaging and ^{99m}Tc-Labeled annexin to measure apoptosis [127, 128, 131, 132, 135].

Lymph node metastases are recurrent with tonsillar, base of tongue, and nasopharyngeal primaries. Histological lymph node involvement from OCSCC is suboptimal when imaged with PET scan, ultrasound, CT, and MRI. Occult neck lymphadenopathy modifies the treatment plan as it is not detected by clinical examination. Anatomical imaging is not very precise for diagnosing malignant lymphadenopathy and usually relies on size criteria. Therefore, PET scan and ultrasound-guided FNA stage the neck. PET scanning with FDG assesses distant metastases and neck lymphadenopathy. Multiple studies have shown the advantage of PET scan over CT scan and MRI in detecting lymph node involvement by cancer. PET scan has higher sensitivity and specificity than CT scan and MRI, which differentiates active tumor from fibrotic changes and, therefore, is useful in detecting recurrent HNC post-treatment [131, 132].

In situations where no primary site is identified with conventional cross-sectional imaging, PET and CT combination is recommended for imaging. This combination is also recommended to detect residual disease post 12 weeks of nonsurgical treatment [136].

Probing

Probing is an invasive technique. A probe used to make measurements inside a tumor provides real-time information about a tumor. An example includes an oxygen-sensitive needle probe of Eppendorf pO_2 inserted into the tumor, which gives access to real-time measurements and provides the possibility to repeat measurements during treatment [137, 138].

Tumor Biopsy

For diagnostic biopsy, part of a tumor is taken out and used to study various aspects of the tumor, including the presence of the HPV virus. The tumor cells taken out can be cultured in vitro, staining of tumor tissue sections with toluidine blue is considered helpful for the detection of a local recurrence or a new lesion [132] by viewing under a microscope. Unknown primary malignancy is revealed through panendoscopy of random biopsies of HNC sites such as nasopharynx, tonsil, sinus, and base of tongue. Histological diagnosis is performed for all patients and tumors that are evident during the examination of the oral cavity, and the oropharyngeal cavity is subjected to biopsy. The tumor cells or tissues can be used to study the levels of specific proteins, RNA, or DNA of a tumor [139]. However, avoiding needle or excisional biopsies of neck lymph nodes is recommended as it can potentially alter the lymphatics and compromise the outcome of subsequent node dissection.

Pathology/Immunohistochemistry

Tumor tissue is sliced into thin sections and fixed onto a glass slide to study them under a microscope. Different staining protocols using fluorescent dye-labeled antibodies help visualize various markers inside or around tumor cells. Multiple small slices of tumors from different patients can be stained on the same slide to perform tissue microarray (TMA).

A combination of PCR and p16-immunohistochemistry (IHC) can be used for detection of HPV. p16-IHC has excellent specificity, acceptable sensitivity, and good predictive value for the diagnosis of HPV-induced HNC [7]. The most common diagnostic tests are summarized in Fig. 1.11.

Possible Delay in Diagnosis Early diagnosis and treatment improve the chances of survival in any malignancy. Regardless of the location and easy visibility of HNC, numerous patients are diagnosed only at an advanced stage. Less education and lack of awareness about the symptoms lead to delayed diagnosis and these factors together contribute to advancement in the disease and higher morbidity and mortality rates [24, 74, 114, 151–153].

Agarwal et al. (2018) studied various reasons associated with delay in diagnosis, and the factors included older age, rural background, illiteracy, joint family, poor socioeconomic status, further distance from the hospital, tobacco chewing, insufficient knowledge, and fear of the disease. Improving health coverage and awareness of available health services may prevent the delay in diagnosis and treatment [152].

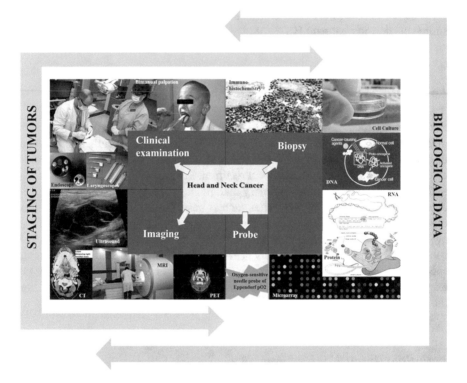

Fig. 1.11 Methods to diagnose head and neck tumor. (Source of images [140–150])

Staging System

A staging system was established by the American Joint Committee on Cancer (AJCC) that incorporates three aspects of tumor growth, including the extent of the primary tumor (T), the involvement of regional lymph nodes (N), and metastasis (M). The TNM staging system (Table 1.4) guides the initial treatment decisions, and is mostly based on clinical examinations and defines the anatomic extent of the tumor. In addition, the TNM staging systems incorporate imaging techniques (e.g., cortical involvement upgrades the stage to T4). Data for pathological staging derived from operative findings and histopathological review are documented separately. The tumor size and its spread from the place of origin is divided into stages of a cancer. Cancer staging varies with the type of cancer, yet the common system of staging is given in the Table 1.5 [154]. Also, based on the appearance of the cancerous cells under a microscope they are graded as discussed in Table 1.6. In general, the T stage is relatively similar for each subdivision of HNC, then differs based on

Table 1.4 Grading system

The stage of cancer (TNM system)	Description
T: Tumor	Characteristics of tumor, for instance its size, growth at the site of its beginning, its presence or growth into nearby tissues
T0	No evidence of a primary tumor
TX	Tumor can't be measured
Tis	Carcinoma in situ or precancer are cancerous cells growing in the most superficial layer of tissue and not into deeper tissues
Tn (e.g., T1, T2, T3, and T4)	The size of the tumor and expanse of its spread into neighboring structures. Higher T number indicates larger tumor and its increased growth in nearby tissues
N: Nodes	Cancer spread into nearby lymph nodes
NX	The adjacent lymph nodes cannot be evaluated
N0	Adjacent lymph nodes do not contain cancer
Nn (e.g. N1, N2, and N3)	Indicates the size, location, and/or the number of nearby lymph nodes. Higher N number indicate increased spread of cancer to nearby lymph nodes
M: Metastasis	Cancer spread into distant parts of the body
M0	No evidence of distant cancer spread
M1	Spread of cancer to distant organs or tissues

Table 1.5 Cancer staging

Cancer stages	Description
0	Site of initiation of carcinoma in situ that has not spread
I	Small cancer that has not spread
II	Grown cancer that hasn't spread
III	Large cancer that could have spread to the nearby tissues and/or the lymph nodes
IV	Metastatic cancer spread from its sites of initiation to a distant body location in the body

Source: Ref. [154]
Based on the appearance of the cancerous cells under a microscope they are graded

Table 1.6 Cancer grading

Cancer grading	Description
Grade 1	Tumor cells and tissues appear similar to healthy cells and tissues. These are called well-differentiated tumors and are considered low grade.
Grade 2	Cells and tissues are slightly abnormal and are called moderately differentiated. These are intermediate grade tumors.
Grade 3	Appearance of cancer cells and tissues is very abnormal. These cancers no longer have an architectural structure or pattern and are considered poorly differentiated. These tumors are considered high grade.
Grade 4	The undifferentiated cancers with most abnormal looking cells. These cells characteristically grow and spread faster than lower grade tumors and are the highest grade.

Table 1.7 Head and neck cancer staging

Stage	Description
0	The tumor growing in situ at the site of initiation in a region of the head and neck, with absence of cancer cells in deeper layers of tissue, nearby structures, lymph nodes or distant sites.
I	The tumor with size 2 cm across or smaller at the site of initiation with no cancer cells existing in nearby structures, lymph nodes, or distant sites.
II	The head and neck tumor measures 2–4 cm across with presence of no cancer cells in nearby structures, lymph nodes, or distant sites.
III	Tumor larger than 4 cm across, with presence of no cancer cells in nearby structures, lymph nodes, or distant sites. *Or* Tumor can be of any size but has not grown into nearby structures or distant sites. *Or* Tumor smaller than 3 cm across with cancer cells present in one lymph node located on the same side of the head or neck as the primary tumor.
IVA	The head and neck cancer of any size growing into nearby structures. Cancer cells may not be present in the lymph nodes, or may have spread to one lymph node, which is located on the same side of the head or neck as the primary tumor and is smaller than 3 cm across. However, cancer not spread to distant sites. *Or* Tumor is any size and may or may not have invaded nearby structures. Cancer cells present in one lymph node, located on the same side of the head or neck as the primary tumor and measuring 3–6 cm across. Cancer cells present in one lymph node on the opposite side of the head or neck and measuring less than 6 cm across. Cancer cells are present in two or more lymph nodes, all smaller than 6 cm across and located on either side of the head or neck.
IVB	Tumor has invaded deeper areas and/or tissues in head and neck. Cancer cells may or may not have spread to lymph nodes and has not spread to distant sites. *Or* Tumor of any size which may or may not have grown into other structures. It has spread to one or more lymph nodes larger than 6 cm across, but has not spread to distant sites.
IVC	Cancer cells have spread to distant sites. The head and neck cancer tumor is any size and may or may not have spread to the lymph nodes.

Source: Ref. [155]

anatomical considerations. At N stage the spread of cancer to nearby nodes has been observed. The M stage indicates metastasis which is uniform throughout. The HNC stages, its TNM staging, and its grouping are provided in Tables 1.7, 1.8, and 1.9. Based on AJCC system in 1997, around two-thirds of patients with HNC are diagnosed with the advanced disease stages III or IV (locoregionally advanced HNC) and one-third with early stages I or II [132].

Table 1.8 TNM staging for head and neck cancer

Tumor (T)	
Lip and oral cavity (C00–C06)	
TX	Primary tumor cannot be assessed
T0	No evidence of primary tumor
Tis	Carcinoma in situ
T1	Tumor 2 cm or less in greatest dimension
T2	Tumor more than 2 cm but not more than 4 cm in greatest dimension
T3	Tumor more than 4 cm in greatest dimension
T4	Lip tumor enters through the cortical bone, inferior alveolar nerve, floor of mouth, or skin of face (i.e., chin or nose)
T4a	Oral cavity tumor invades through cortical bone, into deep (extrinsic) muscle of tongue (genioglossus, hyoglossus, palatoglossus, and styloglossus), maxillary sinus, or skin of face
T4b	Tumor invades masticator space, pterygoid plates, or skull base, and/or encases internal carotid artery
Major salivary glands (C07–C08)	
TX	Primary tumor cannot be assessed
T0	No evidence of primary tumor
T1	Tumor 2 cm or less in greatest dimension without extraparenchymal extension[a]
T2	Tumor more than 2 cm but not more than 4 cm in greatest dimension without extraparenchymal extension[a]
T3	Tumor more than 4 cm in greatest dimension and/or having extraparenchymal extension[a]
T4a	Tumor invades skin, mandible, ear canal, and/or facial nerve
T4b	Tumor invades skull base and/or pterygoid plates and/or encases carotid artery
Oropharynx (C09–10)	
TX	Primary tumor cannot be assessed
T0	No evidence of primary tumor
Tis	Carcinoma in situ
T1	Tumor 2 cm or less in greatest dimension
T2	Tumor more than 2 cm but not more than 4 cm in greatest dimension
T3	Tumor more than 4 cm in greatest dimension
T4a	Tumor invades the larynx, deep/extrinsic muscle of tongue, medial pterygoid, hard palate, or mandible
T4b	Tumor invades lateral pterygoid muscle, pterygoid plates, lateral nasopharynx, or skull base or encases carotid artery
Nasopharynx (C11)	
TX	Primary tumor cannot be assessed
T0	No evidence of primary tumor
Tis	Carcinoma in situ
T1	Tumor confined to the nasopharynx
T2	Tumor extends to soft tissues
T2a	Tumor extends to the oropharynx and/or the nasal cavity without parapharyngeal extension[b]

(continued)

Table 1.8 (continued)

T2b	Any tumor with parapharyngeal extension[b]
T3	Tumor involves bony structures and/or paranasal sinuses
T4	Tumor with intracranial extension and/or involvement of cranial nerves, infratemporal fossa, hypopharynx, orbit, or masticator space

Hypopharynx (C12–C13)

TX	Primary tumor cannot be assessed
T0	No evidence of primary tumor
Tis	Carcinoma in situ
T1	Tumor limited to one subsite of hypopharynx and 2 cm or less in greatest dimension
T2	Tumor invades more than one subsite of hypopharynx or an adjacent site, or measures more than 2 cm but not more than 4 cm in greatest dimension without fixation of hemilarynx
T3	Tumor measures more than 4 cm in greatest dimension or with fixation of hemilarynx
T4a	Tumor invades thyroid/cricoid cartilage, hyoid bone, thyroid gland, esophagus, or central compartment soft tissue
T4b	Tumor invades prevertebral fascia, encases carotid artery, or involves mediastinal structures

Primary tumor (T): Sinuses (C30)

Paranasal sinuses – maxillary

TX	Primary tumor cannot be assessed
T0	No evidence of primary tumor
Tis	Carcinoma in situ
T1	Tumor limited to maxillary sinus mucosa with no erosion or destruction of bone
T2	Tumor causing bone erosion or destruction including extension into hard palate and/or middle nasal meatus, except extension to the posterior wall of maxillary sinus and pterygoid plates
T3	Tumor invades any of the following: bone of posterior wall of maxillary sinus, subcutaneous tissues, floor or medial wall of orbit, pterygoid fossa, ethmoid sinuses
T4a	Tumor invades anterior orbital contents, skin of cheek, pterygoid plates, infratemporal fossa, cribriform plate, sphenoid or frontal sinuses
T4b	Tumor invades any of the following: orbital apex, dura, brain, middle cranial fossa, cranial nerves other than maxillary division of trigeminal nerve V2, nasopharynx, or clivus

Paranasal sinuses: nasal cavity and ethmoid sinus

TX	Primary tumor cannot be assessed
T0	No evidence of primary tumor
Tis	Carcinoma in situ
T1	Tumor restricted to any one subsite, with or without bony invasion
T2	Tumor invading two subsites in a single region or extending to involve an adjacent region within the nasoethmoidal complex, with or without bony invasion
T3	Tumor extends to invade the medial wall or floor of the orbit, maxillary sinus, palate, or cribriform plate
T4a	Tumor invades any of the following: anterior orbital contents, skin of nose or cheek, minimal extension to anterior cranial fossa, pterygoid plates, sphenoid or frontal sinuses

Table 1.8 (continued)

T4b	Tumor invades any of the following: orbital apex, dura, brain, middle cranial fossa, cranial nerves other than maxillary division of trigeminal nerve V2, nasopharynx, or clivus

Larynx (C32)

Glottic

TX	Primary tumor cannot be assessed
T0	No evidence of primary tumor
Tis	Carcinoma in situ
T1	Tumor limited to the vocal cord with normal mobility
T1a	Tumor limited to one vocal cord
T1b	Tumor involves both vocal cords
T2	Tumor extends to supraglottis and/or subglottis, or with impaired vocal cord mobility
T3	Tumor limited to larynx with vocal cord fixation, and/or invades paraglottic space, and/or minor thyroid cartilage erosion (e.g., inner cortex)
T4a	Tumor invades through the thyroid cartilage and/or invades tissues beyond the larynx
T4b	Tumor invades prevertebral space, encases carotid artery, or invades mediastinal structures

Supraglottic

TX	Primary tumor cannot be assessed
T0	No evidence of primary tumor
Tis	Carcinoma in situ
T1	Tumor limited to one subsite of supraglottis with normal vocal cord mobility
T2	Tumor invades mucosa of more than one adjacent subsite of supraglottis or glottis or region outside the supraglottis without fixation of the larynx
T3	Tumor limited to larynx with vocal cord fixation and/or invades any of the following: post-cricoid area, pre-epiglottic tissues, paraglottic space, and/or minor thyroid cartilage erosion (e.g., inner cortex)
T4a	Tumor invades through the thyroid cartilage and/or invades tissue beyond the larynx
T4b	Tumor invades prevertebral space, encases carotid artery, or invades mediastinal structures

Regional lymph nodes (N)

Lip and oral cavity, oropharynx, larynx, hypopharynx, major salivary glands, and paranasal sinuses

NX	Regional lymph nodes cannot be assessed
N0	No regional lymph node metastasis
N1	Metastasis in a single ipsilateral lymph node, 3 cm or less in greatest dimension
N2	Metastasis in a single ipsilateral lymph node, more than 3 cm but not more than 6 cm in greatest dimension; or in multiple ipsilateral lymph nodes, none more than 6 cm in greatest dimension; or in bilateral or contralateral lymph nodes, none more than 6 cm in greatest dimension
N2a	Metastasis in a single ipsilateral lymph node more than 3 cm but not more than 6 cm in greatest dimension
N2b	Metastasis in multiple ipsilateral lymph nodes, none more than 6 cm in greatest dimension

(continued)

Table 1.8 (continued)

N2c	Metastasis in bilateral or contralateral lymph nodes, none more than 6 cm in greatest dimension
N3	Metastasis in a lymph node more than 6 cm in greatest dimension
Nasopharynx	
NX	Regional lymph nodes cannot be assessed
N0	No regional lymph node metastasis
N1	Unilateral metastasis in lymph node(s), 6 cm or less in greatest dimension, above the supraclavicular fossa
N2	Bilateral metastasis in lymph node(s), 6 cm or less in greatest dimension, above the supraclavicular fossa
N3	Metastasis in a lymph node >6 cm, and/or to supraclavicular fossa
N3a	Greater than 6 cm in dimension
N3b	Extension to the supraclavicular fossa
Metastasis (M)	
All head and neck sites	
MX	Distant metastasis cannot be assessed
M0	No distant metastasis
M1	Distant metastasis

Source: Ref. [156]

[a]Extraparenchymal extension is clinical or macroscopic evidence of invasion of soft tissues. Microscopic evidence alone does not constitute extraparenchymal extension for classification purposes

[b]Parapharyngeal extension denotes posterolateral infiltration of tumor beyond the pharyngobasilar fascia

Table 1.9 TNM stage grouping for head and neck cancer

Stage	T	N	M
Lip and oral cavity (C00–C06)			
0	Tis	N0	M0
I	T1	N0	M0
II	T2	N0	M0
III	T3	N0	M0
	T1	N1	
	T2	N1	
	T3	N1	
IVA	T4a	N0	M0
	T4a	N1	
	T1	N2	
	T2	N2	
	T3	N2	
	T4a	N2	
IVB	Any T	N3	M0
	T4b	Any N	

Table 1.9 (continued)

Stage	T	N	M
Major salivary glands (C07–08)			
I	T1	N0	M0
II	T2	N0	M0
III	T3	N0	M0
	T1	N1	
	T2	N1	
	T3	N1	
IVA	T4a	N0	M0
	T4a	N1	
	T1	N2	
	T2	N2	
	T3	N2	
	T4a	N2	
IVB	T4b	Any N	M0
	Any T	N3	
IVC	Any T	Any N	M1
Oropharynx (C09–C10) and hypopharynx (C12–C13)			
0	Tis	N0	M0
I	T1	N0	M0
II	T2	N0	M0
III	T3	N0	M0
	T1	N1	
	T2	N1	
	T3	N1	
IVA	T4a	N0	M0
	T4a	N1	
	T1	N2	
	T2	N2	
	T3	N2	
	T4a	N2	
IVB	T4b	Any N	M0
	Any T	N3	
IVC	Any T	Any N	M1
Nasopharynx (C11)			
0	Tis	N0	M0
I	T1	N0	M0
IIA	T2a	N0	M0
IIB	T1	N1	M0
	T2	N1	
	T2a	N1	
	T2b	N0	
	T2b	N1	

(continued)

Table 1.9 (continued)

Stage	T	N	M
III	T1	N2	M0
	T2a	N2	
	T2b	N2	
	T3	N0	
	T3	N1	
	T3	N2	
IVA	T4	N0	M0
	T4	N1	
	T4	N2	
IVB	Any T	N3	M0
IVC	Any T	Any N	M1
Nasal cavity and paranasal sinuses (C30)			
0	Tis	N0	M0
I	T1	N0	M0
II	T2	N0	M0
III	T3	N0	M0
	T1	N1	
	T2	N1	
	T3	N1	
IVA	T4a	N0	M0
	T4a	N1	
	T1	N2	
	T2	N2	
	T3	N2	
	T4a	N2	
IVB	T4b	Any N	M0
	Any T	N3	
IVC	Any T	Any N	M1
Larynx (supraglottic, glottic, subglottic) (C32)			
0	Tis	N0	M0
I	T1	N0	M0
II	T2	N0	M0
III	T3	N0	M0
	T1	N1	
	T2	N1	
	T3	N1	
IVA	T4a	N0	M0
	T4a	N1	
	T1	N2	
	T2	N2	
	T3	N2	
	T4a	N2	
IVB	T4b	Any N	M0
	Any T	N3	
IVC	Any T	Any N	M1

Source: Ref. [156]

Prevention

There is no proven way to prevent HNC completely, yet HNC is potentially preventable. Prevention is the primary potential strategy for long-term disease control, whereas to improve mortality in the short term, early detection and treatment may have limited potential. The spread of information regarding the risk factors for HNC in the general public through governmental supported programs would promote health [18, 132].

Diverse factors cause different types of HNC. The risk can be lowered by practicing healthy habits that include discontinuing the use of tobacco in any form and circumventing consumption of alcohol, as these are the two major factors responsible for the varied types of HNC.

Vaccines exist to protect against HPV strains associated with HNC. HPV vaccines (Cervarix and Gardasil) are now available, which can help reduce the incidence of various HNC in young adult women with prior exposure to HPV [38]. However, the vaccination of HPV has not been incorporated in the national immunization program of several countries. In Australia, the HPV vaccination program for females aged 12–13 years was introduced in 2007, but there is a dispute about using the HPV vaccine in Australian men. HPV vaccination may decrease the future incidence of these cancers [18, 157]. HPV infection can also be circumvented by limiting the number of sexual partners, as having several partners increases the risk of HPV infection and condoms do not provide complete protection from HPV.

Using a lip balm with an adequate sun protection factor (SPF) reduces the risk of lip cancer. Maintaining and taking proper care of dentures reduces the HNC risk as poorly fitted dentures can trap cancer-causing substances, such as tobacco and alcohol.

Several studies have reported that regular consumption of a diet rich in complex carbohydrates, vegetable oil, fish, fruits, vegetables, phytoestrogens, and lean meat decreases the risk of oral cavity cancer by 50%, and it has also been observed that consumption of fruits and green leafy vegetables decreases the risk of HNC by twofold in comparison to consumption of butter and pulses [18, 20, 38, 115, 158–160]. Zheng et al. (1996) reported that incorporation of dark yellow vegetables and liver in the regular diet reduces the risk of salivary gland cancer [80].

Dark-yellow vegetables contain high levels of carotenoids (β-carotene), a major vitamin A precursor, while liver contains high levels of retinol. Supplementation with a high dose of retinol has been reported to reduce the incidence of second primary cancers in patients with HNC [161]. Rowe et al. (1970) reported that vitamin A deficiency increases the risk of salivary gland carcinogenesis [162]. Dark-yellow vegetables are also high in vitamin C and many other carotenoids; they are efficient antioxidants, which can prevent damage to chromosomes, enzymes, and cell membranes caused by the peroxidation of free radicals [163]. Dietary vitamin C, phenols, aromatic isothiocyanates, and flavones have reports of inhibiting carcinogenesis in experimental studies [80, 163, 164]. Antioxidants protect the cellular and molecular damage caused by ROS and RNS [13].

At present, preventive measures are not considered in the general public due to a lack of awareness about HNC and the lack of cancer prevention programs [165]. Governments should take the initiative to eradicate the causes as was done in Taiwan, whose government initiated a Betel Nut Control Program long ago to crack down on betel nut chewing, by offering a subsidy to farmers growing alternative crops [166]. Additionally, the Taiwanese Bureau of National Health Insurance announced the plan to impose a health tax on betel nuts [166]. Canada has banned the sale of areca nut products [26]. The US FDA has also issued an import alert and banned interstate traffic of areca nut [26]. Developing countries have a higher need to take serious steps toward spreading awareness regarding the risk factors of HNC as this cancer is prevalent amongst low socioeconomic groups.

Treatment

The treatments used for HNC include surgery, radiation therapy (RT), chemotherapy (CT), targeted therapy (TT), and immunotherapy (IT) [45, 167]. The type of treatment used for various HNCs depends on the type and stage of the cancer, possible side effects, and the patient's overall health. Based on the indications, a combination of treatments is often used.

Surgery This process removes some surrounding healthy tissue along with the tumor. More than one operation would be conducted based on the patient's condition [118].

Radiation Therapy (RT) This treatment is mostly recommended instead of surgery. This therapy is also used sometimes after surgery to destroy remaining cancer cells [118].

Chemotherapy (ChT) This therapy is used before or after surgery or in combination with radiation therapy. Cisplatin and Fluorouracil (5-FU) are ChT drugs used to treat HNC [118].

Targeted Therapy (TT) Regardless of the advanced therapies for the treatment of HNSCC, survival rates, functional outcomes, and toxicities of therapy remain poorly understood [168]. Targeted agents currently either approved or under investigation for HNSCC include epidermal growth factor receptor (EGFR) monoclonal antibodies (cetuximab, panitumumab, zalutumumab, and nimotuzumab), EGFR tyrosine kinase inhibitors (gefitinib, erlotinib, lapatinib, afatinib, and dacomitinib), vascular endothelial growth factor receptor (VEGFR) inhibitors (bevacizumab, sorafenib, sunitinib, and vandetanib) and various inhibitors of other pathways such as phosphatidylinositol 30 kinase (PI3K)/AKT/mammalian target of rapamycin (mTOR), MET, and insulin-like growth factor receptor (IGF-1R). Clinical trials are evaluating these emerging agents and their combinations for treating HNSCC [168].

Immunotherapy (IT)   Immunotherapy is an option for patients with advanced HNC.

Diet   A significant difference among the survival of undernourished HNC patients (7.5%) and adequately nourished patients (57.5%) undergoing radiotherapy at 2 years was reported by Brookes (1985) [18, 169].

Stagewise Treatment for HNC

The treatment of early-stage HNCs involves both surgery and definitive RT. Both surgery and definitive RT provide comparable control of local tumor. They both appear to offer equivalent local tumor control. Yet, the type of treatment is chosen based on several factors as site of tumor, the outcome of the treatment, accessibility to treatment expertise, patients' health, and their preference. All these factors need to be evaluated for enhancing the treatment outcome in patients. Surgery involves removal of the primary tumor with or without nodal lymph dissection and is preferred for treatment of oral cavity cancers at an early stage, while definitive RT is favored when patients refuse surgery or when the tumor is medically inoperable and present in hypopharynx, supraglottic, and glottic larynx cancer. In such locations definitive RT provide an improved functional outcome in comparison to surgical approaches. Patients detected with residual disease post-RT are advised to undergo a rescue surgery and patients with presence of close or positive margin, lymphovascular or perineural invasion or identification of a positive lymph node upstaging the tumor are recommended a post-operative RT [126].

ChT is another treatment recommended for HNC. During ChT, the patient is administered with cisplatin and require intravenous infusion capacity accompanied with adequate IV hydration and antiemetics. Sufficient hydration, nutrition, and analgesia must be maintained before, during, and post completion of ChT. Throughout treatment it is essential to monitor the blood counts and health of the patient as ChT produces several side effects. The late treatment-related toxicities such as xerostomia, dysphagia, speech dysfunction, gastric tube dependence, tracheostomy dependence, neuropathies, depression, and cosmetic disfigurement have a significant impact on psychosocial well-being of the patient and therefore necessary care must be provided [126].

Early Stage HNC

Early-stage HNC (stage I and II) is curable in 60–95% of patients with local treatment [170]. Rate of cure is dependent on the size and location of the tumor and the ability to deliver the necessary treatment. Nearly all head and neck tumors are treated via surgical procedures, with the exception of nasopharyngeal carcinoma as surgery for it is very complicated due to its anatomic location and hence RT is used for its treatment [171]. Therefore, the choice of RT versus surgery for stage I and stage II HNC relies on several reasons such as tumor location, the probability for long-term illness due to treatment, physician's skill for the treatment, preference of the patient, comorbidities, and prior history of radiation or expected need for future radiation [118].

Surgery or RT can be used to treat oral cavity tumors. Patients treated with oral cavity tumors recover slowly from surgery with relatively proper function and thereby exhibits low morbidity in comparison to RT, as it exhibits side effects such as acute mucositis, tongue discomfort, dental decay, and possible long-term diet changes [118].

Early-stage tumors in the oropharynx are more frequently treated with RT because surgery generally causes more morbidity than RT. Hence, even though RT exhibits risks such as xerostomia, mild to moderate swallowing dysfunction, this method is considered [118].

Surgery for tumors of the nasopharynx is not easy; therefore, stage I or II (relatively uncommon) are treated with RT alone [118].

Stage III/IV Cancers

Patients with stage III or IV cancers of HNC (locoregionally advanced HNC) suffer from large or locally progressive T3 or T4 tumors or involve lymph nodes within the neck. Notably, about 60% of HNC patients are diagnosed with locoregionally advanced stage III and IV tumor [172, 173]. Among the two stages, a large number are diagnosed with stage IV (stage IVA) tumors [118]. Stage IV HNC patients with metastatic and locoregionally advanced HNC are generally not curable, and patients have an average survival period of about 6 months but then the nonmetastatic stage IV HNC is curable [118].

The treatment of locoregionally advanced HNC is somewhat controversial and is reliant upon the surgeon, institution, and the readiness of a patient to lose essential organs such as the tongue, mandible, pharynx, and larynx [118]. Survival outcomes appear to be better for patients undergoing primary surgery of stage III and IV tumors, often involving postoperative radiation than that for patients receiving radiotherapy only. ChT is integrated into the treatment of most stage III and IV nasopharyngeal tumors, whereas stage III/IV larynx and hypopharynx cancers are treated using sequential or concomitant ChT and RT instead of surgery [118].

In RT, altered fraction radiation implies methodologies such as hyperfractionation RT (HRT – divides the daily doses into small fractions without shortening the duration of treatment) and accelerated RT (ART – deliver a course of radiation in a short period with high daily doses). HRT for treatment of oropharynx cancer has been found to improve locoregional control and survival as against standard fraction radiation. However, HRT exhibits significantly higher side effects. ART has not exhibited consistent benefit that HRT has shown [118].

Combined therapy employing ChT and RT began in the late 1970s to early 1980s. Presurgical ChT almost always led to dramatic tumor responses. There is a slight survival benefit that has been demonstrated with cisplatin and 5-FU as against the locoregional therapy alone [118].

In the 1980s, simultaneous delivery of ChT and RT (concomitant chemoradiotherapy – CRT) was investigated for overcoming radiation resistance in HNC. Patients with HNC not capable of being surgically removed were subjected to randomized trials with RT alone versus the same RT with ChT. Initial studies generally utilized single-agent ChT, but later, multiagent ChT (MCT) was utilized. MCT has been found to exhibit greater overall survival benefit than single-agent ChT. CRT can be used as a rescue tool only with the elimination of surgery. Patients undergoing primary RT will have the potential for cure with rescue surgery. Likewise, few patients, especially those with early-stage HNC who had surgery only, are rescued with RT or CRT [118].

Metastatic Disease

Patients with locoregionally recurrent, incurable, or metastatic HNC have a poor prognosis and have an average survival of 3–4 months without ChT and approximately 5–6 months with ChT [174]. Several single-agent ChT drugs such as cisplatin, carboplatin, paclitaxel, docetaxel, 5-FU, and methotrexate exhibit 15–25% response rates [118, 175]. Combination ChT generally includes cisplatin/carboplatin and paclitaxel/docetaxel, or 5FU, and this treatment increase the response rates to 30–35%. However, the survival rate remains the same, whether it is a single-agent or multi-agent ChT [118].

New treatments are under evaluation for HNC, including various biologically TT. EGFR is overexpressed in the majority of HNC. Hence EGFR is used as a target for the treatment of HNC, either using monoclonal antibodies directed against EGFR or key downstream targets of EGFR. HNC patients generally overexpress p53 or express mutated p53. Therefore, p53 is also considered as the target for gene therapy. Adenovirus is used as a vector, which can be made replication-competent or deficient, to deliver a mutant or wild-type p53 for gene therapies. Based on efficacy and feasibility of utilizing p53 gene transfer observed in phase I and phase II studies, large-scale phase III trials have been conducted to test the efficacy of gene transfer therapy when added to standard ChT for locoregionally advanced head neck cancer [118].

Perspective

The epidemiology of HNC shows a higher percentage incidence of HNC compared to other cancers in the respective continent in areas with developing nations. The main reason could be the overlap of HNC symptoms with indications of regular oral ailments, which are either ignored by the individual or the medical practitioner. The delay is mostly due to a lack of awareness about the symptoms, which results in delayed diagnosis resulting in higher morbidity and mortality rates. The reason can also be the increased usage of carcinogens due to a lack of awareness. Amongst the various HNCs, lip and oral cavity cancer account for the maximum number of cases, which could be due to the most prevalent lifestyle habits such as smoking tobacco and drinking alcohol. As many individuals in developing countries consume tobacco or alcohol in the crude form, and do not follow a regular oral routine, which might prove to be a lot more dangerous than the usage of their refined products, which are used in developed nations. The workers not provided with masks to protection against the occupational dust is also a reason for the increase in incidence of HNC.

In order to reduce the rate of occurrence of HNC, it becomes essential to increase awareness in the developing countries about maintaining oral health, the detriments of using tobacco and alcohol on health, the various exposomes, and their severity in causing HNC. As this cancer is mostly detected at the last stages, its symptoms and ways of prevention can be sent across as a tele-message to individuals in their respective native language, through displays at schools, advertisements in television and movie theatres.

References

1. Black RJ, Bray F, Ferlay J, Parkin DM. Cancer incidence and mortality in the European Union: cancer registry data and estimates of national incidence for 1990. Eur J Cancer. 1997;33(7):1075–107.
2. Hoffman HT, Karnell LH, Funk GF, Robinson RA, Menck HR. The National Cancer Data Base report on cancer of the head and neck. Arch Otolaryngol Head Neck Surg. 1998;124(9):951–62.
3. Levi F, Lucchini F, La Vecchia C, Negri E. Trends in mortality from cancer in the European Union, 1955-94. Lancet. 1999;354(9180):742–3.
4. Stoyanov GS, Kitanova M, Dzhenkov DL, Ghenev P, Sapundzhiev N. Demographics of head and neck cancer patients: a single institution experience. Cureus. 2017;9(7):e1418.
5. Royster HP. Surgical diagnosis in cancer of the head and neck. Surg Clin North Am. 1952;32(6):1599–616.
6. Lynch P.J. CBhcolb. https://upload.wikimedia.org/wikipedia/commons/5/51/Head_lateral_mouth_anatomy.jpg.
7. Shaikh MH, Khan AI, Sadat A, Chowdhury AH, Jinnah SA, Gopalan V, et al. Prevalence and types of high-risk human papillomaviruses in head and neck cancers from Bangladesh. BMC Cancer. 2017;17(1):792.
8. Siegel RL, Miller KD, Jemal A. Cancer statistics, 2020. CA Cancer J Clin. 2020;70(1):7–30.
9. NIH. National cancer institute 2020. Available from: https://seer.cancer.gov/statfacts/html/lip.html.
10. Sankaranarayanan R, Masuyer E, Swaminathan R, Ferlay J, Whelan S. Head and neck cancer: a global perspective on epidemiology and prognosis. Anticancer Res. 1998;18(6B):4779–86.
11. Addala L, Pentapati CK, Reddy Thavanati PK, Anjaneyulu V, Sadhnani MD. Risk factor profiles of head and neck cancer patients of Andhra Pradesh, India. Indian J Cancer. 2012;49(2):215–9.
12. Turner MC, Nieuwenhuijsen M, Anderson K, Balshaw D, Cui Y, Dunton G, et al. Assessing the exposome with external measures: commentary on the state of the science and research recommendations. Annu Rev Public Health. 2017;38:215–39.
13. Khalili J. Oral cancer: risk factors, prevention and diagnostic. Exp Oncol. 2008;30(4):259–64.
14. Khan Z, Tonnies J, Muller S. Smokeless tobacco and oral cancer in South Asia: a systematic review with meta-analysis. J Cancer Epidemiol. 2014;2014:394696.
15. Gupta PC, Ray CS. Epidemiology of betel quid usage. Ann Acad Med Singap. 2004;33(4 Suppl):31–6.

16. Proia NK, Paszkiewicz GM, Nasca MA, Franke GE, Pauly JL. Smoking and smokeless tobacco-associated human buccal cell mutations and their association with oral cancer – a review. Cancer Epidemiol Biomark Prev. 2006;15(6):1061–77.
17. Gupta PC, Sinor PN, Bhonsle RB, Pawar VS, Mehta HC. Oral submucous fibrosis in India: a new epidemic? Natl Med J India. 1998;11(3):113–6.
18. Singh SP, Eisenberg R, Hoffman G. An overview and comparative evaluation of head and neck cancer risk factors in India and Australia. Int J Otolaryngol Head Neck Surg. 2018;7(5):254–67.
19. Elwood JM, Pearson JC, Skippen DH, Jackson SM. Alcohol, smoking, social and occupational factors in the aetiology of cancer of the oral cavity, pharynx and larynx. Int J Cancer. 1984;34(5):603–12.
20. Warnakulasuriya S. 14 – Food, nutrition and oral cancer. In: Wilson M, editor. Food constituents and oral health. Cambridge: Woodhead Publishing; 2009. p. 273–95.
21. Garavello W, Bertuccio P, Levi F, Lucchini F, Bosetti C, Malvezzi M, et al. The oral cancer epidemic in central and eastern Europe. Int J Cancer. 2010;127(1):160–71.
22. Gupta B, Johnson NW, Kumar N. Global epidemiology of head and neck cancers: a continuing challenge. Oncology. 2016;91(1):13–23.
23. Gupta N, Gupta R, Acharya AK, Patthi B, Goud V, Reddy S, et al. Changing trends in oral cancer – a global scenario. Nepal J Epidemiol. 2016;6(4):613–9.
24. Warnakulasuriya S. Global epidemiology of oral and oropharyngeal cancer. Oral Oncol. 2009;45(4–5):309–16.
25. Boffetta P, Hecht S, Gray N, Gupta P, Straif K. Smokeless tobacco and cancer. Lancet Oncol. 2008;9(7):667–75.
26. Pankaj C. Areca nut or betel nut control is mandatory if India wants to reduce the burden of cancer especially cancer of the oral cavity. Int J Head Neck Surg. 2010;1(1):17–20.
27. Mahboubi E. The epidemiology of oral cavity, pharyngeal and esophageal cancer outside of North America and Western Europe. Cancer. 1977;40(4 Suppl):1879–86.
28. Sapkota A, Gajalakshmi V, Jetly DH, Roychowdhury S, Dikshit RP, Brennan P, et al. Smokeless tobacco and increased risk of hypopharyngeal and laryngeal cancers: a multicentric case-control study from India. Int J Cancer. 2007;121(8):1793–8.
29. Mahdavifar N, Ghoncheh M, Mohammadian-Hafshejani A, Khosravi B, Salehiniya H. Epidemiology and inequality in the incidence and mortality of nasopharynx cancer in Asia. Osong Public Health Res Perspect. 2016;7(6):360–72.
30. Yu MC, Yuan JM. Epidemiology of nasopharyngeal carcinoma. Semin Cancer Biol. 2002;12(6):421–9.
31. Horn-Ross PL, Ljung BM, Morrow M. Environmental factors and the risk of salivary gland cancer. Epidemiology. 1997;8(4):414–9.
32. La Vecchia C, Tavani A, Franceschi S, Levi F, Corrao G, Negri E. Epidemiology and prevention of oral cancer. Oral Oncol. 1997;33(5):302–12.
33. Maier H, Sennewald E, Heller GF, Weidauer H. Chronic alcohol consumption – the key risk factor for pharyngeal cancer. Otolaryngol Head Neck Surg. 1994;110(2):168–73.
34. Tuyns AJ, Esteve J, Raymond L, Berrino F, Benhamou E, Blanchet F, et al. Cancer of the larynx/hypopharynx, tobacco and alcohol: IARC international case-control study in Turin and Varese (Italy), Zaragoza and Navarra (Spain), Geneva (Switzerland) and Calvados (France). Int J Cancer. 1988;41(4):483–91.
35. Guenel P, Chastang JF, Luce D, Leclerc A, Brugere J. A study of the interaction of alcohol drinking and tobacco smoking among French cases of laryngeal cancer. J Epidemiol Community Health. 1988;42(4):350–4.
36. Laforest L, Luce D, Goldberg P, Begin D, Gerin M, Demers PA, et al. Laryngeal and hypopharyngeal cancers and occupational exposure to formaldehyde and various dusts: a case-control study in France. Occup Environ Med. 2000;57(11):767–73.
37. Blot WJ, McLaughlin JK, Winn DM, Austin DF, Greenberg RS, Preston-Martin S, et al. Smoking and drinking in relation to oral and pharyngeal cancer. Cancer Res. 1988;48(11):3282–7.

38. Warnakulasuriya S. Causes of oral cancer – an appraisal of controversies. Br Dent J. 2009;207(10):471–5.
39. Smith EM, Rubenstein LM, Haugen TH, Pawlita M, Turek LP. Complex etiology underlies risk and survival in head and neck cancer human papillomavirus, tobacco, and alcohol: a case for multifactor disease. J Oncol. 2012;2012:571862.
40. Perdomo S, Martin Roa G, Brennan P, Forman D, Sierra MS. Head and neck cancer burden and preventive measures in Central and South America. Cancer Epidemiol. 2016;44(Suppl 1):S43–52.
41. Gillison ML, Koch WM, Capone RB, Spafford M, Westra WH, Wu L, et al. Evidence for a causal association between human papillomavirus and a subset of head and neck cancers. J Natl Cancer Inst. 2000;92(9):709–20.
42. Näsman A, Attner P, Hammarstedt L, Du J, Eriksson M, Giraud G, et al. Incidence of human papillomavirus (HPV) positive tonsillar carcinoma in Stockholm, Sweden: an epidemic of viral-induced carcinoma? Int J Cancer. 2009;125(2):362–6.
43. Mehanna H, Beech T, Nicholson T, El-Hariry I, McConkey C, Paleri V, et al. Prevalence of human papillomavirus in oropharyngeal and nonoropharyngeal head and neck cancer – systematic review and meta-analysis of trends by time and region. Head Neck. 2013;35(5):747–55.
44. Mehanna H, Evans M, Beasley M, Chatterjee S, Dilkes M, Homer J, et al. Oropharyngeal cancer: United Kingdom national multidisciplinary guidelines. J Laryngol Otol. 2016;130(S2):S90–S6.
45. Chi AC, Day TA, Neville BW. Oral cavity and oropharyngeal squamous cell carcinoma – an update. CA Cancer J Clin. 2015;65(5):401–21.
46. Chang ET, Adami HO. The enigmatic epidemiology of nasopharyngeal carcinoma. Cancer Epidemiol Biomark Prev. 2006;15(10):1765–77.
47. Lawal AO, Adisa AO, Kolude B, Adeyemi BF. Malignant salivary gland tumours of the head and neck region: a single institutions review. Pan Afr Med J. 2015;20:121.
48. Levi F, Pasche C, La Vecchia C, Lucchini F, Franceschi S, Monnier P. Food groups and risk of oral and pharyngeal cancer. Int J Cancer. 1998;77(5):705–9.
49. Kreimer AR, Randi G, Herrero R, Castellsague X, La Vecchia C, Franceschi S, et al. Diet and body mass, and oral and oropharyngeal squamous cell carcinomas: analysis from the IARC multinational case-control study. Int J Cancer. 2006;118(9):2293–7.
50. Lucenteforte E, Garavello W, Bosetti C, La Vecchia C. Dietary factors and oral and pharyngeal cancer risk. Oral Oncol. 2009;45(6):461–7.
51. Forrest J, Campbell P, Kreiger N, Sloan M. Salivary gland cancer: an exploratory analysis of dietary factors. Nutr Cancer. 2008;60(4):469–73.
52. Dasanayake AP, Silverman AJ, Warnakulasuriya S. Mate drinking and oral and oro-pharyngeal cancer: a systematic review and meta-analysis. Oral Oncol. 2010;46(2):82–6.
53. Otoh EC, Johnson NW, Danfillo IS, Adeleke OA, Olasoji HA. Primary head and neck cancers in North Eastern Nigeria. West Afr J Med. 2004;23(4):305–13.
54. da Lilly-Tariah OB, Somefun AO, Adeyemo WL. Current evidence on the burden of head and neck cancers in Nigeria. Head Neck Oncol. 2009;1:14.
55. Yu MC, Ho JH, Lai SH, Henderson BE. Cantonese-style salted fish as a cause of nasopharyngeal carcinoma: report of a case-control study in Hong Kong. Cancer Res. 1986;46(2):956–61.
56. Ning JP, Yu MC, Wang QS, Henderson BE. Consumption of salted fish and other risk factors for nasopharyngeal carcinoma (NPC) in Tianjin, a low-risk region for NPC in the People's Republic of China. J Natl Cancer Inst. 1990;82(4):291–6.
57. Armstrong RW, Imrey PB, Lye MS, Armstrong MJ, Yu MC, Sani S. Nasopharyngeal carcinoma in Malaysian Chinese: salted fish and other dietary exposures. Int J Cancer. 1998;77(2):228–35.
58. Her C. Nasopharyngeal cancer and the Southeast Asian patient. Am Fam Physician. 2001;63(9):1776–82.
59. Jia WH, Luo XY, Feng BJ, Ruan HL, Bei JX, Liu WS, et al. Traditional Cantonese diet and nasopharyngeal carcinoma risk: a large-scale case-control study in Guangdong, China. BMC Cancer. 2010;10:446.

60. Zou XN, Lu SH, Liu B. Volatile N-nitrosamines and their precursors in Chinese salted fish – a possible etological factor for NPC in China. Int J Cancer. 1994;59(2):155–8.
61. Huang DP, Ho JH, Webb KS, Wood BJ, Gough TA. Volatile nitrosamines in salt-preserved fish before and after cooking. Food Cosmet Toxicol. 1981;19(2):167–71.
62. Hildesheim A, West S, DeVeyra E, De Guzman MF, Jurado A, Jones C, et al. Herbal medicine use, Epstein-Barr virus, and risk of nasopharyngeal carcinoma. Cancer Res. 1992;52(11):3048–51.
63. Divaris K, Olshan AF, Smith J, Bell ME, Weissler MC, Funkhouser WK, et al. Oral health and risk for head and neck squamous cell carcinoma: the Carolina Head and Neck Cancer Study. Cancer Causes Control. 2010;21(4):567–75.
64. Meyer MS, Joshipura K, Giovannucci E, Michaud DS. A review of the relationship between tooth loss, periodontal disease, and cancer. Cancer Causes Control. 2008;19(9):895–907.
65. Holmes L Jr, DesVignes-Kendrick M, Slomka J, Mahabir S, Beeravolu S, Emani SR. Is dental care utilization associated with oral cavity cancer in a large sample of community-based United States residents? Community Dent Oral Epidemiol. 2009;37(2):134–42.
66. Zheng TZ, Boyle P, Hu HF, Duan J, Jian PJ, Ma DQ, et al. Dentition, oral hygiene, and risk of oral cancer: a case-control study in Beijing, People's Republic of China. Cancer Causes Control. 1990;1(3):235–41.
67. Albrecht M, Banoczy J, Dinya E, Tamas G Jr. Occurrence of oral leukoplakia and lichen planus in diabetes mellitus. J Oral Pathol Med. 1992;21(8):364–6.
68. van Leeuwen MT, Grulich AE, McDonald SP, McCredie MR, Amin J, Stewart JH, et al. Immunosuppression and other risk factors for lip cancer after kidney transplantation. Cancer Epidemiol Biomark Prev. 2009;18(2):561–9.
69. Li AC, Warnakulasuriya S, Thompson RP. Neoplasia of the tongue in a patient with Crohn's disease treated with azathioprine: case report. Eur J Gastroenterol Hepatol. 2003;15(2):185–7.
70. Zhao H, Chu M, Huang Z, Yang X, Ran S, Hu B, et al. Variations in oral microbiota associated with oral cancer. Sci Rep. 2017;7(1):11773.
71. Faggiano F, Partanen T, Kogevinas M, Boffetta P. Socioeconomic differences in cancer incidence and mortality. IARC Sci Publ. 1997;138:65–176.
72. Conway DI, Petticrew M, Marlborough H, Berthiller J, Hashibe M, Macpherson LM. Socioeconomic inequalities and oral cancer risk: a systematic review and meta-analysis of case-control studies. Int J Cancer. 2008;122(12):2811–9.
73. McDonald JT, Johnson-Obaseki S, Hwang E, Connell C, Corsten M. The relationship between survival and socio-economic status for head and neck cancer in Canada. J Otolaryngol Head Neck Surg. 2014;43:2.
74. Tiyuri A, Mohammadian-Hafshejani A, Iziy E, Gandomani H, Salehiniya H. The incidence and mortality of lip and oral cavity cancer and its relationship to the 2012 Human Development Index of Asia. BMRAT. 2017;4(02):1147–65.
75. Wake M. The urban/rural divide in head and neck cancer – the effect of atmospheric pollution. Clin Otolaryngol Allied Sci. 1993;18(4):298–302.
76. Dietz A, Senneweld E, Maier H. Indoor air pollution by emissions of fossil fuel single stoves: possibly a hitherto underrated risk factor in the development of carcinomas in the head and neck. Otolaryngol Head Neck Surg. 1995;112(2):308–15.
77. Pintos J, Franco EL, Kowalski LP, Oliveira BV, Curado MP. Use of wood stoves and risk of cancers of the upper aero-digestive tract: a case-control study. Int J Epidemiol. 1998;27(6):936–40.
78. Williams RR, Stegens NL, Goldsmith JR. Associations of cancer site and type with occupation and industry from the Third National Cancer Survey Interview. J Natl Cancer Inst. 1977;59(4):1147–85.
79. Flanders WD, Rothman KJ. Occupational risk for laryngeal cancer. Am J Public Health. 1982;72(4):369–72.
80. Zheng W, Shu XO, Ji BT, Gao YT. Diet and other risk factors for cancer of the salivary glands: a population-based case-control study. Int J Cancer. 1996;67(2):194–8.

81. Paget-Bailly S, Guida F, Carton M, Menvielle G, Radoi L, Cyr D, et al. Occupation and head and neck cancer risk in men: results from the ICARE study, a French population-based case-control study. J Occup Environ Med. 2013;55(9):1065–73.
82. Comba P, Barbieri PG, Battista G, Belli S, Ponterio F, Zanetti D, et al. Cancer of the nose and paranasal sinuses in the metal industry: a case-control study. Br J Ind Med. 1992;49(3):193–6.
83. Binazzi A, Ferrante P, Marinaccio A. Occupational exposure and sinonasal cancer: a systematic review and meta-analysis. BMC Cancer. 2015;15:49.
84. Cauvin JM, Guenel P, Luce D, Brugere J, Leclerc A. Occupational exposure and head and neck carcinoma. Clin Otolaryngol Allied Sci. 1990;15(5):439–45.
85. Dietz A, Ramroth H, Urban T, Ahrens W, Becher H. Exposure to cement dust, related occupational groups and laryngeal cancer risk: results of a population based case-control study. Int J Cancer. 2004;108(6):907–11.
86. Pukkala E, Soderholm AL, Lindqvist C. Cancers of the lip and oropharynx in different social and occupational groups in Finland. Eur J Cancer B Oral Oncol. 1994;30B(3):209–15.
87. Gustavsson P, Jakobsson R, Johansson H, Lewin F, Norell S, Rutkvist LE. Occupational exposures and squamous cell carcinoma of the oral cavity, pharynx, larynx, and oesophagus: a case-control study in Sweden. Occup Environ Med. 1998;55(6):393–400.
88. Boukheris H, Curtis RE, Land CE, Dores GM. Incidence of carcinoma of the major salivary glands according to the WHO classification, 1992 to 2006: a population-based study in the United States. Cancer Epidemiol Biomark Prev. 2009;18(11):2899–906.
89. Langevin SM, McClean MD, Michaud DS, Eliot M, Nelson HH, Kelsey KT. Occupational dust exposure and head and neck squamous cell carcinoma risk in a population-based case-control study conducted in the greater Boston area. Cancer Med. 2013;2(6):978–86.
90. Elwood JM. Wood exposure and smoking: association with cancer of the nasal cavity and paranasal sinuses in British Columbia. Can Med Assoc J. 1981;124(12):1573–7.
91. Purdue MP, Järvholm B, Bergdahl IA, Hayes RB, Baris D. Occupational exposures and head and neck cancers among Swedish construction workers. Scand J Work Environ Health. 2006;32(4):270–5.
92. Straif K, Benbrahim-Tallaa L, Baan R, Grosse Y, Secretan B, El Ghissassi F, et al. A review of human carcinogens – Part C: Metals, arsenic, dusts, and fibres. Lancet Oncol. 2009;10(5):453–4.
93. Menvielle G, Fayosse A, Radoi L, Guida F, Sanchez M, Carton M, et al. The joint effect of asbestos exposure, tobacco smoking and alcohol drinking on laryngeal cancer risk: evidence from the French population-based case-control study, ICARE. Occup Environ Med. 2016;73(1):28–33.
94. Carton M, Barul C, Menvielle G, Cyr D, Sanchez M, Pilorget C, et al. Occupational exposure to solvents and risk of head and neck cancer in women: a population-based case-control study in France. BMJ Open. 2017;7(1):e012833.
95. Schottenfeld D, Fraumeni JF Jr. Cancer epidemiology and prevention. New York: Oxford University Press; 2006.
96. Land CE, Saku T, Hayashi Y, Takahara O, Matsuura H, Tokuoka S, et al. Incidence of salivary gland tumors among atomic bomb survivors, 1950-1987. Evaluation of radiation-related risk. Radiat Res. 1996;146(1):28–36.
97. Dong C, Hemminki K. Second primary neoplasms among 53 159 haematolymphoproliferative malignancy patients in Sweden, 1958-1996: a search for common mechanisms. Br J Cancer. 2001;85(7):997–1005.
98. Perea-Milla Lopez E, Minarro-Del Moral RM, Martinez-Garcia C, Zanetti R, Rosso S, Serrano S, et al. Lifestyles, environmental and phenotypic factors associated with lip cancer: a case-control study in southern Spain. Br J Cancer. 2003;88(11):1702–7.
99. Vukadinovic M, Jezdic Z, Petrovic M, Medenica LM, Lens M. Surgical management of squamous cell carcinoma of the lip: analysis of a 10-year experience in 223 patients. J Oral Maxillofac Surg. 2007;65(4):675–9.

100. Ariyawardana A, Johnson NW. Trends of lip, oral cavity and oropharyngeal cancers in Australia 1982-2008: overall good news but with rising rates in the oropharynx. BMC Cancer. 2013;13:333.
101. Belsky JL, Takeichi N, Yamamoto T, Cihak RW, Hirose F, Ezaki H, et al. Salivary gland neoplasms following atomic radiation: additional cases and reanalysis of combined data in a fixed population, 1957-1970. Cancer. 1975;35(2):555–9.
102. Spitz MR, Tilley BC, Batsakis JG, Gibeau JM, Newell GR. Risk factors for major salivary gland carcinoma. A case-comparison study. Cancer. 1984;54(9):1854–9.
103. Khlifi R, Hamza-Chaffai A. Head and neck cancer due to heavy metal exposure via tobacco smoking and professional exposure: a review. Toxicol Appl Pharmacol. 2010;248(2):71–88.
104. Llewellyn CD, Linklater K, Bell J, Johnson NW, Warnakulasuriya S. An analysis of risk factors for oral cancer in young people: a case-control study. Oral Oncol. 2004;40(3):304–13.
105. Hussein AA, Helder MN, de Visscher JG, Leemans CR, Braakhuis BJ, de Vet HCW, et al. Global incidence of oral and oropharynx cancer in patients younger than 45 years versus older patients: a systematic review. Eur J Cancer. 2017;82:115–27.
106. Russell JL, Chen NW, Ortiz SJ, Schrank TP, Kuo YF, Resto VA. Racial and ethnic disparities in salivary gland cancer survival. JAMA Otolaryngol Head Neck Surg. 2014;140(6):504–12.
107. Dahlstrom KR, Little JA, Zafereo ME, Lung M, Wei Q, Sturgis EM. Squamous cell carcinoma of the head and neck in never smoker-never drinkers: a descriptive epidemiologic study. Head Neck. 2008;30(1):75–84.
108. Subapriya R, Thangavelu A, Mathavan B, Ramachandran CR, Nagini S. Assessment of risk factors for oral squamous cell carcinoma in Chidambaram, Southern India: a case-control study. Eur J Cancer Prev. 2007;16(3):251–6.
109. Gheit T, Anantharaman D, Holzinger D, Alemany L, Tous S, Lucas E, et al. Role of mucosal high-risk human papillomavirus types in head and neck cancers in Central India. Int J Cancer. 2017;141(1):143–51.
110. Tsao SW, Tsang CM, Lo KW. Epstein-Barr virus infection and nasopharyngeal carcinoma. Philos Trans R Soc Lond B Biol Sci. 2017;372(1732):20160270.
111. King GN, Healy CM, Glover MT, Kwan JT, Williams DM, Leigh IM, et al. Increased prevalence of dysplastic and malignant lip lesions in renal-transplant recipients. N Engl J Med. 1995;332(16):1052–7.
112. Tavani A, Gallus S, La Vecchia C, Talamini R, Barbone F, Herrero R, et al. Diet and risk of oral and pharyngeal cancer. An Italian case-control study. Eur J Cancer Prev. 2001;10(2):191–5.
113. Petridou E, Zavras AI, Lefatzis D, Dessypris N, Laskaris G, Dokianakis G, et al. The role of diet and specific micronutrients in the etiology of oral carcinoma. Cancer. 2002;94(11):2981–8.
114. Llewellyn CD, Johnson NW, Warnakulasuriya S. Factors associated with delay in presentation among younger patients with oral cancer. Oral Surg Oral Med Oral Pathol Oral Radiol Endod. 2004;97(6):707–13.
115. Freedman ND, Park Y, Subar AF, Hollenbeck AR, Leitzmann MF, Schatzkin A, et al. Fruit and vegetable intake and head and neck cancer risk in a large United States prospective cohort study. Int J Cancer. 2008;122(10):2330–6.
116. Talamini R, Vaccarella S, Barbone F, Tavani A, La Vecchia C, Herrero R, et al. Oral hygiene, dentition, sexual habits and risk of oral cancer. Br J Cancer. 2000;83(9):1238–42.
117. Preston-Martin S, Henderson BE, Bernstein L. Medical and dental x rays as risk factors for recently diagnosed tumors of the head. Natl Cancer Inst Monogr. 1985;69:175–9.
118. Brockstein B, Masters G. Head and neck cancer. New York: Springer-Verlag New York Inc.; 2003.
119. Diz P, Meleti M, Diniz-Freitas M, Vescovi P, Warnakulasuriya S, Johnson NW, et al. Oral and pharyngeal cancer in Europe: incidence, mortality and trends as presented to the Global Oral Cancer Forum. Transl Res Oral Oncol. 2017;2:2057178X17701517.
120. Epstein JB, Kish RV, Hallajian L, Sciubba J. Head and neck, oral, and oropharyngeal cancer: a review of medicolegal cases. Oral Surg Oral Med Oral Pathol Oral Radiol. 2015;119(2):177–86.

121. Cancer Research UK. Together we will beat cancer. 2018 [updated 10 May 2018]. Available from: https://www.cancerresearchuk.org/about-cancer/mouth-cancer/symptoms.
122. Koivunen P, Rantala N, Hyrynkangas K, Jokinen K, Alho OP. The impact of patient and professional diagnostic delays on survival in pharyngeal cancer. Cancer. 2001;92(11):2885–91.
123. Argiris A, Karamouzis MV, Raben D, Ferris RL. Head and neck cancer. Lancet. 2008;371(9625):1695–709.
124. Davies L, Welch HG. Epidemiology of head and neck cancer in the United States. Otolaryngol Head Neck Surg. 2006;135(3):451–7.
125. Mehanna H, Paleri V, West CM, Nutting C. Head and neck cancer – Part 1: Epidemiology, presentation, and prevention. BMJ. 2010;341:c4684.
126. WHO Expert Committee on the Selection UoEMaWHO. The selection and use of essential medicines: report of the WHO Expert Committee, 2013 (including the 18th WHO model list of essential medicines and the 4th WHO model list of essential medicines for children), WHO technical report series; no. 985. Geneva: World Health Organization; 2014.
127. Rumboldt Z, Gordon L, Gordon L, Bonsall R, Ackermann S. Imaging in head and neck cancer. Curr Treat Options in Oncol. 2006;7(1):23–34.
128. Abraham J. Imaging for head and neck cancer. Surg Oncol Clin N Am. 2015;24(3):455–71.
129. Knappe M, Louw M, Gregor RT. Ultrasonography-guided fine-needle aspiration for the assessment of cervical metastases. Arch Otolaryngol Head Neck Surg. 2000;126(9):1091–6.
130. Righi PD, Kopecky KK, Caldemeyer KS, Ball VA, Weisberger EC, Radpour S. Comparison of ultrasound-fine needle aspiration and computed tomography in patients undergoing elective neck dissection. Head Neck. 1997;19(7):604–10.
131. Brockstein B, Masters G. Head and neck cancer. New York: Springer Science & Business Media; 2006.
132. Argiris A, Eng C. Epidemiology, staging, and screening of head and neck cancer. Cancer Treat Res. 2003;114:15–60.
133. Cancer.net. 2018. Available from: https://www.cancer.net/cancer-types/nasal-cavity-and-paranasal-sinus-cancer/diagnosis.
134. Knowles SM, Wu AM. Advances in immuno-positron emission tomography: antibodies for molecular imaging in oncology. J Clin Oncol. 2012;30(31):3884–92.
135. Nimmagadda S, Ford EC, Wong JW, Pomper MG. Targeted molecular imaging in oncology: focus on radiation therapy. Semin Radiat Oncol. 2008;18(2):136–48.
136. Lewis-Jones H, Colley S, Gibson D. Imaging in head and neck cancer: United Kingdom National Multidisciplinary Guidelines. J Laryngol Otol. 2016;130(S2):S28–31.
137. Nordsmark M, Overgaard J. A confirmatory prognostic study on oxygenation status and locoregional control in advanced head and neck squamous cell carcinoma treated by radiation therapy. Radiother Oncol. 2000;57(1):39–43.
138. Bratasz A, Pandian RP, Deng Y, Petryakov S, Grecula JC, Gupta N, et al. In vivo imaging of changes in tumor oxygenation during growth and after treatment. Magn Reson Med. 2007;57(5):950–9.
139. Tanay A, Regev A. Scaling single-cell genomics from phenomenology to mechanism. Nature. 2017;541(7637):331–8.
140. (https://creativecommons.org/licenses/by/3.0) DCB.
141. (https://creativecommons.org/licenses/by/2.0) kCB.
142. (https://creativecommons.org/licenses/by-sa/4.0) PCB-S.
143. (https://creativecommons.org/licenses/by-sa/4.0) NCB-S.
144. (https://creativecommons.org/licenses/by-sa/4.0) mCB-S.
145. (https://creativecommons.org/licenses/by-sa/3.0) SCB-S.
146. (https://creativecommons.org/licenses/by-sa/3.0) NDCB-S.
147. https://www.59mdw.af.mil/News/Photos/igphoto/2000074686/.
148. CDC (Centers for Disease Control and Prevention) – Public Health Image Library (PHIL) – ID#:10189.

149. Goodyear M. p. Transverse plane enhancing CT scan viewed in the caudo-cephalic direction showing a right tonsillar enhancing squamous cell carcinoma (HPV positive). 2017.
150. Institute NC. Oncogenes. p. This graphic illustrates the stages of how a normal cell is converted to a cancer cell, when an oncogene becomes activated.
151. Albano PM, Lumang-Salvador C, Orosa J 3rd, Racelis S, Leano M, Angeles LM, et al. Overall survival of Filipino patients with squamous cell carcinoma of the head and neck: a single-institution experience. Asian Pac J Cancer Prev. 2013;14(8):4769–74.
152. Agarwal N, Singh D, Verma M, Sharma S, Spartacus RK, Chaturvedi M. Possible causes for delay in diagnosis and treatment in head and neck cancer: an institutional study. Int J Commun Med Public Health. 2018;5(6):2291–5.
153. McGurk M, Chan C, Jones J, O'Regan E, Sherriff M. Delay in diagnosis and its effect on outcome in head and neck cancer. Br J Oral Maxillofac Surg. 2005;43(4):281–4.
154. NHS. 2018. Available from: https://www.nhs.uk/common-health-questions/operations-tests-and-procedures/what-do-cancer-stages-and-grades-mean/.
155. Cancer Treatment Centers of America. 2020 [09.06.2020]. Available from: https://www.cancercenter.com/cancer-types/head-and-neck-cancer/stages.
156. Shah NP, Workman RB Jr, Coleman RE. PET and PET/CT in head and neck cancer. In: Workman Jr RB, Coleman RE, editors. PET/CT essentials for clinical practice. New York: Springer; 2006.
157. Shefer A, Markowitz L, Deeks S, Tam T, Irwin K, Garland SM, et al. Early experience with human papillomavirus vaccine introduction in the United States, Canada and Australia. Vaccine. 2008;26(Suppl 10):K68–75.
158. Sinha R, Anderson DE, McDonald SS, Greenwald P. Cancer risk and diet in India. J Postgrad Med. 2003;49(3):222–8.
159. Negri E, Franceschi S, Bosetti C, Levi F, Conti E, Parpinel M, et al. Selected micronutrients and oral and pharyngeal cancer. Int J Cancer. 2000;86(1):122–7.
160. Potter JD, Steinmetz K. Vegetables, fruit and phytoestrogens as preventive agents. IARC Sci Publ. 1996;139:61–90.
161. Hong WK, Lippman SM, Itri LM, Karp DD, Lee JS, Byers RM, et al. Prevention of second primary tumors with isotretinoin in squamous-cell carcinoma of the head and neck. N Engl J Med. 1990;323(12):795–801.
162. Rowe NH, Grammer FC, Watson FR, Nickerson NH. A study of environmental influence upon salivary gland neoplasia in rats. Cancer. 1970;26(2):436–44.
163. Steinmetz KA, Potter JD. Vegetables, fruit, and cancer. II. Mechanisms. Cancer Causes Control. 1991;2(6):427–42.
164. Block G. Vitamin C and cancer prevention: the epidemiologic evidence. Am J Clin Nutr. 1991;53(1 Suppl):270S–82S.
165. Bhattacharjee A, Chakraborty A, Purkaystha P. Prevalence of head and neck cancers in the north east-an institutional study. Indian J Otolaryngol Head Neck Surg. 2006;58(1):15–9.
166. IARC Working Group on the Evaluation of Carcinogenic Risks to Humans. Betel-quid and areca-nut chewing and some areca-nut derived nitrosamines. IARC Monogr Eval Carcinog Risks Hum. 2004;85:1–334.
167. Steuer CE, El-Deiry M, Parks JR, Higgins KA, Saba NF. An update on larynx cancer. CA Cancer J Clin. 2017;67(1):31–50.
168. Dorsey K, Agulnik M. Promising new molecular targeted therapies in head and neck cancer. Drugs. 2013;73(4):315–25.
169. Brookes GB. Nutritional status – a prognostic indicator in head and neck cancer. Otolaryngol Head Neck Surg. 1985;93(1):69–74.
170. Worsham MJ. Identifying the risk factors for late-stage head and neck cancer. Expert Rev Anticancer Ther. 2011;11(9):1321–5.
171. Yeh SA. Radiotherapy for head and neck cancer. Semin Plast Surg. 2010;24(2):127–36.

172. Kim DH, Kim WT, Lee JH, Ki YK, Nam JH, Lee BJ, et al. Analysis of the prognostic factors for distant metastasis after induction chemotherapy followed by concurrent chemoradiotherapy for head and neck cancer. Cancer Res Treat. 2015;47(1):46–54.
173. Lee JH, Song JH, Lee SN, Kang JH, Kim MS, Sun DI, et al. Adjuvant postoperative radiotherapy with or without chemotherapy for locally advanced squamous cell carcinoma of the head and neck: the importance of patient selection for the postoperative chemoradiotherapy. Cancer Res Treat. 2013;45(1):31–9.
174. Brockstein B, Vokes E. Treatment of metastatic and recurrent head and neck cancer UpToDate: UpToDate; 2013. Available from: uptodate.com/contents/treatment-of-metastatic-and-recurrent-head-and-neck-cancer/print.
175. Molin Y, Fayette J. Current chemotherapies for recurrent/metastatic head and neck cancer. Anti-Cancer Drugs. 2011;22(7):621–5.

Chapter 2
Potentially Malignant Disorders of the Oral Cavity

Hamzah Alkofahi and Mehdi Ebrahimi

Introduction

Head and neck cancers involving varieties of oral cancers can adversely impact the patients' lifestyle. However, the associated mortality and morbidity rates can be greatly reduced with early detection and treatment of potentially malignant lesions or cancers [1]. As such, early intervention is critical before the malignant transformation of lesions.

Oral cancers can be preceded by visible clinical changes in the oral mucosa representing an intermediate clinical state with increased cancer risk. In 1972, the term "precancer" has been accredited for the first time by WHO (World Health Organization). This term was further classified into (i) lesions and (ii) conditions. With a progressive understanding of the premalignancy process, in 2007, the term "Oral Potentially Malignant Disorders (OPMDs)" was introduced by an expert panel from WHO [2]. Later in 2017, this terminology was included in the WHO classification of head and neck tumors [3].

Other terminologies have been also reported in the literature (i.e., precancer, premalignant, preneoplastic, carcinoma prone, epithelial precursor, intraepithelial neoplasia, and intraepithelial carcinoma) and referred to the transformation of "oral

H. Alkofahi
Division of Plastic & Reconstructive Surgery, Department of Surgery, Stanford University School of Medicine, Stanford, CA, USA

Department of Oral and Maxillofacial Surgery, Jordanian Royal Medical Services, Irbid, Jordan

M. Ebrahimi (✉)
Prince Philip Dental Hospital, The University of Hong Kong, Pok Fu Lam, Hong Kong, China
e-mail: ebrahimi@connect.hku.hk

© Springer Nature Switzerland AG 2021
R. El Assal et al. (eds.), *Early Detection and Treatment of Head & Neck Cancers*, https://doi.org/10.1007/978-3-030-69852-2_2

mucosa" to Oral Squamous Cell Carcinoma (OSCC). OSCC is a potential threat that significantly compromises the head and neck and systemic health. For OPMDs, a global prevalence rate at 4.47% (95% CI = 2.43–7.08) has been estimated at a higher rate in Asians and the male gender [4]. The concept of denoting some lesions or disorders of the oral mucosa as "precancerous" is based on the coexisting similarities with cancerous lesions evidenced by clinical presentations, morphological and cytological observations, and genomic or molecular alterations in OPMDs [1].

According to WHO, a precancerous lesion is defined as "a morphologically altered tissue in which oral cancer is more likely to occur than in its normal counterpart." Examples include (1) oral leukoplakia (OL), (2) oral erythroplakia (OE), (3) sublingual keratosis, and (4) chronic hyperplastic candidiasis. However, not all potential lesions will transform into malignancy. In general, whitish lesions occur more commonly than red lesions and they are associated with a lower risk of malignant transformation.

A precancerous condition is also defined by WHO as "a generalized state associated with a significantly increased risk of cancer." However, they are not necessarily preceded by the specific lesion. A common example includes oral submucous fibrosis (OSMF). Other less common examples with lesser risk are lichen planus, sideroblastic dysphagia, tylosis, dyskeratosis congenita, and smoking keratosis. Table 2.1 summarizes the clinically relevant OPMDs, their subtypes, anatomical locations, and the available cumulative malignant transformation rates. This chapter provides a general overview of the most common OPMDs, followed by a detailed discussion about the available screening methods that would aid in the early detection of OPMDs and malignant changes. This includes conventional (i.e., staining, light-based detection systems, optical diagnostic technologies), and recent promising molecular biomarkers analysis techniques.

Oral Potentially Malignant Disorders (OPMDs)

Leukoplakia

Oral Leukoplakia (OL) (*leuko* = white; *plakia* = patch) is the most common oral precancerous lesion. OL is defined as a white patch or plaque that could not be related to a specific diagnosis [7]. In most cases, the cause of oral white lesions is evident, which could be a fungal infection, trauma, leukoedema, white sponge nevus, or chronic irritation. Therefore, the diagnosis can only be reached when other white lesions are excluded.

The global prevalence of oral leukoplakia was estimated between 1.49% and 2.60% [8] with a malignance transformation rate ranging from 0.1% to 17.5% [9]. Although leukoplakia can occur at any age, it often occurs in male individuals under the age of 40 [10]. The significant difference in the worldwide incidence of OL could be related to age, habitual risk factors, and ethnic diversities. The main

Table 2.1 Characteristics of OPMDs

Disorders	Clinical features	Locations	Cumulative malignant transformation rate (99% CI)
Leukoplakia	Generally asymptomatic white plaque that cannot be rubbed off	Cheeks, lips, gingiva	8.6% (5.1–13.0%)
Erythroplakia	A symptomatic predominantly red patch with a well-defined margin	Mouth floor, tongue, retromolar pad, soft palate	33.1% (13.6–56.2%)
Proliferative verrucous leukoplakia (PVL)	Multifocal corrugated white patch or plaque with a high recurrence rate	Gingivae, alveolar process, palate	49.5% (26.7–72.4%)
Viadent leukoplakia	White patch or plaque	Gingivae, buccal and labial vestibule	No data
Candida leukoplakia	Firm, white leathery plaques	Cheeks, lips, palate	No data
Smokeless tobacco keratosis	White plaque	Buccal or labial vestibule	No data
Palatal keratosis associated with reverse smoking	White patches and plaques	Palate, tongue 83.3% dysplasia	No data
Verrucous hyperplasia	The extensive thick white plaque	Buccal mucosa	No data
Oral verrucous carcinoma	The extensive thick white plaque	Buccal mucosa	No data
Dyskeratosis congenita	Oral leukoplakia	Buccal mucosa, tongue, oropharynx	No data
Actinic cheilosis	Diffuse, poorly defined atrophic, erosive, ulcerative, or keratotic plaques	Lower lip	No data
Keratoacanthoma	Firm, sessile non-tender nodule + a central plug of keratin	Lips, tongue, sublingual region	No data
Oral submucous fibrosis	Mucosal rigidity Buccal mucosa, retromolar area, restricted mouth opening	Tongue, soft palate	5.2% (2.9–8.0%)
Oral lichenoid lesions	White-and red lesions with a reticular, striated appearance	Localized next to allergenic material	3.8% (1.6–7.0%)
Oral lichen planus	Asymptomatic, reticular, annular, linear, erosive, atrophic, bullous, ulcerative, popular, plaque-like	Posterior buccal mucosa, tongue, gingivae, palate, vermilion border	1.4% (0.9–1.9%)
Discoid lupus erythematosus	White plaques with elevated borders, radiating white striae, and telangiectasia	Cheeks, lips, palate	No data
Epidermolysis bullosa	Bullae and vesicle formation following mild trauma	Cheeks, tongue, palate	No data
Verruciform xanthoma	A well-demarcated mass with a yellow-white or red color and a papillary or verruciform surface	Gingivae, tongue, buccal mucosa, vestibular mucosa, the floor of the mouth	No data
Graft-versus-host disease	Atrophy, erythema, erosions, ulcers, lichenoid lesions	Cheeks, tongue, lips, buccal & labial vestibule	No data

Compiled from Refs. [5, 6]

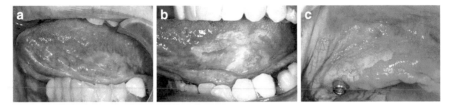

Fig. 2.1 Forms of leukoplakia. (**a**) A patch of homogeneous leukoplakia with a flat, thin, and uniformly white appearance; (**b**) a carcinoma arising in a patch of nonhomogeneous leukoplakia; (**c**) proliferative verrucous leukoplakia affecting the gingiva and the alveolar and buccal mucosae. (Reproduced with permission from Ref. [11])

etiological factor is still unknown; however, many predisposing factors can increase the risk of occurrence of OL (i.e., smoking/smokeless tobacco, alcohol, human papillomavirus, chronic irritation, and electro galvanism) and progression to malignant lesions. Smoking or smokeless tobacco results in a sixfold increased risk of occurrence of OL [11]. Interestingly, tobacco-associated leukoplakias seem to have less malignant potential than leukoplakias found in patients that do not use tobacco [12].

Clinically, OL can be divided into two main distinct forms: (i) homogeneous lesions which are asymptomatic uniformly flat and white patch, and may exhibit shallow fissured-like cracked mud (Fig. 2.1), and (ii) nonhomogeneous varieties. Nonhomogeneous varieties are usually symptomatic and present three clinical subtypes: (1) speckled (e.g., *erythroleukoplakia*), which is a predominantly white form but mixed with red color; (2) nodular, which is small, round, red/white excrescences with irregular borders; and (3) verrucous or exophytic form with the corrugated or wrinkled surface appearance and papillary projections that may be indistinguishable from verrucous carcinoma [11]. Although buccal mucosa is the most frequently affected site, leukoplakia can affect any part of the oral cavity including gingiva, tongue, and floor of the mouth. The highest risk for malignant transformation includes the OL in the soft palate and sublingual area. Microscopically, OL is characterized by (i) para- or ortho-hyperkeratosis (thick surface epithelium caused by keratin secretion) and (ii) acanthosis (thick spinous layer) of the epithelium. The subepithelial lamina propria shows various degrees of chronic inflammatory infiltrates.

Proliferative Verrucous Leukoplakia (PVL) is a distinguished type of OL that appears as multiple, well-defined, wart-like speckled patches with a chance of progression to a more aggressive form of transformation to malignancy such as conventional or verrucous carcinoma. The major clinical criteria for the diagnosis of PVL include (i) OL involving more than two oral sites mostly gingiva, alveolar process, and palate; (ii) presence of verrucous area; (iii) spread during the course of the disease; and (iv) recurrence in a previously treated area [13]. Carrard et al. (2013) [14] introduced useful histologic diagnostic criteria for PVL which include (1) presence of verrucous or wart-like areas, involving more than two oral subsites; (2) minimum size of at least 3 cm of the involved area; (3) disease period of at least 5 years characterized by spreading and enlarging, as well as recurrences in the previously treated area; and, (4) the realization of at least one biopsy to rule out VC or OSCC.

Based on the evidence presented, the features that stand out as significant determinants contributing to the malignant potential of OL include advanced age, female gender, long-lasting lesion exceeding 200 mm^2, nonhomogeneous type (e.g., erythroleukoplakia), coinfection with *Candida Albicans*, and the higher grades of dysplastic changes in the lesion [15]. The progression of the disease and malignant transformation is uneven; therefore, the patients should be followed up closely for changes in the homogeneity, size, and eruption of new lesions. Treatment strategy involves controlling the associated risk factors and various types of surgical interventions (i.e., conventional surgery, laser ablation, cryosurgery, and photodynamic therapy).

The dysplastic progression of OL to malignancy can be occult as downregulation of extracellular matrix (ECM) pathways [16] without any notable clinical changes. However, the current state-of-art knowledge highlights the importance of different dynamic transitional states between epithelial and mesenchymal phenotypes in disease progression and tumorigenesis. A shift from the epithelial state toward the mesenchymal state, in a process known as epithelial–mesenchymal transition (EMT), renders the cells a migratory and invasive behavior by modifying the adhesion molecules expressed by the cells. The current understanding of the EMT pathway and its associated proteins (i.e., Snail, Twist, E-cadherin, N-cadherin, and Vimentin), as well as transitional events need further expansion for better prognosis and tumor management strategies. Interested readers are referred to related literature elsewhere [17, 18].

Erythroplakia

It a fiery red usually velvety, flat, or sometimes depressed lesion with an irregular outline (although well defined) that cannot be characterized as any other specific lesion (Fig. 2.2). Erythroplakia is usually asymptomatic, but some patients may report burning sensation or pain on food intake [19]. Erythroplakia occurs most commonly in the soft palate and floor of the mouth and less commonly in the tongue and buccal mucosa. It is usually a solitary lesion unlike candidiasis or systemic lupus, which mostly has multiple lesions [20].

Although erythroplakia is less common than leukoplakia, it presents a greater potential for malignant transformation [7]. It has been found as part of early invasive oral carcinomas and often presents as "carcinoma *in situ*" or "invasive carcinoma" at the time of biopsy [2, 21]. The worldwide prevalence of erythroplakia from different geographical areas is ranging from 0.02% to 0.8% and affect equally male and female in middle elderly people [20]. The etiology of erythroplakia is unknown; however, there is a strong association with smoking and alcohol consumption [22].

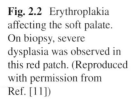

Fig. 2.2 Erythroplakia affecting the soft palate. On biopsy, severe dysplasia was observed in this red patch. (Reproduced with permission from Ref. [11])

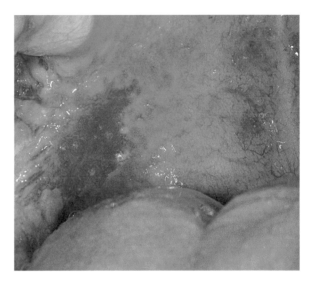

Microscopically, the atrophic epithelial cells become unable to produce keratin which appears clinically as red lesions. The subepithelial connective tissue also shows inflammatory cells. Histopathologically, erythroplakia commonly shows a range of epithelial changes from dysplasia to invasive carcinoma [23]. The risk of malignant transformation is greater with more severe dysplastic changes in an individual lesion [24]. Therefore, a thorough initial clinical examination of signs and symptoms of erythroplakia is essential. This should be along with behavior management and cessation of alcohol/smoking habits followed by biopsy and long-term follow-up to trace possible recurrence. Following a biopsy that determines the nature and extent of the lesion, the excision is the treatment of choice for erythroplakia [25]. Early detection of such lesions may prevent malignant transformation and improve the survival rate and quality of life [26].

Oral Submucous Fibrosis

Oral submucous fibrosis (OSMF) is a chronic irreversible disorder characterized by inflammation and subsequent fibrosis of lamina propria and deeper connective tissues (Fig. 2.3). Early clinical features may include mucosal blanching, burning sensation on exposure to spicy food, and loss of normal pigmentation [27]. The progression of the disease is associated with loss of fibro-elasticity, epithelial atrophy, and a remarkable decrease in mouth opening [28]. Although it can involve any part of the lining mucosa of the upper digestive tract, the buccal mucosa is the most commonly reported site [29]. OSMF is mainly associated with areca nut chewing,

Fig. 2.3 Blanching of buccal mucosa in a case of early OSMF. (Reproduced with permission from Ref. [11])

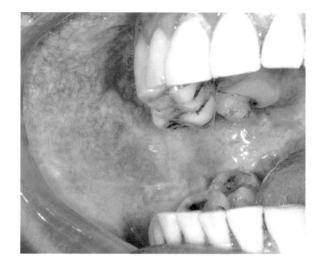

the main component of betel quid [30]. Betel chewing is a habit practiced in southeast Asia and India similar to tobacco chewing in western countries.

The pathogenesis of OSMF is not well understood; however, the disorder is considered to be multifactorial including areca nut chewing, ingestion of chilies, genetic and immunologic processes, and nutritional deficiencies [31, 32]. Oral submucous fibrosis has a high rate of morbidity because it causes a progressive inability to open the mouth, resulting in difficulty eating and consequent nutritional deficiencies.

It is well known for its malignant transformation to squamous cell carcinoma with a conversion rate of 10% to oral squamous cell carcinoma [33]. Various molecular and genetic pathways may induce pathogenesis to malignant form including changes in the cell cycle, DNA, angiogenesis, EMT, and tissue hypoxia [30, 31]. The potential role and activation of genetic pathways have also been postulated including Transforming Growth Factor-β (TGF-β) [31, 34], Interleukin-6 (IL-6) [35], Bone Morphogenetic Protein 7 (BMP7) [36], and collagen isoforms [36].

Histologic findings vary according to the stage of the disease (Fig. 2.3) [37]. OSMF is generally characterized by dense bundles of collagen, thick bands of subepithelial hyalinization extending into the submucosal tissues (and replacing fat or fibrovascular tissue), decreased vascularity, and atrophy of epithelium and underlying muscle [38, 39].

The treatment choice of the patient with OSMF depends on the stage of the disease. The early-stage disease necessitates the education of the patient and habit control. The later stage of the disease is irreversible, and the main aim of treatment is restoring normal mouth functions. The role of different medications has been investigated as potential treatment modalities such as steroid, placental extracts [40], hyaluronidase [41], IFN-gamma [42], lycopene [43], and pentoxifylline [44]. However, surgical intervention is indicated in patients with severe trismus and those with dysplastic or neoplastic changes. Treatment modalities may include simple excision of the fibrous bands, split-thickness skin grafting following bilateral temporalis myotomy or coronoidectomy, and application of laser (i.e., KTP-532 laser and ErCr:YSGG laser) [38, 45, 46].

Diagnosis and Screening of OPMDs

Cancerous lesions are usually preceded by OPMDs [47]; however, due to the nature and inconsistent pattern of OPMDs, the risk of malignant transformation is very difficult to be assessed in individual cases [15, 48]. This unknown risk of malignant transformation is the main reason behind the importance of early diagnosis of OPMDs. Moreover, early detection of cancerous changes would significantly improve the quality of life by reducing the treatment-associated morbidity and mortality rates with improved survival rate up to 82% if localized oral cancer is detected (Fig. 2.4) [49].

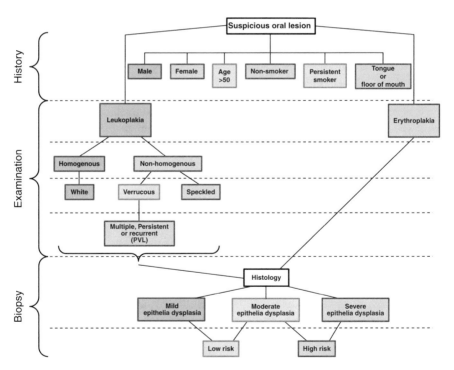

Fig. 2.4 A simple algorithm for clinical risk assessment of oral potentially malignant disorders (OPMDs). The clinician is faced with a suspicious oral lesion, and at each stage of the assessment process, the risk of individual features is illustrated as green (low risk), amber (medium risk), or red (high risk). (Reproduced with permission from Ref. [56])

It is reported that the most malignant transformation upon exposure to carcinogenic stimuli arises during the first 2 years of detection of OPMDs, however, the risk may continue for the next 10–15 years [50, 51]. These risks may induce cytological changes that ultimately lead to malignancy. Supported with recent molecular studies, this phenomenon is known as "field cancerization" and it is proposed for the first time by Slaughter in 1953 [52]. The high-risk individual (i.e., heavy user of tobacco smoke, betel nut chewing, and alcohol consumption) and high-risk OPMDs (i.e., erythroplakia, erythroleukoplakia, proliferative verrucous leukoplakia, and OSMF) should be identified and monitored carefully during follow-up [53].

A systematic intraoral and extraoral visual examination and palpation including head and neck regions is the key to achieve a provisional clinical diagnosis. This is still the most common method for screening and follow-up of OPMDs for potential signs of malignant transformation. It is simple to use and effective with 84% sensitivity and 96% specificity [54]. However, it is only successful in the accessible area and still holds the risk of false-negative results. As such, several investigative adjunctive aids have been developed and applied clinically and in research fields [54, 55]. These are broadly categorized under invasive (i.e., brush cytology, biopsy) and noninvasive techniques (i.e., staining, light-based detection systems, optical diagnostic methods, and molecular biomarkers).

Noninvasive Techniques

Vital Staining

Vital staining refers to the use of dyes to stain oral mucosa tissues for better visualization of OPMDs and malignancy. Different dyes have been applied and investigated such as toluidine blue or methylene blue [57, 58], Rose Bengal staining [59, 60], and Lugol's iodine staining [61]. The oral mucosa is prerinsed with acetic acid followed by water before the application of dye. The result of the test is positive if tissue staining is observed and negative if otherwise. For example, toluidine blue or methylene blue has a high affinity for acidic components (i.e., nucleic acid) and it appears dark (positive) or pale royal blue (doubtful) upon staining [62–64].

Vital staining is a simple, cheap, and convenient method with the ability to define clinically unapparent lesions. It can also be used to assess the extent of OPMDs for incisional biopsy. However, the disadvantages are the possibility of staining benign inflammatory lesions and failure in some cancerous and dysplastic lesions. Therefore, due to a high percentage of false-positive results [65], it is applied with other adjunct methods to confirm the test results (i.e., cytology and light-based detection methods) [66].

Light-Based Detection Systems

Chemiluminescence

Chemiluminescence is the emission of light (luminescence) with specific wavelengths (430, 540, and 580 nm) for the visual distinction between the normal and abnormal tissues. Commercially available chemiluminescence techniques include ViziLite, ViziLite Plus, Microlux/DL, and Orascoptic DK. ViziLite™ is the most commonly used system, which includes (i) ViziLite (OralLite), a disposable chemiluminescence light stick; and (ii) ViziLite Blue Oral Lesion Identification and Marking System, which is a three-component swab system used as an adjunct to the ViziLite Test [67]. To use ViziLite, first, the patient is instructed to rinse his mouth with 1% citric acid to clean the attached glycoproteins and dehydrate the mucosa, then the light source is applied. If the appearance of the epithelium is lightly bluish-white the test result is considered negative while a positive result indicates distinctly white (acetowhite) epithelial appearance [68]. However, according to the literature, there is not enough evidence to support the application of chemiluminescence techniques for discrimination between inflammatory, traumatic, OPMDs, and malignant lesions [69–71].

Tissue Autofluorescence

Tissue autofluorescence is a phenomenon where endogenous fluorophores in cells produce a fluorescent emission upon exposure to the light of a specific wavelength (365 nm) [72]. Due to the changes in tissue architecture and concentrations of fluorophores, the abnormal mucosal tissues alter the absorption and scattering properties of light [73]. As a result of the loss of autofluorescence, the abnormal tissues appear dark while normal tissues demonstrate a pale green fluorescence [74]. Although this system may assist in the screening of OPMDs and oral cancer, it cannot differentiate between them [75]. Furthermore, the results should be interpreted carefully due to the frequent report of false-positive results. For example, conditions such as mucosal pigmentations, ulcerations, gingivitis, irritation, and hematoma may reduce the fluorescence and results in a dark appearance. As such, the suspicious positive lesions need to be followed up with great caution [76].

Photodynamic Techniques

This is an alternative minimally invasive approach for diagnosis as well as treatment of OPMDs and other oral cancers. The photodynamic technique is a cold photochemical process and there is no heat production. Therefore, it is a safe technique compared to the thermal laser method and other invasive approaches due to the minimum risk of damage to underlying and surrounding tissues and vital structures [77].

Three fundamental elements of this technique include tissue oxygen, a photosensitizer (PS), and visible light of a specific wavelength [78]. Here, the PS is activated upon light exposure that results in a series of photochemical and photobiological reactions based on the type of the light source. For diagnostic purposes, the PS is activated using a light source of a short wavelength. The excited electrons undergo "internal conversion" and release their energy in the form of fluorescence light that is applied for visualization of the lesion [79]. For therapeutic applications, the PS is activated using a light source of a long wavelength. The excited PS undergo "intersystem crossing" that results in type I or II reaction with the concurrent release of reactive oxygen species for therapeutic purposes [79].

Results of the systemic and critical review indicate that photodynamic therapy is an effective noninvasive management protocol for the treatment of OPMDs [80–82]. The common PS applied are aminolevulinic acid (ALA), meta-tetrahydroxyphenylchlorin, Foscan, hematoporphyrin derivatives, Photofrin, Photosan, methylene blue, and chlorine-e6. Application of laser light (e.g., wavelength: 420–660 nm and power density: 50–500 mW/cm^2) for appropriate duration (i.e., 1–15 min with a 7-day interval between sessions) resulted in 23.58–100% complete response rate [77, 80, 82]. According to the literature, the most promising method is the topical application of 20% ALA with a diode laser as the optimal choice of the light source [81]. Further randomized clinical studies with both interim and long-term follow-ups are required to verify the validity of this approach in the management of OPMDs.

Optical Diagnostic Technologies

Novel technologies in optical-based diagnostic systems and reagents are promising alternative adjuncts to histopathological and microscopical studies for the diagnosis and screening of precancerous (i.e., OPMDs) and cancerous lesions. These systems are capable of tracing minor changes within the tissue with real-time imaging results. Examples include Raman spectroscopy, diffuse reflectance spectroscopy, optical coherence tomography, confocal laser microscopy, high-resolution microendoscopy, and narrow-band imaging [83]. However, due to technical limitations, limited penetration depth, and high cost, there is no strong literature on their application for OPMDs. Furthermore, their reliability as a potential alternative to other screening methods needs further studies [84–87].

Recently, the advances in nanotechnology and nanoparticles (i.e., nanobeads, gold nanoarray, nano-bio-chips) offer high detection sensitivity with higher image contrast and resolution. This allows early detection and more accurate monitoring of potential intraepithelial malignant changes [88]. Moreover, the nano-based diagnostic methods can offer an analysis of biomarkers at a nano-scale with molecular targeted imaging and the possibility of intraoperative identification of surgical margins [88]. However, the application of this technology for the potential detection of precancerous and cancerous lesions is in the early developmental phase. Further studies are required to successfully transfer these technologies to clinical practice.

Prognostic Molecular Biomarkers

Treatment planning for the management of OPMDs depends on the estimated risk of malignant changes and healthcare regulations as per the target population. Lesions with low-risk ranking may be treated with habit change, oral hygiene instruction, and close monitoring. However, high-risk lesions undergo invasive approaches (i.e., surgery or laser) and tight follow-up to observe for recurrences [89, 90]. Unfortunately, despite advancement in oral oncology, no significant improvement is observed in the survival rate of oral squamous cell carcinoma which is mainly related to late diagnosis [91].

In this context, the ideal approach would be an individualized treatment plan based on accurate identification of prognostic molecular biomarkers for malignant transformation. This could offer individualized management protocol (i.e., diagnosis, risk assessment, noninvasive and invasive interventions, and follow-up) for OPMDs and other malignant lesions and help in reducing worldwide cancer incidence rate [92, 93].

P53 (a product of the tumor suppressor gene *TP53* that plays an essential role in cell cycle regulation, apoptosis, and DNA repair [94]) is the most frequently reported immunohistochemical biomarker. However, conflicting literature is seen concerning the association between p53 and malignant transformation of OPMD [95].

The next most commonly investigated biomarker is Ki-67 protein which is expressed in the cell nucleus during mitosis [96]. As such, Ki-67 was suggested to be an important indicator of the level of aggressiveness in different tumors [97, 98]. According to the literature, overexpression of Ki-67 was associated with malignant transformation in about 50% of the studies, however, it is not an independent predictor factor of malignant transformation in OPMDs [99].

Podoplanin is another potential independent predictor of OPMD malignant transformation and a promising biomarker for clinical application [99]. It is a transmembrane glycoprotein that can induce oral tumorigenesis following transcriptional activation by ErbB3-binding protein-1 (Ebp1) [100]. Furthermore, through the downregulation of E-cadherin, podoplanin can increase epithelial–mesenchymal transition (EMT) [17, 101]. Moreover, it is also associated with platelet aggregation that results in the induction of cell migration and malignant progression [102]. However, further studies are required to establish sound knowledge about its role in malignant transformation.

Other promising prognostic biomarkers under investigations are DNA ploidy [103–105], abnormal DNA content (DNA aneuploidy) [106, 107], increased epidermal growth factor receptor (EGFR) gene copy numbers [108, 109], and loss of heterozygosity (LOH) in 3p/9p [110, 111].

With continuous research in the field of cytology and genomics, several contemporary biomarkers have been discovered. However, their detailed information and application in clinical practice are questionable [112]. The current evidence regarding the prognostic value of molecular biomarkers for monitoring OPMDs malignant transformation is equivocal [113]. Therefore, to date, no single biomarker has proved to be of real clinical value [56, 99]. Future well-designed longitudinal studies in different populations would help to fill the knowledge gap regarding the prognostic value of biomarkers in malignant transformation of OPMD. Furthermore, the importance of ethnic diversity and demographic factors are to be considered during the study of prognostic biomarkers for OPMD. This is because different populations are exposed to different risk factors that impact the rate and extent of malignant transformation. To avoid possible publication bias, it is important to adhere to international guidelines in study design and reporting the findings such as Strengthening the Reporting of Observational Studies in Epidemiology (STROBE) [114] for observational studies and Consolidated Standards of Reporting Trials (CONSORT) [115] for clinical trials.

Invasive Detection Techniques

Incisional Biopsy

According to the current knowledge, surgical incisional biopsy and histopathological microscopic evaluation still remain the gold standard for confirmation of the clinical diagnosis of OPMDs [53, 116]. This minimized the risk of misclassification, exclude any occult malignant transformation, determine the presence of epithelial dysplasia, and help in proper management. However, there is a chance of bias or misdiagnosis due to sampling error during the biopsy procedure. As such, the standard biopsy should involve all readable areas of the lesion (i.e., both white and red patches) to ascertain the presence of epithelial dysplasia or squamous cell carcinoma [53]. Further, it should allow a standard three-grading system of epithelial dysplasia (i.e., mild, moderate, or severe) according to WHO guidelines for pathology reporting or a two-grading system (i.e., low risk and high risk) according to Kujan et al. [117]. It has also been suggested that a two-tier system may be more reproducible and clinically translatable for better management [118].

Oral Brush Cytology (OBC)

OBC is a minimally invasive, simple, safe, and relatively painless procedure for harvesting sample cells from the suspicious lesion of the oral mucosa [119]. Upon the early application of oral cytology in 1963, the available techniques for OBC have been improved remarkably. Recently, the modern techniques for OBC have been the focus of many studies due to their potential role for screening and early detection of OPMDs and oral cancer as well as oral biomarkers [47, 66].

Two main types of brush techniques are conventional exfoliative cytology (i.e., Cytobrush, OralCDx, Toothbrush) and liquid-based cytology (i.e., Cytobrush, Orcellex). For example, the OralCDx® method is a computer-assisted transepithelial sample analysis of the cytological fragments that detects abnormal cells in all epithelial layers of the oral mucosa [120]. However, any suspicious lesion will need the scalpel biopsy for confirmation.

Table 2.2 Available techniques for the clinical detection and diagnosis of OPMDs and oral cancer

Categories	Techniques	Sensitivity (%)	Specificity (%)	Advantages	Disadvantages	Indications
Vital staining	Toluidine blue, Tolonium chloride	38–100	9–100	Sensitive; chair-side; rapid; low-cost	High false-positive rates, the possibility of failure, contraindication in iodine allergy	Help in defining the abnormal unseen area and assessing the site of excision for biopsy
	Methylene blue staining	90–91.4	66.6–69		No data	Poor literature and unknown efficacy in the detection of OPMD
	Rose Bengal staining	90–100	73.7–89.09		No data	
	Lugol's iodine staining	87.5–94.7	83.8–84.2	No data	No data	No data
Light-based detection systems	Chemiluminescence ViziLite	71–100	0–84.6	effective; rapid; chair-side, simple	Low specificity, the necessity of a dark environment, high initial set-up cost, inability to objectively measure visualization results	Could improve the visualization of white through tissue reflectance
	Chemiluminescence ViziLite Plus	77.3	27.8			
	Chemiluminescence Microlux/DL	77.8–94.3	70.7–99.6			
	Chemiluminescence Orascoptic DK	NA	NA			
	VELscope	30–100	15–100	Rapid; chair-side; easy to operate	Moderate false-positive rates	Help better identification of OPMD
	Photodynamic diagnosis	79–100	50–99	Real-time; cost-effective	Strict patient management; high false-positive rates	Rarely applied method in the clinic

Optical diagnostic technologies	Raman spectroscopy	97.44–100	77–100	Real-time	Weak signal; time-consuming, relatively slow speed of spectrum acquisitions	The difficulty of capturing weak tissue Raman signals
	Elastic scattering spectroscopy	72–98	68–75	Real-time	No data	Rarely applied
	Diffuse reflectance spectroscopy	76–100	76–97	Simple; Low-cost; Real-time	No data	Help detection of abnormal tissue morphology of the oral mucosa.
	Narrow-band imaging	84.62–96	88.2–100	Real-time; Easy to manage	Moderate false-positive rates	May enhance the visualization of the mucosa surface and microvasculature
	Optical coherence tomography	73–100	78–98	Real-time; High sensitivity; High specificity	Need a histopathologist to interpret and assess; examines only a very small area at a time	For assessing and imaging OPMD ex vivo or in vivo
	Confocal laser endomicroscopy	80	100	Real-time; "Optical biopsy"		For 3D imaging of the mucosa
	Confocal reflectance microscopy	73	88			
Oral brush cytology	Conventional exfoliative (i.e., OralCDx), Liquid-based cytology (i.e., Orcellex)	91	91	Ability to detect large or multiple lesions, the ability to access "the basement membrane collecting cells from all three epithelial layers of the oral mucosa. The liquid-based cytology offers a better cytological morphology"	Possibility of failure in detecting smaller or less obvious lesions, difficulties in detecting lesion with necrosis or blood clot	Microscopic assessment and interpretation of sample cells
Molecular biomarker analysis	Podoplanin, p53, Ki-67, EGFR, DNA aneuploidy, LOH, miRNA	No data	No data	Rapid; Easy to operate, minimally invasive (blood), noninvasive (saliva)	Early developmental phase, lack of solid knowledge about the validity	For early detection and dynamic monitoring of OPMD using biomarkers from blood or saliva

Compiled from Refs. [99, 122]

The introduction of liquid-based cytology added more value to conventional OBC techniques. This method offers a clean background with good quality of cell morphology and staining [66]. Given the relatively high values of specificity and sensitivity of OBC, this method seems to be the most accurate of all adjunctive techniques [66, 121]. However, further well-designed studies are required to evaluate the accuracy of this method and other combined adjunctive techniques [47].

A systematic review and meta-analysis of 41 cross-sectional studies on different screening methods of OPMDs failed to suggest any reliable alternative to the conventional incisional biopsy method [66]. Therefore, scalpel biopsy remains the gold standard method of diagnosis and screening. However, OBC has shown promise as a potential alternative adjunctive method (Table 2.2).

Conclusion

Accurate prediction of malignant changes in OPMDs is the main goal of current studies. The ultimate goal is to minimize the morbidity and mortality rate and improve the survival rate and the quality of life of the patients. Despite technological advances in recent years, the available adjunctive technologies show poor diagnostic accuracy and high false-positive results, therefore, up to date, the gold standard for diagnosis of OPMDs is still the incisional biopsy and histological assessment. Oral brush cytology with the use of liquid-based technology has shown promising results, however, predicting the malignant transformation of OPMDs constitutes a clinical challenge. More recently, the research into the field of genomics and molecular biology for determining the prognostic biomarkers of malignant transformation holds a big hope for the future.

References

1. Dhanuthai K, Rojanawatsirivej S, Thosaporn W, Kintarak S, Subarnbhesaj A, Darling M, Kryshtalskyj E, Chiang C-P, Shin H-I, Choi S-Y, Lee S-S, Aminishakib P. Oral cancer: a multicenter study. Med Oral Patol Oral Cir Bucal. 2018;23:e23–9. https://doi.org/10.4317/medoral.21999.
2. Warnakulasuriya S, Johnson NW, van der Waal I. Nomenclature and classification of potentially malignant disorders of the oral mucosa. J Oral Pathol Med. 2007;36:575–80. https://doi.org/10.1111/j.1600-0714.2007.00582.x.
3. Müller S. Update from the 4th edition of the World Health Organization of head and neck tumours: tumours of the oral cavity and mobile tongue. Head Neck Pathol. 2017;11:33–40. https://doi.org/10.1007/s12105-017-0792-3.
4. Mello FW, Miguel AFP, Dutra KL, Porporatti AL, Warnakulasuriya S, Guerra ENS, Rivero ERC. Prevalence of oral potentially malignant disorders: a systematic review and meta-analysis. J Oral Pathol Med. 2018;47:633–40. https://doi.org/10.1111/jop.12726.
5. Iocca O, Sollecito TP, Alawi F, Weinstein GS, Newman JG, De Virgilio A, Di Maio P, Spriano G, Pardiñas López S, Shanti RM. Potentially malignant disorders of the oral cavity and

oral dysplasia: a systematic review and meta-analysis of malignant transformation rate by subtype. Head Neck. 2020;42:539–55. https://doi.org/10.1002/hed.26006.

6. Mortazavi H, Baharvand M, Mehdipour M. Oral potentially malignant disorders: an overview of more than 20 entities. J Dent Res Dent Clin Dent Prospects. 2014;8:6–14. https://doi.org/10.5681/joddd.2014.002.

7. van der Waal I. Potentially malignant disorders of the oral and oropharyngeal mucosa; terminology, classification and present concepts of management. Oral Oncol. 2009;45:317–23. https://doi.org/10.1016/j.oraloncology.2008.05.016.

8. Petti S. Pooled estimate of world leukoplakia prevalence: a systematic review. Oral Oncol. 2003;39:770–80. https://doi.org/10.1016/S1368-8375(03)00102-7.

9. Kumar Srivastava V. To study the prevalence of premalignancies in teenagers having betel, gutkha, khaini, tobacco chewing, beedi and ganja smoking habit and their association with social class and education status. Int J Clin Pediatr Dent. 2014;7:86–92. https://doi.org/10.5005/jp-journals-10005-1243.

10. Vazquez-Alvarez R, Fernandez-Gonzalez F, Gandara-Vila P, Reboiras-Lopez D, Garcia-Garcia A, Gandara-Rey J. Correlation between clinical and pathologic diagnosis in oral leukoplakia in 54 patients. Med Oral Patol Oral Cir Bucal. 2010;15:e832–8. https://doi.org/10.4317/medoral.15.e832.

11. Warnakulasuriya S. Clinical features and presentation of oral potentially malignant disorders. Oral Surg Oral Med Oral Pathol Oral Radiol. 2018;125:582–90. https://doi.org/10.1016/j.oooo.2018.03.011.

12. Haya-Fernández MC, Bagán JV, Murillo-Cortés J, Poveda-Roda R, Calabuig C. The prevalence of oral leukoplakia in 138 patients with oral squamous cell carcinoma. Oral Dis. 2004;10:346–8. https://doi.org/10.1111/j.1601-0825.2004.01031.x.

13. Cerero-Lapiedra R, Baladé-Martínez D, Moreno-López L-A, Esparza-Gómez G, Bagán JV. Proliferative verrucous leukoplakia: a proposal for diagnostic criteria. Med Oral Patol Oral Cir Bucal. 2010;15:e839–45. http://www.ncbi.nlm.nih.gov/pubmed/20173704.

14. Carrard VC, Brouns EREA, van der Waal I. Proliferative verrucous leukoplakia; a critical appraisal of the diagnostic criteria. Med Oral Patol Oral Cir Bucal. 2013;18:e411–3. https://doi.org/10.4317/medoral.18912.

15. Warnakulasuriya S, Ariyawardana A. Malignant transformation of oral leukoplakia: a systematic review of observational studies. J Oral Pathol Med. 2016;45:155–66. https://doi.org/10.1111/jop.12339.

16. Farah CS, Fox SA. Dysplastic oral leukoplakia is molecularly distinct from leukoplakia without dysplasia. Oral Dis. 2019;25:1715–23. https://doi.org/10.1111/odi.13156.

17. Nieto MA, Huang RY-J, Jackson RA, Thiery JP. EMT: 2016. Cell. 2016;166:21–45. https://doi.org/10.1016/j.cell.2016.06.028.

18. Liu P-F, Kang B-H, Wu Y-M, Sun J-H, Yen L-M, Fu T-Y, Lin Y-C, Liou H-H, Lin Y-S, Sie H-C, Hsieh I-C, Tseng Y-K, Shu C-W, Hsieh Y-D, Ger L-P. Vimentin is a potential prognostic factor for tongue squamous cell carcinoma among five epithelial–mesenchymal transition-related proteins. PLoS One. 2017;12:e0178581. https://doi.org/10.1371/journal.pone.0178581.

19. Holmstrup P. Oral erythroplakia-what is it? Oral Dis. 2018;24:138–43. https://doi.org/10.1111/odi.12709.

20. Reichart PA, Philipsen HP. Oral erythroplakia – a review. Oral Oncol. 2005;41:551–61. https://doi.org/10.1016/j.oraloncology.2004.12.003.

21. Lapthanasupkul P, Poomsawat S, Punyasingh J. A clinicopathologic study of oral leukoplakia and erythroplakia in a Thai population. Quintessence Int. 2007;38:e448–55. http://www.ncbi.nlm.nih.gov/pubmed/17823667.

22. Villa A, Villa C, Abati S. Oral cancer and oral erythroplakia: an update and implication for clinicians. Aust Dent J. 2011;56:253–6. https://doi.org/10.1111/j.1834-7819.2011.01337.x.

23. van der Waal I. Potentially malignant disorders of the oral and oropharyngeal mucosa; present concepts of management. Oral Oncol. 2010;46:423–5. https://doi.org/10.1016/j.oraloncology.2010.02.016.

24. Warnakulasuriya S, Reibel J, Bouquot J, Dabelsteen E. Oral epithelial dysplasia classification systems: predictive value, utility, weaknesses and scope for improvement. J Oral Pathol Med. 2008;37:127–33. https://doi.org/10.1111/j.1600-0714.2007.00584.x.
25. Yang SW, Lee YS, Chang LC, Hsieh TY, Chen TA. Outcome of excision of oral erythroplakia. Br J Oral Maxillofac Surg. 2015;53:142–7. https://doi.org/10.1016/j.bjoms.2014.10.016.
26. Mignogna MD, Fedele S. Oral cancer screening: 5 minutes to save a life. Lancet. 2005;365:1905–6. https://doi.org/10.1016/S0140-6736(05)66635-4.
27. Zain RB, Ikeda N, Gupta PC, Warnakulasuriya S, van Wyk CW, Shrestha P, Axéll T. Oral mucosal lesions associated with betel quid, areca nut and tobacco chewing habits: consensus from a workshop held in Kuala Lumpur, Malaysia, November 25–27, 1996. J Oral Pathol Med. 1999;28:1–4. https://doi.org/10.1111/j.1600-0714.1999.tb01985.x.
28. Cox SC, Walker DM. Oral submucous fibrosis. A review. Aust Dent J. 1996;41:294–9. https://doi.org/10.1111/j.1834-7819.1996.tb03136.x.
29. Paissat DK. Oral submucous fibrosis. Int J Oral Surg. 1981;10:307–12. https://doi.org/10.1016/s0300-9785(81)80026-9.
30. Chattopadhyay A, Ray JG. Molecular pathology of malignant transformation of oral submucous fibrosis. J Environ Pathol Toxicol Oncol. 2016;35:193–205. https://doi.org/10.1615/JEnvironPatholToxicolOncol.2016014024.
31. Pant I, Rao SG, Kondaiah P. Role of areca nut induced JNK/ATF2/Jun axis in the activation of TGF-β pathway in precancerous Oral Submucous Fibrosis. Sci Rep. 2016;6:34314. https://doi.org/10.1038/srep34314.
32. Hernandez BY, Zhu X, Goodman MT, Gatewood R, Mendiola P, Quinata K, Paulino YC. Betel nut chewing, oral premalignant lesions, and the oral microbiome. PLoS One. 2017;12:e0172196. https://doi.org/10.1371/journal.pone.0172196.
33. Lian I-B, Tseng Y-T, Su C-C, Tsai K-Y. Progression of precancerous lesions to oral cancer: results based on the Taiwan National Health Insurance Database. Oral Oncol. 2013;49:427–30. https://doi.org/10.1016/j.oraloncology.2012.12.004.
34. Haque MF, Harris M, Meghji S, Barrett AW. Immunolocalization of cytokines and growth factors in oral submucous fibrosis. Cytokine. 1998;10:713–9. https://doi.org/10.1006/cyto.1997.0342.
35. Chang M-C, Wu H-L, Lee J-J, Lee P-H, Chang H-H, Hahn L-J, Lin B-R, Chen Y-J, Jeng J-H. The induction of prostaglandin E2 production, interleukin-6 production, cell cycle arrest, and cytotoxicity in primary oral keratinocytes and KB cancer cells by areca nut ingredients is differentially regulated by MEK/ERK activation. J Biol Chem. 2004;279:50676–83. https://doi.org/10.1074/jbc.M404465200.
36. Khan I, Agarwal P, Thangjam GS, Radhesh R, Rao SG, Kondaiah P. Role of TGF-β and BMP7 in the pathogenesis of oral submucous fibrosis. Growth Factors. 2011;29:119–27. https://doi.org/10.3109/08977194.2011.582839.
37. Agarwal RK, Hebbale M, Mhapuskar A, Tepan M. Correlation of ultrasonographic measurements, histopathological grading, and clinical staging in oral submucous fibrosis. Indian J Dent Res. 2017;28:476–81. https://doi.org/10.4103/ijdr.IJDR_517_16.
38. Canniff JP, Harvey W, Harris M. Oral submucous fibrosis: its pathogenesis and management. Br Dent J. 1986;160:429–34. https://doi.org/10.1038/sj.bdj.4805876.
39. Kadani M, Satish BNVS, Maharudrappa B, Prashant KM, Hugar D, Allad U, Prabhu PS. Evaluation of plasma fibrinogen degradation products and total serum protein concentration in oral submucous fibrosis. J Clin Diagn Res. 2014;8:ZC54–7. https://doi.org/10.7860/JCDR/2014/9061.4385.
40. Sur TK, Biswas TK, Ali L, Mukherjee B. Anti-inflammatory and anti-platelet aggregation activity of human placental extract. Acta Pharmacol Sin. 2003;24:187–92. http://www.ncbi.nlm.nih.gov/pubmed/12546729.
41. Kakar PK, Puri RK, Venkatachalam VP. Oral submucous fibrosis – treatment with hyalase. J Laryngol Otol. 1985;99:57–9. https://doi.org/10.1017/s0022215100096286.

42. Haque MF, Meghji S, Nazir R, Harris M. Interferon gamma (IFN-gamma) may reverse oral submucous fibrosis. J Oral Pathol Med. 2001;30:12–21. https://doi.org/10.1034/j.1600-0714 .2001.300103.x.
43. Kumar A, Bagewadi A, Keluskar V, Singh M. Efficacy of lycopene in the management of oral submucous fibrosis. Oral Surg Oral Med Oral Pathol Oral Radiol Endod. 2007;103:207–13. https://doi.org/10.1016/j.tripleo.2006.07.011.
44. Liu J, Chen F, Wei Z, Qiu M, Li Z, Dan H, Chen Q, Jiang L. Evaluating the efficacy of pentoxifylline in the treatment of oral submucous fibrosis: a meta-analysis. Oral Dis. 2018;24:706–16. https://doi.org/10.1111/odi.12715.
45. Nayak DR, Mahesh SG, Aggarwal D, Pavithran P, Pujary K, Pillai S. Role of KTP-532 laser in management of oral submucous fibrosis. J Laryngol Otol. 2009;123:418–21. https://doi.org/10.1017/S0022215108003642.
46. Chaudhry Z, Gupta SR, Oberoi SS. The efficacy of ErCr:YSGG laser fibrotomy in management of moderate oral submucous fibrosis: a preliminary study. J Maxillofac Oral Surg. 2014;13:286–94. https://doi.org/10.1007/s12663-013-0511-x.
47. Alsarraf AH, Kujan O, Farah CS. The utility of oral brush cytology in the early detection of oral cancer and oral potentially malignant disorders: a systematic review. J Oral Pathol Med. 2018;47:104–16. https://doi.org/10.1111/jop.12660.
48. Fitzpatrick SG, Hirsch SA, Gordon SC. The malignant transformation of oral lichen planus and oral lichenoid lesions. J Am Dent Assoc. 2014;145:45–56. https://doi.org/10.14219/jada.2013.10.
49. Gómez I, Seoane J, Varela-Centelles P, Diz P, Takkouche B. Is diagnostic delay related to advanced-stage oral cancer? A meta-analysis. Eur J Oral Sci. 2009;117:541–6. https://doi.org/10.1111/j.1600-0722.2009.00672.x.
50. Silverman S, Gorsky M, Lozada F. Oral leukoplakia and malignant transformation. A follow-up study of 257 patients. Cancer. 1984;53:563–8. https://doi.org/10.1002/1097-014 2(19840201)53:3<563::aid-cncr2820530332>3.0.co;2-f.
51. Warnakulasuriya S, Kovacevic T, Madden P, Coupland VH, Sperandio M, Odell E, Møller H. Factors predicting malignant transformation in oral potentially malignant disorders among patients accrued over a 10-year period in South East England. J Oral Pathol Med. 2011;40:677–83. https://doi.org/10.1111/j.1600-0714.2011.01054.x.
52. Torezan LAR, Festa-Neto C. Cutaneous field cancerization: clinical, histopathological and therapeutic aspects. An Bras Dermatol. 2013;88:775–86. https://doi.org/10.1590/abd1806-4841.20132300.
53. Warnakulasuriya S. Oral potentially malignant disorders: a comprehensive review on clinical aspects and management. Oral Oncol. 2020;102:104550. https://doi.org/10.1016/j.oraloncology.2019.104550.
54. Downer MC, Moles DR, Palmer S, Speight PM. A systematic review of test performance in screening for oral cancer and precancer. Oral Oncol. 2004;40:264–73. https://doi.org/10.1016/j.oraloncology.2003.08.013.
55. Awan KH, Morgan PR, Warnakulasuriya S. Assessing the accuracy of autofluorescence, chemiluminescence and toluidine blue as diagnostic tools for oral potentially malignant disorders – a clinicopathological evaluation. Clin Oral Investig. 2015;19:2267–72. https://doi.org/10.1007/s00784-015-1457-9.
56. Speight PM, Khurram SA, Kujan O. Oral potentially malignant disorders: risk of progression to malignancy. Oral Surg Oral Med Oral Pathol Oral Radiol. 2018;125:612–27. https://doi.org/10.1016/j.oooo.2017.12.011.
57. Seoane Lestón J, Diz Dios P. Diagnostic clinical aids in oral cancer. Oral Oncol. 2010;46:418–22. https://doi.org/10.1016/j.oraloncology.2010.03.006.
58. Lingen MW, Kalmar JR, Karrison T, Speight PM. Critical evaluation of diagnostic aids for the detection of oral cancer. Oral Oncol. 2008;44:10–22. https://doi.org/10.1016/j.oraloncology.2007.06.011.

59. Du G-F, Li C-Z, Chen H-Z, Chen X-M, Xiao Q, Cao Z-G, Shang S-H, Cai X. Rose Bengal staining in detection of oral precancerous and malignant lesions with colorimetric evaluation: a pilot study. Int J Cancer. 2007;120:1958–63. https://doi.org/10.1002/ijc.22467.
60. Mittal N, Palaskar S, Shankari M. Rose Bengal staining – diagnostic aid for potentially malignant and malignant disorders: a pilot study. Indian J Dent Res. 2012;23:561–4. https://doi.org/10.4103/0970-9290.107326.
61. Chaudhari A, Hegde-Shetiya S, Shirahatti R, Agrawal D. Comparison of different screening methods in estimating the prevalence of precancer and cancer amongst male inmates of a jail in Maharashtra, India. Asian Pac J Cancer Prev. 2013;14:859–64. https://doi.org/10.7314/apjcp.2013.14.2.859.
62. Pallagatti S, Sheikh S, Aggarwal A, Gupta D, Singh R, Handa R, Kaur S, Mago J. Toluidine blue staining as an adjunctive tool for early diagnosis of dysplastic changes in the oral mucosa. J Clin Exp Dent. 2013;5:e187–91. https://doi.org/10.4317/jced.51121.
63. Riaz A, Shreedhar B, Kamboj M, Natarajan S. Methylene blue as an early diagnostic marker for oral precancer and cancer. Springerplus. 2013;2:95. https://doi.org/10.1186/2193-1801-2-95.
64. Gandolfo S, Pentenero M, Broccoletti R, Pagano M, Carrozzo M, Scully C. Toluidine blue uptake in potentially malignant oral lesions in vivo: clinical and histological assessment. Oral Oncol. 2006;42:89–95. https://doi.org/10.1016/j.oraloncology.2005.06.016.
65. Driemel O, Kunkel M, Hullmann M, von Eggeling F, Müller-Richter U, Kosmehl H, Reichert TE. Diagnosis of oral squamous cell carcinoma and its precursor lesions. J Dtsch Dermatol Ges. 2007;5:1095–100. https://doi.org/10.1111/j.1610-0387.2007.06397.x.
66. Macey R, Walsh T, Brocklehurst P, Kerr AR, Liu JLY, Lingen MW, Ogden GR, Warnakulasuriya S, Scully C. Diagnostic tests for oral cancer and potentially malignant disorders in patients presenting with clinically evident lesions. Cochrane Database Syst Rev. 2015;2015(5):CD010276. https://doi.org/10.1002/14651858.CD010276.pub2.
67. Sambandham T, Masthan KMK, Kumar MS, Jha A. The application of vizilite in oral cancer. J Clin Diagn Res. 2013;7:185–6. https://doi.org/10.7860/JCDR/2012/5163.2704.
68. Rajmohan M, Rao UK, Joshua E, Rajasekaran ST, Kannan R. Assessment of oral mucosa in normal, precancer and cancer using chemiluminescent illumination, toluidine blue supravital staining and oral exfoliative cytology. J Oral Maxillofac Pathol. 2012;16:325–9. https://doi.org/10.4103/0973-029X.102476.
69. McIntosh L, McCullough MJ, Farah CS. The assessment of diffused light illumination and acetic acid rinse (Microlux/DL) in the visualisation of oral mucosal lesions. Oral Oncol. 2009;45:e227–31. https://doi.org/10.1016/j.oraloncology.2009.08.001.
70. Awan KH, Morgan PR, Warnakulasuriya S. Utility of chemiluminescence (ViziLite™) in the detection of oral potentially malignant disorders and benign keratoses. J Oral Pathol Med. 2011;40:541–4. https://doi.org/10.1111/j.1600-0714.2011.01048.x.
71. Rashid A, Warnakulasuriya S. The use of light-based (optical) detection systems as adjuncts in the detection of oral cancer and oral potentially malignant disorders: a systematic review. J Oral Pathol Med. 2015;44:307–28. https://doi.org/10.1111/jop.12218.
72. Farah CS, McIntosh L, Georgiou A, McCullough MJ. Efficacy of tissue autofluorescence imaging (VELscope) in the visualization of oral mucosal lesions. Head Neck. 2012;34:856–62. https://doi.org/10.1002/hed.21834.
73. Bhatia N, Lalla Y, Vu AN, Farah CS. Advances in optical adjunctive AIDS for visualisation and detection of oral malignant and potentially malignant lesions. Int J Dent. 2013;2013:194029. https://doi.org/10.1155/2013/194029.
74. Balevi B. Evidence-based decision making: should the general dentist adopt the use of the VELscope for routine screening for oral cancer? J Can Dent Assoc. 2007;73:603–6. http://www.ncbi.nlm.nih.gov/pubmed/17868507.
75. Moro A, Di Nardo F, Boniello R, Marianetti TM, Cervelli D, Gasparini G, Pelo S. Autofluorescence and early detection of mucosal lesions in patients at risk for oral cancer. J Craniofac Surg. 2010;21:1899–903. https://doi.org/10.1097/SCS.0b013e3181f4afb4.

76. Mercadante V, Paderni C, Campisi G. Novel non-invasive adjunctive techniques for early oral cancer diagnosis and oral lesions examination. Curr Pharm Des. 2012;18:5442–51. https://doi.org/10.2174/138161212803307626.
77. Figueira JA, Veltrini VC. Photodynamic therapy in oral potentially malignant disorders-critical literature review of existing protocols. Photodiagn Photodyn Ther. 2017;20:125–9. https://doi.org/10.1016/j.pdpdt.2017.09.007.
78. Hopper C. Photodynamic therapy: a clinical reality in the treatment of cancer. Lancet Oncol. 2000;1:212–9. https://doi.org/10.1016/s1470-2045(00)00166-2.
79. Zhu TC, Finlay JC. The role of photodynamic therapy (PDT) physics. Med Phys. 2008;35:3127–36. https://doi.org/10.1118/1.2937440.
80. Li Y, Wang B, Zheng S, He Y. Photodynamic therapy in the treatment of oral leukoplakia: a systematic review. Photodiagn Photodyn Ther. 2019;25:17–22. https://doi.org/10.1016/j.pdpdt.2018.10.023.
81. Jin X, Xu H, Deng J, Dan H, Ji P, Chen Q, Zeng X. Photodynamic therapy for oral potentially malignant disorders. Photodiagn Photodyn Ther. 2019;28:146–52. https://doi.org/10.1016/j.pdpdt.2019.08.005.
82. Gondivkar SM, Gadbail AR, Choudhary MG, Vedpathak PR, Likhitkar MS. Photodynamic treatment outcomes of potentially-malignant lesions and malignancies of the head and neck region: a systematic review. J Investig Clin Dent. 2018;9:e12270. https://doi.org/10.1111/jicd.12270.
83. Wu C, Gleysteen J, Teraphongphom NT, Li Y, Rosenthal E. In-vivo optical imaging in head and neck oncology: basic principles, clinical applications and future directions. Int J Oral Sci. 2018;10:10. https://doi.org/10.1038/s41368-018-0011-4.
84. Stephen MM, Jayanthi JL, Unni NG, Kolady PE, Beena VT, Jeemon P, Subhash N. Diagnostic accuracy of diffuse reflectance imaging for early detection of pre-malignant and malignant changes in the oral cavity: a feasibility study. BMC Cancer. 2013;13:278. https://doi.org/10.1186/1471-2407-13-278.
85. Green B, Tsiroyannis C, Brennan PA. Optical diagnostic systems for assessing head and neck lesions. Oral Dis. 2016;22:180–4. https://doi.org/10.1111/odi.12398.
86. Krishna H, Majumder SK, Chaturvedi P, Sidramesh M, Gupta PK. In vivo Raman spectroscopy for detection of oral neoplasia: a pilot clinical study. J Biophotonics. 2014;7:690–702. https://doi.org/10.1002/jbio.201300030.
87. Green B, Cobb ARM, Brennan PA, Hopper C. Optical diagnostic techniques for use in lesions of the head and neck: review of the latest developments. Br J Oral Maxillofac Surg. 2014;52:675–80. https://doi.org/10.1016/j.bjoms.2014.06.010.
88. Chen X-J, Zhang X-Q, Liu Q, Zhang J, Zhou G. Nanotechnology: a promising method for oral cancer detection and diagnosis. J Nanobiotechnology. 2018;16:52. https://doi.org/10.1186/s12951-018-0378-6.
89. Wetzel SL, Wollenberg J. Oral potentially malignant disorders. Dent Clin N Am. 2020;64:25–37. https://doi.org/10.1016/j.cden.2019.08.004.
90. Dancyger A, Heard V, Huang B, Suley C, Tang D, Ariyawardana A. Malignant transformation of actinic cheilitis: a systematic review of observational studies. J Investig Clin Dent. 2018;9:e12343. https://doi.org/10.1111/jicd.12343.
91. Miller KD, Siegel RL, Lin CC, Mariotto AB, Kramer JL, Rowland JH, Stein KD, Alteri R, Jemal A. Cancer treatment and survivorship statistics, 2016. CA Cancer J Clin. 2016;66:271–89. https://doi.org/10.3322/caac.21349.
92. Foy J-P, Bertolus C, Saintigny P. Oral cancer prevention worldwide: challenges and perspectives. Oral Oncol. 2019;88:91–4. https://doi.org/10.1016/j.oraloncology.2018.11.008.
93. Warnakulasuriya S. Potentially malignant disorders of the oral cavity. In: Textbook of oral cancer. Cham: Springer; 2020. p. 141–58. https://doi.org/10.1007/978-3-030-32316-5_12.
94. Vogelstein B, Lane D, Levine AJ. Surfing the p53 network. Nature. 2000;408:307–10. https://doi.org/10.1038/35042675.

95. Goldstein I, Marcel V, Olivier M, Oren M, Rotter V, Hainaut P. Understanding wild-type and mutant p53 activities in human cancer: new landmarks on the way to targeted therapies. Cancer Gene Ther. 2011;18:2–11. https://doi.org/10.1038/cgt.2010.63.

96. Scholzen T, Gerdes J. The Ki-67 protein: from the known and the unknown. J Cell Physiol. 2000;182:311–22. https://doi.org/10.1002/(SICI)1097-4652(200003)182:3<311:: AID-JCP1>3.0.CO;2-9.

97. Pelosi G, Massa F, Gatti G, Righi L, Volante M, Birocco N, Maisonneuve P, Sonzogni A, Harari S, Albini A, Papotti M. Ki-67 evaluation for clinical decision in metastatic lung carcinoids: a proof of concept. Clin Pathol. 2019;12:2632010X19829259. https://doi.org/10.117 7/2632010X19829259.

98. Niotis A, Tsiambas E, Fotiades PP, Ragos V, Polymeneas G. Ki-67 and topoisomerase IIa proliferation markers in colon adenocarcinoma. J BUON. 2018;23:24–7. http://www.ncbi. nlm.nih.gov/pubmed/30722108.

99. Mello FW, Melo G, Guerra ENS, Warnakulasuriya S, Garnis C, Rivero ERC. Oral potentially malignant disorders: a scoping review of prognostic biomarkers. Crit Rev Oncol Hematol. 2020;153:102986. https://doi.org/10.1016/j.critrevonc.2020.102986.

100. Mei Y, Zhang P, Zuo H, Clark D, Xia R, Li J, Liu Z, Mao L. Ebp1 activates podoplanin expression and contributes to oral tumorigenesis. Oncogene. 2014;33:3839–50. https://doi. org/10.1038/onc.2013.354.

101. Martin-Villar E, Megias D, Castel S, Yurrita MM, Vilaro S, Quintanilla M. Podoplanin binds ERM proteins to activate RhoA and promote epithelial-mesenchymal transition. J Cell Sci. 2006;119:4541–53. https://doi.org/10.1242/jcs.03218.

102. Suzuki-Inoue K, Osada M, Ozaki Y. Physiologic and pathophysiologic roles of interaction between C-type lectin-like receptor 2 and podoplanin: partners from in utero to adulthood. J Thromb Haemost. 2017;15:219–29. https://doi.org/10.1111/jth.13590.

103. Danielsen HE, Pradhan M, Novelli M. Revisiting tumour aneuploidy – the place of ploidy assessment in the molecular era. Nat Rev Clin Oncol. 2016;13:291–304. https://doi. org/10.1038/nrclinonc.2015.208.

104. Zaini ZM, McParland H, Møller H, Husband K, Odell EW. Predicting malignant progression in clinically high-risk lesions by DNA ploidy analysis and dysplasia grading. Sci Rep. 2018;8:15874. https://doi.org/10.1038/s41598-018-34165-5.

105. Siebers TJH, Bergshoeff VE, Otte-Höller I, Kremer B, Speel EJM, van der Laak JAWM, Merkx MAW, Slootweg PJ. Chromosome instability predicts the progression of premalignant oral lesions. Oral Oncol. 2013;49:1121–8. https://doi.org/10.1016/j.oraloncology.2013.09.006.

106. Bradley G, Odell EW, Raphael S, Ho J, Le LW, Benchimol S, Kamel-Reid S. Abnormal DNA content in oral epithelial dysplasia is associated with increased risk of progression to carcinoma. Br J Cancer. 2010;103:1432–42. https://doi.org/10.1038/sj.bjc.6605905.

107. Nayak S, Goel MM, Makker A, Bhatia V, Chandra S, Kumar S, Agarwal SP. Fibroblast growth factor (FGF-2) and its receptors FGFR-2 and FGFR-3 may be putative biomarkers of malignant transformation of potentially malignant oral lesions into oral squamous cell carcinoma. PLoS One. 2015;10:e0138801. https://doi.org/10.1371/journal.pone.0138801.

108. Poh CF, Zhu Y, Chen E, Berean KW, Wu L, Zhang L, Rosin MP. Unique FISH patterns associated with cancer progression of oral dysplasia. J Dent Res. 2012;91:52–7. https://doi. org/10.1177/0022034511425676.

109. Taoudi Benchekroun M, Saintigny P, Thomas SM, El-Naggar AK, Papadimitrakopoulou V, Ren H, Lang W, Fan Y-H, Huang J, Feng L, Lee JJ, Kim ES, Hong WK, Johnson FM, Grandis JR, Mao L. Epidermal growth factor receptor expression and gene copy number in the risk of oral cancer. Cancer Prev Res (Phila). 2010;3:800–9. https://doi.org/10.1158/1940-6207. CAPR-09-0163.

110. Foy J-P, Bertolus C, Ortiz-Cuaran S, Albaret M-A, Williams WN, Lang W, Destandau S, De Souza G, Sohier E, Kielbassa J, Thomas E, Deneuve S, Goudot P, Puisieux A, Viari A, Mao L, Caux C, Lippman S, Saintigny P. Immunological and classical subtypes of oral premalignant lesions. Onco Targets Ther. 2018;7:e1496880. https://doi.org/10.108 0/2162402X.2018.1496880.

111. William WN, Papadimitrakopoulou V, Lee JJ, Mao L, Cohen EEW, Lin HY, Gillenwater AM, Martin JW, Lingen MW, Boyle JO, Shin DM, Vigneswaran N, Shinn N, Heymach JV, Wistuba II, Tang X, Kim ES, Saintigny P, Blair EA, Meiller T, Gutkind JS, Myers J, El-Naggar A, Lippman SM. Erlotinib and the risk of oral cancer. JAMA Oncol. 2016;2:209. https://doi.org/10.1001/jamaoncol.2015.4364.
112. Sarode GS, Sarode SC, Maniyar N, Sharma N, Yerwadekar S, Patil S. Recent trends in predictive biomarkers for determining malignant potential of oral potentially malignant disorders. Oncol Rev. 2019;13:424. https://doi.org/10.4081/oncol.2019.424.
113. El-Sakka H, Kujan O, Farah CS. Assessing miRNAs profile expression as a risk stratification biomarker in oral potentially malignant disorders: a systematic review. Oral Oncol. 2018;77:57–82. https://doi.org/10.1016/j.oraloncology.2017.11.021.
114. von Elm E, Altman DG, Egger M, Pocock SJ, Gøtzsche PC, Vandenbroucke JP. The strengthening the reporting of observational studies in epidemiology (STROBE) statement: guidelines for reporting observational studies. Int J Surg. 2014;12:1495–9. https://doi.org/10.1016/j.ijsu.2014.07.013.
115. Moher D, Hopewell S, Schulz KF, Montori V, Gøtzsche PC, Devereaux PJ, Elbourne D, Egger M, Altman DG. CONSORT 2010 explanation and elaboration: updated guidelines for reporting parallel group randomised trials. Int J Surg. 2012;10:28–55. https://doi.org/10.1016/j.ijsu.2011.10.001.
116. McCullough MJ, Prasad G, Farah CS. Oral mucosal malignancy and potentially malignant lesions: an update on the epidemiology, risk factors, diagnosis and management. Aust Dent J. 2010;55(Suppl 1):61–5. https://doi.org/10.1111/j.1834-7819.2010.01200.x.
117. Kujan O, Oliver RJ, Khattab A, Roberts SA, Thakker N, Sloan P. Evaluation of a new binary system of grading oral epithelial dysplasia for prediction of malignant transformation. Oral Oncol. 2006;42:987–93. https://doi.org/10.1016/j.oraloncology.2005.12.014.
118. Ranganathan K, Kavitha L. Oral epithelial dysplasia: classifications and clinical relevance in risk assessment of oral potentially malignant disorders. J Oral Maxillofac Pathol. 2019;23:19–27. https://doi.org/10.4103/jomfp.JOMFP_13_19.
119. Mehrotra R, Gupta A, Singh M, Ibrahim R. Retraction: application of cytology and molecular biology in diagnosing premalignant or malignant oral lesions. Mol Cancer. 2012;11:57. https://doi.org/10.1186/1476-4598-11-57.
120. Casparis S, Borm JM, Tomic MA, Burkhardt A, Locher MC. Transepithelial brush biopsy – oral CDx® – a noninvasive method for the early detection of precancerous and cancerous lesions. J Clin Diagn Res. 2014;8:222–6. https://doi.org/10.7860/JCDR/2014/7659.4065.
121. Lingen MW, Tampi MP, Urquhart O, Abt E, Agrawal N, Chaturvedi AK, Cohen E, D'Souza G, Gurenlian J, Kalmar JR, Kerr AR, Lambert PM, Patton LL, Sollecito TP, Truelove E, Banfield L, Carrasco-Labra A. Adjuncts for the evaluation of potentially malignant disorders in the oral cavity: diagnostic test accuracy systematic review and meta-analysis-a report of the American Dental Association. J Am Dent Assoc. 2017;148:797–813.e52. https://doi.org/10.1016/j.adaj.2017.08.045.
122. Liu D, Zhao X, Zeng X, Dan H, Chen Q. Non-invasive techniques for detection and diagnosis of oral potentially malignant disorders. Tohoku J Exp Med. 2016;238:165–77. https://doi.org/10.1620/tjem.238.165.

Chapter 3
Diagnosis and Management of Intraoral Epithelial Dysplasia

M. Anthony Pogrel

Introduction

According to the American Cancer Society, there are over 53,000 new cases of oral and oropharyngeal cancers diagnosed in 2020 in the United States alone. Oral cancer, along with melanoma, is one of the two types of cancer which, for unknown reasons, are increasing in frequency [1]. Oral cancer rarely develops from normal epithelium, but rather emerges from a preliminary dysplastic phase; therefore, if it could be eliminated at the dysplastic phase, the subsequent cancer would not develop.

Dysplasia is a histological term denoting abnormalities and disordered growth in the epithelium and the basal layer. Traditionally, this has been graded histologically as (i) mild dysplasia, (ii) moderate dysplasia, (iii) severe dysplasia (Fig. 3.1), and (iv) carcinoma in situ.

The possible transformation rates to squamous cell carcinoma for these lesions are unknown. It is also unknown whether a dysplasia has to progress from one stage to the next or whether it can transform from mild or moderate dysplasia directly into carcinoma. Estimates for the transformation rate into squamous cell carcinoma from mild dysplasia range from 10% to 20% over a five-year period, whereas for moderate or severe dysplasia, transformation rates range from 35% to 50% [2]. Lesions in the floor of the mouth (Fig. 3.2) are more prone to malignant transformation, possibly due the presence of more carcinogenic byproducts pooled in the floor of the mouth [3]. Many attempts have been made to predict features of dysplastic lesions that may signal progression to carcinoma. For example, there appears to be overexpression of metalloproteinases 1 and 9, overexpression of MRNA (as

M. A. Pogrel (✉)
Department of Oral and Maxillofacial Surgery, University of California, San Francisco, San Francisco, CA, USA
e-mail: tony.pogrel@ucsf.edu

© Springer Nature Switzerland AG 2021
R. El Assal et al. (eds.), *Early Detection and Treatment of Head & Neck Cancers*, https://doi.org/10.1007/978-3-030-69852-2_3

Fig. 3.1 Histopathology of severe epithelial dysplasia showing hyperchromatism of the nuclei, pleomorphism, and an irregular but intact basement membrane (hematoxylin and eosin staining; 40x magnification)

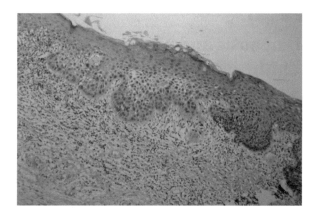

Fig. 3.2 Mild dysplasia in the floor of the mouth, which is known to have a high propensity for malignant transformation

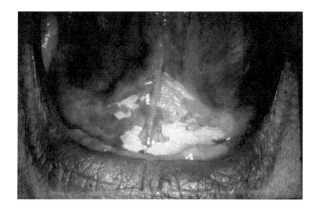

measured by reverse transcription), and expression of Ki-67 on immunohistochemistry in lesions that progress to carcinoma. Genomic markers with aberrations noted on microassay have also been evaluated as a way of predicating transformation [4]. However, at present none of these features have shown consistent reliability or predictability.

Another issue is that there is no standardization for the diagnosis of oral dysplasia. It has been shown that there is not reliable consistency in the grading of a histological specimen between oral and maxillofacial pathologists; there is not even consistent grading when one oral and maxillofacial pathologist evaluates the same specimen 30 days apart [5].

Clinically, the appearance of dysplasia lacks uniformity. It can present as a white patch, or leukoplakia (Fig. 3.3a), which is the mildest form of dysplasia with a low malignant transformation rate, on the order of 2–5%. It can also appear as a speckled red and white lesion, commonly called erythroleukoplakia (Fig. 3.3b), which has a more sinister prognosis, with a higher malignant transformation rate ranging from 20% to 30% [6]. However, the mucosa can clinically appear perfectly normal and yet still be dysplastic on histopathological examination, making clinical detection a challenge.

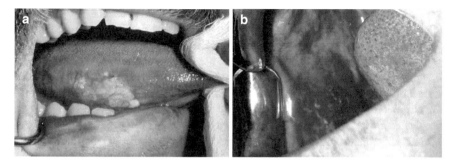

Fig. 3.3 Clinical appearance of dysplasia lacks uniformity. (**a**) A typical patch of homogenous white leukoplakia on the right lateral tongue. Histologically, this is often mild dysplasia. (**b**) A speckled area of erythroleukoplakia, known to have a higher malignant transformation rate than leukoplakia

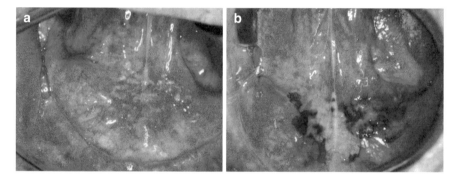

Fig. 3.4 Staining of leukoplakia with toluidine blue. (**a**) Leukoplakia in the floor of the mouth. (**b**) Leukoplakia lesion after staining with toluidine blue. Note the areas retaining the blue dye. These are the areas which are most likely to show dysplastic changes, and they will be biopsied

Aids in the Diagnosis of Oral Dysplasia

Over the years, many techniques have been proposed to enable oral dysplasia to be diagnosed more predictably and, therefore, treated more predictably.

A. *Toluidine blue*. Toluidine blue is a vital stain, which essentially stains nuclei near the cell surface. Because this often applies to dysplastic tissue, staining the mucosa with toluidine blue will show areas of possible dysplasia. The technique involves first removing the surface mucin with sodium bicarbonate or 1% acetic acid, then staining the area with 1% toluidine blue, and then gently de-staining with 1% acetic acid. Any areas that continue to retain the stain are more likely to be dysplastic and are the areas that should be biopsied (Fig. 3.4). The stained area can also be decolorized naturally by first staining it and then sending the patient away for an hour or two to have a drink. The mucosa will naturally decolorize, and any areas retaining the stain are considered suspicious [7]. This technique has been subject to extensive studies, with valid results [8]. It is recommended as a technique to determine which areas should be biopsied for the most accurate results. However, inflammatory and granulomatous reactions will also give a positive result with toluidine blue. In Europe, a similar staining technique utilizing Lugol's iodine, signaling loss of glycogen, has also been employed with similarly meaningful results [9].

B. *Brush test (Oral CDx)*. This technique involves utilizing cytology to look for dysplastic cells. Cytology has been used very successfully for early diagnosis of cervical cancer; however, it has always presented problems when used on the oral mucosa. This is because the oral mucosa is contaminated by saliva, food, and other debris as well as because the basal layer is placed more deeply and is more difficult to get meaningful material from. However, a recently developed brush technique that can reach down to the basement membrane, coupled with a computerized examination system, has enabled more accurate cytology to be performed [10, 11] (Fig. 3.5). The problem with this technique, however, is that it can rarely be used as a substitute for formal biopsy; it tends to be more useful as a preliminary test before the biopsy is carried out. Thus, it does not typically save time or eliminate procedures. It has also been suggested that a simple toothbrush, used without a computerized examination system, can achieve similar results [12].

C. *ViziLite*. This technique utilizes chemiluminescence and tissue reflectance with the claim that the light emitted by a chemical reaction in a darkened room will show dysplastic areas better than direct examination in ambient light. This technique has also been used in conjunction with toluidine blue [13]. Despite claims, it appears this technique may be no better than direct examination under ambient light [14].

D. *Fluorescent light*. This approach utilizes fluorescent light to examine the oral mucosa. The concept is that normal tissues will reflect back the fluorescent light, whereas dysplastic and malignant tissues will absorb it; therefore, in normal tissues, there will be no reflectance, and the area will appear dark [15, 16]. However, it is not clear if this technique offers improvement over direct exami-

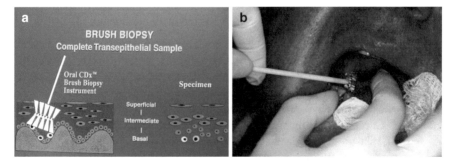

Fig. 3.5 Brush test. (**a**) The diagrammatic illustration of the brush biopsy technique with a (**b**) clinical slide of the brush being applied to the tissues

nation with a good headlight. This technique does detect an increased blood supply to the area, so it would detect both dysplastic tissue and inflammatory tissue, leading to false positives in the latter case.

Special Emphasis on Other Differential Diagnosis

Proliferative Verrucous Leukoplakia

Proliferative verrucous leukoplakia is a specific condition first diagnosed in 1985 by Hansen et al. [17]. It is a specific form of leukoplakia, which is diagnosable both clinically (Fig. 3.6) and histologically. When left untreated, the lesion will almost inevitably progress through stages of verrucous hyperplasia to verrucous carcinoma and on to squamous cell carcinoma. Fairly radical surgery is required to remove this lesion, and reconstruction may involve both hard and soft tissue grafting. Even then, the lesion can be difficult to eliminate, and recurrences may occur many years later. When the lesion forms around the gingiva (Fig. 3.6b), it is particularly troublesome to remove since it tends to spread through the periodontal ligament [18], and carrying out a gingivectomy or other localized procedure is ineffective. Only a subapical

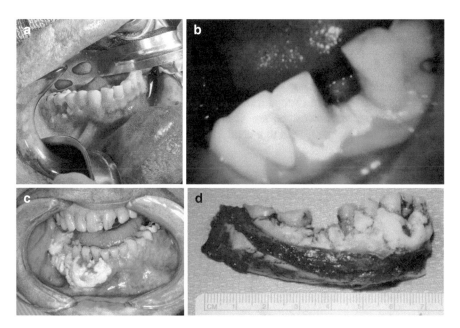

Fig. 3.6 Proliferative verrucous leukoplakia. (**a**) The typical verrucous appearance of PVL in the oral cavity. (**b**) PVL specifically around the regions of gingival margin. (**c**, **d**) A more proliferative type of verrucous leukoplakia that can only be eliminated by an "en bloc" marginal resection of the mandible

resection of the tissues to include the teeth in a block of bone can be successful (Fig. 3.6c, d).

Lichen Planus

Controversy exists as to whether intraoral lichen planus, which affects 0.2–0.3% of the population and is more common in women, should be considered a premalignant condition. Current knowledge suggests the reticular form of lichen planus (Fig. 3.7a) is probably not premalignant, but the atrophic (Fig. 3.7b) or ulcerative forms (Fig. 3.7c) may be premalignant with a transformation rate in the region of 1–2% [19, 20]. Efforts should therefore be made to treat lichen planus in the ulcerative or atrophic presentations. The treatment most often involves steroids or other immune modulators, with surgical or laser excision for isolated lesions where indicated. Lichen Planus is currently classified by WHO as a Potentially Malignant Disease (PMD) rather than a Premalignant Disease.

Treatment of Intraoral Dysplasia

Traditionally, the treatment of intraoral dysplasia has been surgical following biopsy confirmation of the diagnosis. Where possible, wide margins are advised, although this can sometimes involve skin or mucosal grafting for reconstruction. However, the evidence that this technique improves the final results and lowers the incidence of subsequent oral cancer development has been difficult to prove, although some multi-center studies from Europe have finally produced reasonable evidence that early surgical intervention can be beneficial in the long term [21, 22]. Surgical treatment should remove the tissues to a depth of at least 2–3 mm below the basement membrane (Fig. 3.8).

A surgical laser, such as the carbon dioxide laser with a wavelength of 10.6 μm, has been advocated for removal of oral dysplasia when it is in the form of leukoplakia or erythroleukoplakia. It is acceptable to use the laser as a surgical scalpel to

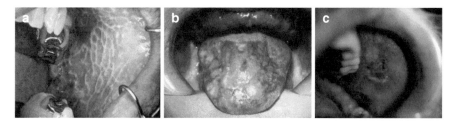

Fig. 3.7 Forms of intraoral lichen planus. (**a**) Reticular lichen planus, which is normally benign. (**b, c**) Atrophic and ulcerative lichen planus, which may have malignant potentials

Fig. 3.8 A surgically removed specimen of erythroleukoplakia showing excision to a depth of 2–3 mm to give the optimal conditions for a cure

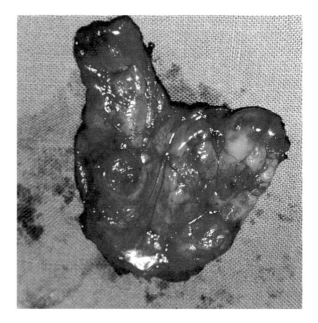

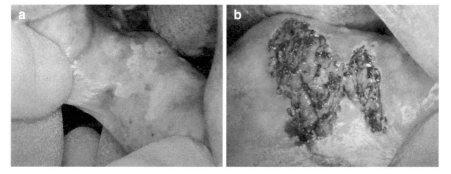

Fig. 3.9 Areas of (**a**) filmy leukoplakia treated by (**b**) surface vaporization with a carbon dioxide laser. This technique has a high incidence of recurrence and may unmask an underlying malignancy

remove a surgical specimen, although it does make it more difficult for the oral and maxillofacial pathologist since they have to compensate for the laser disruption of the surgical margin, which usually extends to the thickness of three cells. In addition, when the laser is used to "wipe over" or vaporize the area, it does not penetrate deeply; therefore, there is often a recurrence of the dysplasia (Fig. 3.9). There have also been reported cases of oral cancer developing in an area which has been "wiped" or superficially vaporized with the surgical carbon dioxide laser, which is more worrying [23, 24]. Although allegations have been made that the laser may be stimulating the formation of oral cancer, it seems more likely that the cancer was already present within the dysplastic tissue and was merely unmasked by removing the more superficial layers of epithelium, strengthening the case for a deeper excision [23, 24].

For very extensive areas of leukoplakia, or for particularly mild or moderate dysplasia, a protocol of "wait and see" with biopsies where indicated may have to be adopted. The rationale of this approach is that with regular examination, any malignant change can be diagnosed early, leading to a favorable prognosis.

How to Avoid the Development of Dysplasia and Oral Cancer

Smoking

Among known habits that increase the incidence of oral cancer is smoking. Cigars and pipes burn hotter in the mouth and may be more harmful than cigarettes for the oral mucosa, although the lungs may be protected. The use of smokeless tobacco in the form of chewing tobacco or snuff remains controversial. There is no doubt that this causes changes in the mucosa and will cause hyperplasia and verrucous-type lesions, and recent studies have shown the progression to oral cancer from some of these lesions [25].

Drinking

Hard liquor is understood to encourage oral cancer, likely by dehydration and eventual atrophy of the oral mucosa, making it more susceptible to carcinogens in the diet. In addition, although that drinking and smoking are two independent risk factors, they might synergistically to increase risk oral cancer.

Chewing

Betel nut chewing as practiced on the Indian subcontinent is a known cause of submucosal fibrosis of the oral cavity, a premalignant condition that can lead to oral cancer. It has been shown that it is the areca oil within the betel nuts which is the primary irritant [26].

Vitamin Imbalance

The early studies with vitamin A and its derivatives showed that high doses of vitamin A would cause leukoplakia and other intraoral dysplastic lesions to regress [27–33]. However, as soon as the therapy was discontinued, the lesions recurred.

Additionally, vitamin A caused extreme thinning and cracking of the mucosa as well as other systemic side effects which were unacceptable for most patients. It is unknown whether this treatment would have led to a decrease in the subsequent development of oral cancer, but at the moment, vitamin A is not utilized for this purpose. However, the vegetable equivalent of vitamin A is beta carotene, and this is better tolerated and has been recommended as a method of preventing oral lesions and possibly recurrences if lesions have already been treated [29–32]. The carotenoids and their related flavonoids are best utilized as beta carotene from carrots, sweet potatoes, lettuce, and kale among others [28]. Four carrot sticks per day is adequate, as any more will actually cause the skin to turn orange. Beta carotene is also available in the form of a carotene-rich drink and is also available in tablet form. Folic acid (vitamin B9) may also decrease the risk of oral cancer, and this is found in spinach, asparagus, bean, peas, and lentils [34]. Alcohol creates acetaldehyde, which inhibits folic acid, possibly another reason why alcohol may promote oral cancer.

Oncogenic Viruses

Although over 50% of oropharyngeal carcinomas are human papilloma virus (HPV)-positive for viral DNA, the number in the oral cavity appears to be much lower. If one looks at P16, which is a surrogate marker for HPV, about 25% of oral carcinomas are positive, but if one looks for viral DNA, only about 5% are positive. The difference in these two numbers has not been adequately explained. Almost all of the oral malignancies that are HPV-positive occur in the floor of the mouth and may be related to microtrauma or even to ectopic salivary or tonsillar tissue. It does not, therefore, appear that HPV is a major cause of intraoral epithelial dysplasia or oral malignancy [35]. However, it is possible that potentially malignant lesions such as proliferative verrucous leukoplakia could have a viral etiology [18].

Surprising Good Side Effects of Medications

Certain medications that have been commonly used have shown to have the beneficial effect of lowering the incidence of oral cancer and, therefore, likely a lower incidence of dysplasia. Among these medications are nicotinamide [36], aspirin [37, 38], and metformin [39, 40]. In addition, a large Veterans Administration System study showed that sodium valproate, as given for petite mal and seizure disorders, may result in a lower incidence of head and neck cancer [41, 42]. The mechanism for the positive influence of these medications on the prevention of primary oral cancer and its recurrence is not clear, but it may involve their anti-inflammatory effects.

Conclusion

Despite years of cancer research, little progress has been made toward understanding the clinical behaviors and the underlying molecular biology of oral dysplasia. This unfortunate circumstance most likely underlies the overall lack of improvement in 5-year survival rates for oral cancer in general. In the future, this problem can be addressed on multiple fronts including prognostic and treatment response-specific biomarker development using both canonical molecular signatures and non-canonical methods such as digital histomorphometric analysis done with the aid of artificial intelligence/machine learning, creation of biosensors to provide real-time surveillance for those early biomarkers that correlate with disease that is likely to be progressive, detailed prospective studies to correlate clinical progression with molecular progression in relation to biomarker development, and finally, increased understanding of the clinical phenotypes in correlation with molecular genotypes which eventually results in targetable drug targets. Cancer has a knack of finding a way to win and defeat any treatment aimed to control it. Targeting treatment of dysplasia should prove more effective because the underlying molecular mechanisms responsible for genetic replication and control are not as disturbed, compared to cancer, and thus treatment evasion is bound to be less likely.

References

1. Campbell BR, Netterville JL, Sinard RJ, Mannion K, Rohde SL, Langerman A, Kim YJ, Lewis JS, Lang Kuhs KA. Early onset oral tongue cancer in the United States: a literature review. Oral Oncol. 2018;87:1–7.
2. Reibel J. Prognosis of oral pre-malignant lesions: significance of clinical, histopathological, and molecular biological characteristics. Crit Rev Oral Biol Med. 2003;14:47–62.
3. Rock LD, Rosin MP, Zhang L, Chan B, Shariati B, Laronde DM. Characterization of epithelial oral dysplasia in non smokers: first steps towards precision medicine. Oral Oncol. 2018;78:119–25.
4. Smith J, Rattay T, McConkey C, Helliwell T, Mehanna H. Biomarkers in dysplasia of the oral cavity: a systematic review. Oral Oncol. 2009;45:647–53.
5. Warnakulasuriya S, Reibel J, Bouquot J, Dabelsteen E. Oral epithelial dysplasia classification systems: predictive value, utility, weaknesses and scope for improvement. J Oral Pathol Med. 2008;37:127–33.
6. Awadallah M, Idle M, Patel K, Kademani D. Management update of potentially premalignant oral epithelial lesions. Oral Surg Oral Med Oral Pathol Oral Radiol. 2018;125:628–36.
7. Silverman S Jr, Migliorati C, Barbosa J. Toluidine blue staining in the detection of oral precancerous and malignant lesions. Oral Surg Oral Med Oral Pathol. 1984;57:379–82.
8. Chainani-Wu N, Madden E, Cox D, Sroussi H, Epstein J, Silverman S Jr. Toluidine blue aids in detection of dysplasia and carcinoma in suspicious oral lesions. Oral Dis. 2015;21:879–85.
9. Elimairi I, Altay MA, Abdoun O, Elmairi A, Tozoglu S, Baur DA, Quereshy F. Clinical relevance of the utilization of vital Lugol's Iodine staining in detection and diagnosis of oral cancer and dysplasia. Clin Oral Investig. 2017;21:589–95.
10. Casparis S, Borm JM, Tomic MA, Burkhardt A, Locher MC. Transepithelial brush biopsy-Oral CDx-A non invasive method for the early detection of precancerous and cancerous lesions. J Clin Diagn Res. 2014;8:222–6.

11. Sciubba JJ, Larian B. Oral squamous cell carcinoma; early detection and improved 5 year survival in 102 patients. Gen Dent. 2018;66:e11–6.
12. Mehrotra R, Singh MK, Pandya S, Singh M. The use of an oral brush biopsy without computer-assisted analysis in the evaluation of oral lesions: a study of 94 patients. Oral Surg Oral Med Oral Pathol Oral Radiol Endod. 2008;106:246–53.
13. Sambandham T, Masthan KM, Kumar MS, Jha A. The application of vizilite in oral cancer. J Clin Diagn Res. 2013;7:185–6.
14. Oh ES, Laskin DM. Efficacy of the Vizilite system in the identification of oral lesions. J Oral Maxillofac Surg. 2007;65:424–6.
15. Yamamoto N, Kawaguchi K, Fujihara H, Hasebe M, Kishi Y, Yasukama M, Kumagai K, Hamada Y. Detection accuracy for epithelial dysplasia using an objective autofluoroescence visualization method based on the luminance ratio. Int J Oral Sci. 2017;9(11):e2. https://doi.org/10.1038/ijosNov2017.37.
16. Kikuta S, Iwanaga J, Todoroki K, Shinozaki K, Tanoue R, Nakamura M, Kusukawa J. Clinical application of the illumiscan fluorescence visualization device in detecting oral mucosal lesions. Cureus. 2018;10(8):e3111. https://doi.org/10.7759/cureus.311.
17. Hansen LS, Olson JA, Silverman S Jr. Proliferative verrucous leukoplakia. A long term study of thirty patients. Oral Surg Oral Med Oral Pathol. 1985;60:285–98.
18. Upadhyaya JD, Fitzpatrick SG, Islam MN, Bhattacharyya I, Cohen DM. A retrospective 20 year analysis of proliferative verrucous hyperplasia and its progression to malignancy and association with high risk human papillomavirus. Head Neck Pathol. 2018;12(4):500–10. https://doi.org/10.1007/s12105-018-0893-7.
19. Ingafou M, Leao JC, Porter SR, Scully C. Oral lichen planus: a retrospective study of 690 British patients. Oral Dis. 2006;12:463–8.
20. Speight PM, Khurram SA, Kujan O. Oral potentially malignant disorders:risk of progression to malignancy. Oral Surg Oral Med Oral Pathol Oral Radiol. 2018;125:612–27.
21. Mehanna HM, Rattay T, Smith J, McConkey CC. Treatment and follow up of oral dysplasia-a systematic review and meta-analysis. Head Neck. 2009;31:1600–9.
22. Balasundaram I, Payne KF, Al-Hadad I, Alibhai M, Thomas S, Bhandari R. Is there any benefit in surgery for potentially malignant disorders of the oral cavity? J Oral Pathol Med. 2014;43:239–44.
23. Brouns ER, Baart JA, Karagozoglu KH, Aartman IH, Bloemena E, Van der Waal I. Treatment results of CO_2 laser vaporisation in a cohort of 35 patients with oral leukoplakia. Oral Dis. 2013;19:212–6.
24. Dong Y, Chen Y, Tao Y, Hao Y, Jiang Y, Dan H, Zang X, Chen Q, Zhou Y. Malignant transformation of oral leukoplakiatreated with carbon dioxide laser: a meta-analysis. Lasers Med Sci. 2018;34(1):209–21. https://doi.org/10.1007/s10103-018-2674-7.
25. Gupta S, Gupta R, Sinha DN, Mehrotra R. Relationship between type of smokeless tobacco and risk of cancer: a systematic review. Indian J Med Res. 2018;148:56–76.
26. Avakeri G, Patil SG, Aljabab AS, Lin KC, Merkx MAW, Gao S, Brennan PA. Oral submucous fibrosis: an update on pathophysiology of malignamnt transformation. J Orasl Pathol Med. 2017;46:413–7.
27. Hong WK, Endicott J, Itri LM, Doos W, Batsakis JG, Bell R, Fofonoff S, Byers R, Atkinson EN, Vaughan C, et al. 13-cic-retinoic acid in the treatment of oral leukoplakia. N Engl J Med. 1986;315:1501–5.
28. Piatelli A, Fiorini M, Santinelli A, Rubini C. blc-2 expression and apoptotic bodies in 13-cis-retinoic acid(isotretinoin)-treated oral leukoplakia: a pilot study. Oral Onc. 1999;35:314–20.
29. Sankaranarayanan R, Mathew B, Varghese C, Sudhakaran PR, Menon V, Jayadeep A, Nair MK, Mathews C, Mahalingam TR, Balaram P, Nair PP. Chemoprevention of oral leukoplakia with Vitamin A and beta carotene: an assessment. Oral Onc. 1999;33:231–6.
30. Stich HF, Mathew B, Sankaranarayanan R, Nair MK. Remission of oral precancerous lesions of tobacco/areca nut chewers following administration of beta-carotene or Vitamin A, and maintenance of the protective effect. Cancer Detect Prev. 1991;15:93–8.

31. Stich HF, Brunnemann KD, Mathew B, Sankaranarayanan R, Nair MK. Chemoprevention trials with Vitamin A and beta carotene: some unresolved issues. Prev Med. 1989;18:732–9.
32. Stich HF, Rosin MP, Hornby AP, Mathew B, Sankaranarayanan R, Nair MK. Remission of oral leukoplakias and micronuclei in tobacco/betel quid chewers treated with beta carotene and with beta carotene plus vitamin A. Int J Cancer. 1988;15:195–9.
33. Stich HF, Hornby AP, Mathew B, Sankaranarayanan R, Nair MK. Response of oral leukoplakia to the administration of Vitamin A. Cancer Lett. 1988;40:93–101.
34. Galeone C, Edefonti V, Parpinel M, Leoncini E, Matsuo K, Talamini O, Olshan AF, Zevallos JP, Winn DM, Jayaprakash V, Moysich K, Zhang ZF, Morgenstern H, Levi F, Bosetti C, Kelsey K, Mc Clean M, Schantz S, Yu GP, Boffetta P, Lee YC, Hashibe M, La Vecchia C, Boccia S. Folate intake and the risk of oral cavity and pharyngeal cancer: a pooled analysis within the International Head and neck Cancer Epidemiology Consortium. Int J Cancer. 2015;136:904–14.
35. Hubbers CU, Akgul B. HPV and cancer of the oral cavity. Virulence. 2015;6:244–8.
36. Chen AC, Martin AJ, Choy B, Fernandez-Panas P, Dalziell RA, McKenzie CA, Scolyer RA, Dhillon HM, Vardy JKL, Kricker A, St George G, Chinniah N, Halliday GM, Damian DL. A phase 3 randomized trial of nicotinamide for skin cancer chemoprotection. N Engl J Med. 2015;373:1618–26.
37. Lumley CJ, Kaffenberger TM, Desale S, Tefera E, Han CJ, Rafei H, Maxwell JH. Post diagnosis aspirin use and survival in patients with head and neck cancer. Head Neck. 2018;41(5):1220–6. https://doi.org/10.1002/hed.25518.
38. Zhang X, Feng H, Li Z, Guo J, Li M. Aspirin is involved in the cell cycle arrest, apoptosis, cell migration, and invasionof oral squamous cell carcinoma. Int J Med Sci. 2018;19m12(7):E2029. https://doi.org/10.3390/ijms19072029.
39. Saka Herran C, Jane-Salas C, Estrugo Devesa A, Lopez-Lopez J. Protective effectrs of metformin, statins and anti-indflammatory drugs on head and nrck casncer: a systematic review. Oral Oncol. 2018;85:68–81.
40. Verma A, Rich LJ, Vincent-Chong VK, Seshadri M. Visualizing the effects of metformin on tumor growth, vascularity and metabolism in head and neck cancer. J Oral Pathol Med. 2018;47:484–91.
41. Kang H, Gillespie TW, Goodman M, Brodie SA, Brandes M, Ribeiro M, Ramalingam SS, Shin DM, Khuri FR, Brandes JC. Long term use of valproic acid in US veterans is associated with a reduced risk of smoking-related cases of head and neck cancer. Cancer. 2014;120:1394–400.
42. Lee SH, Nam HJ, Kang HJ, Samuels TL, Johnston N, Lim YC. Valproic acid suppresses the self-renewal and proliferation of head and neck cancer stem cells. Oncol Rep. 2015;34:2065–71.

Chapter 4
Dysphagia in Head and Neck Cancers

Lisa M. Evangelista

Introduction

In the United States, a paradigm shift in oncologic treatments reflects the changing trends of head and neck cancers. Between 1988 and 2004, there has been a 50% decrease in cancers of the larynx and hypopharynx attributed to lower rates of tobacco use. However, cancers of the oropharynx have staggeringly increased across the past few decades. The oropharynx is the most common site for cancers of the head and neck in the United States. The increase in oropharyngeal squamous cell carcinomas is directly related to the human papilloma virus (HPV). HPV-associated oropharyngeal cancers have increased by 225% from 1988 to 2004 [1]. While the survival outlook for HPV-positive cancers is more favorable than HPV-negative cancers, the burden of treatment-related toxicities on functional outcomes remains high.

Advancements in treatments for head and neck cancer have simultaneously focused on improving oncologic cure while achieving improved functional outcomes. Despite efforts to mitigate treatment toxicities that result in dysphagia, the incidence of dysphagia in patients undergoing head and neck cancer treatments continues to increase. Dysphagia may present acutely during and immediately after treatment; however, the cumulative effects of oncologic treatment can result in long-term and progressive dysphagia. The 2-year prevalence of dysphagia and pneumonia development in patients who have undergone treatment for head and neck cancers is 45.3%. Across a 10-year post-treatment period, dysphagia increased by 11.7%. Further studies have evaluated the increasing rate of dysphagia and associated complications following chemoradiation therapy for head and neck cancers.

L. M. Evangelista (✉)
Department of Otolaryngology/Head & Neck Surgery, University of California at Davis Medical Center, Sacramento, CA, USA
e-mail: evangelista@ucdavis.edu

© Springer Nature Switzerland AG 2021
R. El Assal et al. (eds.), *Early Detection and Treatment of Head & Neck Cancers*, https://doi.org/10.1007/978-3-030-69852-2_4

For patients who completed chemoradiation therapy 2–5 years and 5 or more years beyond diagnosis, dysphagia incidence increased from 14.9% to 26%, respectively. Gastrostomy tube placement increased from 2.82% to 3.32%, and the incidence of aspiration pneumonia increased from 3.13% to 6.75% for patients in the same time periods [2]. While significant efforts in treatment paradigms and protocols have been made to minimize poor swallowing outcomes, interventions aimed at reducing rates and severity of dysphagia remain a priority.

Surgical Management

The presence and severity of dysphagia following surgical intervention for head and neck cancers is largely dependent on the type, location, and extent of surgical resection performed. Traditional surgical approaches involved widely ablative surgeries that resulted in poor functional outcomes. Surgical resection and reconstruction may result in perturbations to the swallowing mechanism due to impairments in anatomic and physiologic functioning that result in dysphagia and potential aspiration.

One of the main advancements in surgical approaches for head and neck cancers is the use of transoral robotic surgery (TORS). TORS is a minimally invasive approach in head and neck cancer surgery that uses endoscopic technique for surgical resection [3]. By reducing the need for an open surgical approach such as mandibulotomy or pharyngotomy, the anatomic framework for critical swallowing structures is preserved with TORS. Furthermore, the use of TORS prior to adjuvant chemoradiation therapy may reduce the radiation dose needed when compared radiation dosing delivered in the definitive treatment setting. By limiting the necessary radiation treatment dose, radiation toxicities that result in dysphagia can be mitigated. When compared with intensity-modulated radiation therapy for the treatment of oropharyngeal cancer, rates of feeding tube placement and dependence were lower in patients treated with TORS [4]. With the advent of minimally invasive surgery, use of robotic technology, and advancements in surgical reconstruction, functional outcomes following surgical intervention for head and neck cancers are of growing importance [5].

Oral Cavity Cancers

Surgical resection and reconstruction of oral cavity cancers can render significant dysphagia in the oral preparatory, oral, and pharyngeal phases of the swallow [6]. Surgical resection of the lips, tongue, floor of mouth, alveolar processes, and hard palate can result in the following:

- Poor labial closure resulting in spillage from the mouth
- Premature spillage into the pharynx due to decreased oral containment of the bolus
- Reduced lingual mobility resulting in inefficient anterior-to-posterior transit of the bolus from the oral cavity into the pharynx

- Regurgitation of food and liquid into the nasal cavity from a hard palate defect
- Decreased hyolaryngeal excursion if muscles of the floor of mouth are resected

Oropharyngeal and Nasopharyngeal Cancers

Swallowing dysfunction following surgical resection of the oropharynx and naso-pharynx including the base of tongue, palatine tonsils, pharyngeal tonsils, and velum may include:

- Incomplete velopharyngeal closure resulting in nasal regurgitation
- Impaired pharyngeal motor response resulting in delayed swallow initiation
- Reduced pharyngeal clearance of the bolus due to impaired base of tongue retraction and pharyngeal constriction

Laryngeal and Hypopharyngeal Cancers

Swallowing dysfunction following surgical interventions for cancers of the larynx and hypopharynx are widely dependent on the extent of the surgical resection. Treatment for early-stage laryngeal cancers may not result in significant or pro-longed dysphagia. Surgical interventions for advanced stage cancers of the larynx commonly result in impairments in laryngeal closure and pharyngeal constriction. While most early-stage hypopharyngeal cancers are treated with organ-sparing modalities, advanced hypopharyngeal cancers are treated with a combination of total laryngectomy and pharyngectomy.

Partial laryngectomies, including vertical partial, supraglottic, and supracricoid laryngectomies, may result in the following physiologic impairments and dysphagia symptoms [7]:

- Reduced tongue base retraction resulting in incomplete pharyngeal clearance
- Laryngeal penetration and aspiration due to neoglottic incompetency
- Decreased hyolaryngeal excursion resulting in impaired laryngeal closure and pharyngeal clearance

Total laryngectomy, or complete removal of the larynx, may be performed for advanced stage tumors, persistent disease, or a non-functional larynx [8]. While aspiration is no longer a concern following total laryngectomy due to separation of the trachea from the esophagus, dysphagia continues to be prevalent following total laryngectomy and is experienced by 72% of patients [9]. Physiologic impairments in the swallowing mechanism include:

- Reduced tongue base retraction resulting in incomplete bolus clearance from the neopharynx
- Residue in the neopharynx due to impaired pharyngeal contractility

- Decreased pharyngeal peristalsis attributed to impaired pharyngeal sensation
- Sensation of food sticking in the throat as a result of narrowing or stricture of the neo-pharyngoesophageal segment

Radiation Therapy

Radiation therapy is a common modality used in the treatment of head and neck cancers. Whether used in the definitive or adjuvant treatment settings, patients who undergo radiation therapy may experience early and late-term swallowing complications [10]. It is well documented that there is a radiation dose-dependent relationship to organs involved in swallowing and the severity of dysphagia [11]. With the advent of intensity-modulated radiation therapy, contemporary practices in radiation oncology have aimed to preserve swallowing function by reducing radiation dose to organs at risk in comparison to conventional radiation therapy. Despite advances to reduce toxicities in radiation oncology, dysphagia continues to be a common complication in both the early and late stages of treatment [12].

Early or acute side effects of radiation therapy include xerostomia, mucositis, and dysgeusia.

- Xerostomia, or dry mouth, is the most common side effect of radiation therapy. Dryness of the oral mucosal membranes may persist during and after radiation therapy. During radiation therapy, xerostomia occurs due to atrophy or chronic inflammation of the secretory cells in the salivary glands. Long-term xerostomia may be related to radiation-induced necrosis of the salivary glands resulting in persistent oral dryness. Xerostomia may increase the risk of dental caries, oral candidiasis, and difficulties with chewing and swallowing [13].
- Mucositis is a common tissue injury resulting from radiation therapy (Fig. 4.1). Inflammation to the oral and pharyngeal mucosa may result in severe pain with swallowing. Furthermore, mucositis may result in decreased oral intake and subsequent weight loss [14].
- Dysgeusia, or taste dysfunction, may negatively impact quality of life. Taste alternations may result in decreased oral intake leading to subsequent nutritional compromise [15].
- Edema, or swelling of the tissues of the head and neck, may develop following surgery or radiation therapy (Fig. 4.2). Tissue edema can result in decreased peristalsis and contractility of the muscles involved in swallowing (Fig. 4.3).

The long-term side effects of radiation therapy may result in irreversible consequential injury to the swallowing apparatus. Fibrosis, atrophy, and vascular damage to the muscles involved in swallowing can negatively impact the safety and efficiency of swallowing. Patients with radiation-induced dysphagia may present with complaints of difficulty swallowing, the sensation of tightness of the throat, development of aspiration pneumonia, or the need for alternate methods of nutrition and hydration [16].

Fig. 4.1 Mucositis of the pharynx and larynx

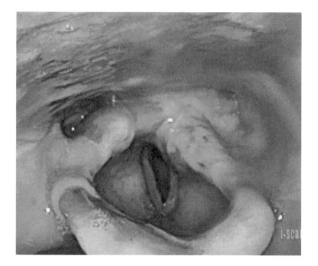

Fig. 4.2 Edema of the larynx following the completion of radiation therapy

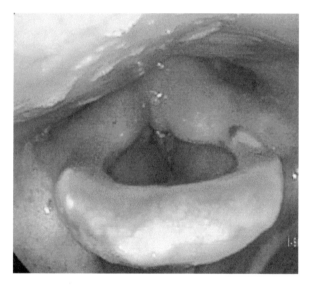

Fibrosis and denervation resulting in muscle atrophy can impact the mobility and contractility of the entire swallowing musculature resulting in the following (Figs. 4.4 and 4.5):

- Reduced oral tongue and base of tongue mobility resulting in inadequate clearance of food from the oral cavity and pharynx
- Impaired airway protection resulting in laryngeal penetration or aspiration
- Diminished pharyngeal constriction yielding incomplete clearance of food from the pharynx and hypopharynx
- Esophaeal stenosis characterized by decreased distention of the pharyngoesophageal segment

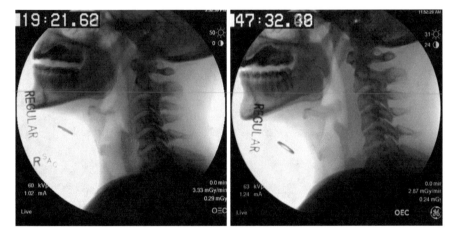

Fig. 4.3 Fluoroscopic comparison of posterior pharyngeal wall edema before and 3 months after radiation therapy

Fig. 4.4 Videofluoroscopic evidence of base of tongue atrophy

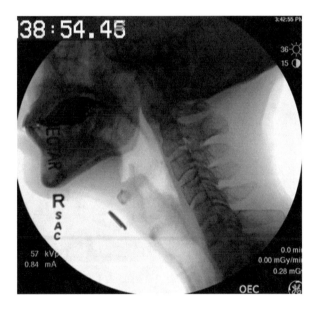

Assessment of Swallowing Disorders in Head and Neck Cancers

A comprehensive assessment of swallowing function includes an in-depth medical history, clinical oral examination, and instrumental diagnostics. Ideally, evaluation of swallowing function should be performed prior to oncologic intervention to determine a patient's baseline function [16].

Fig. 4.5 Denervation
of the larynx following
late toxicities of
radiation therapy

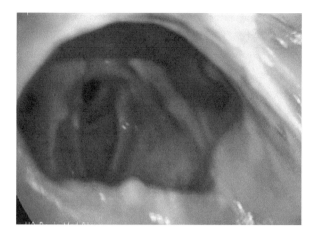

Medical History

A thorough review of the patient's medical chart should be conducted to obtain information regarding a patient's current and previous health history. Pertinent medical history may include:

- Oncologic history including tumor site and stage
- Previous or planned surgical and medical interventions for head and neck cancer(s)
- Previous or existing dysphagia
- Current oral diet, need for diet modifications, or use of alternate methods of nutrition and hydration
- Unintentional weight loss
- Pulmonary status including current or previous history of aspiration pneumonia
- Comorbidities that may negatively impact swallowing function
- Current medications

Clinical Oral Examination

The clinical examination provides information regarding the integrity and function of the oral mechanism. Evaluation of both sensory and motor functions of the oral-facial structures is necessary to determine cranial nerve and muscular pathologies that may impact deglutition.

Assessment of anatomic symmetry and integrity of the oral and facial structures at rest is first initiated. Tasks to elicit sensory and motoric function of the olfactory, trigeminal, facial, glossopharyngeal, vagus, and hypoglossal nerves should be performed (Figs. 4.6, 4.7, and 4.8). Abnormal movements such as flaccidity, spasticity,

Fig. 4.6 Lingual range
of motion

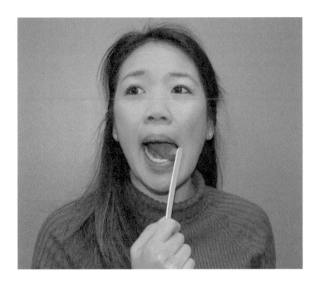

Fig. 4.7 Labial range of
motion with lip protrusion

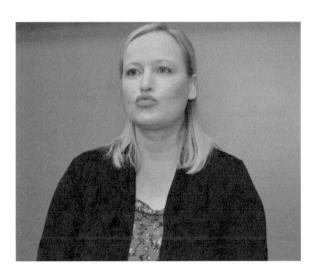

dyskinesia, fasciculation, or tremors resulting from cranial nerve pathology may contribute to dysphagia [17].

Instrumental Evaluation

The use of instrumental diagnostics allows for the structural and physiologic evaluation of the swallowing mechanism. The most common instruments used in the evaluation of swallowing with patients with head and neck cancers are the

Fig. 4.8 Labial range of motion with lip retraction

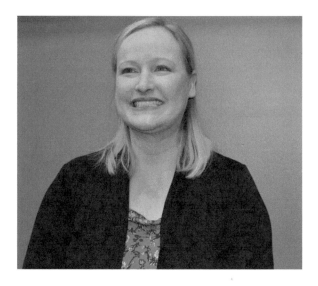

videofluoroscopic swallow study (VFSS) and fiberoptic endoscopic evaluation of swallowing (FEES).

The VFSS allows for visualization of the oral preparatory, oral, pharyngeal, and upper esophageal phases of the swallow. With the use of a radiation technique known as fluoroscopy, anatomical structures and physiologic kinematics of swallowing are visualized (Fig. 4.9). During VFSS, the patient is seated in an upright position. Barium, a radiopaque contrast, in varying consistencies and volumes is administered to evaluate the safety and efficiency of the swallow. Biomechanics in the oral cavity, larynx, pharynx, and upper esophagus can be evaluated in the lateral and anterior-posterior planes (Figs. 4.10 and 4.11) [18].

The analysis of VFSS includes evaluation of structural presentation and physiologic function of the oral cavity, larynx, pharynx, and upper esophagus. While VFSS is a widely used diagnostic method, there continues to be variability in the analysis of swallowing parameters. Over the past two decades, tools have been developed to improve the standardization and objectivity of VFSS analysis. The Penetration-Aspiration Scale, an 8-point interval scale, describes the severity of laryngeal penetration or aspiration and the patient's response to such events [19]. To quantify pharyngeal residue, the Pharyngeal Retention Scale describes volume aggregation of residue in the valleculae and pyriform sinuses following a swallow [20]. Advancements in technology have allowed for a more refined objective evaluation of swallowing biomechanics through the use of computational analysis. Objective measurements of swallowing kinematics allow for quantitative analysis on timing of swallowing gestures and displacement of structures. The use of objective measures mitigates subjective interpretation of normal and pathologic swallowing performance [21].

Fiberoptic endoscopic evaluation of swallowing provides direct visualization of the larynx and pharynx. The FEES examination begins with the insertion of the endoscope into the nasal cavity, over the velum, and into the pharynx (Fig. 4.12).

Fig. 4.9 Videofluoroscopy in radiation suite

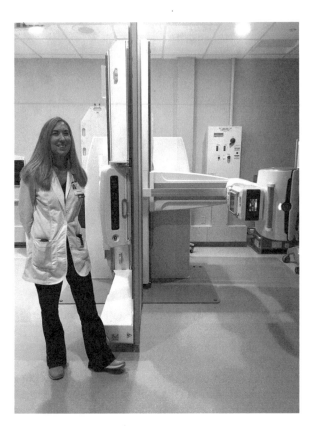

Fig. 4.10 Videofluoroscopic swallow study (lateral view)

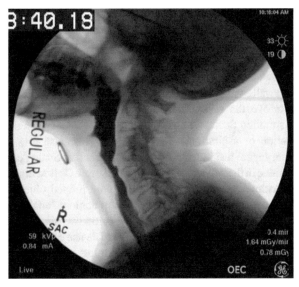

Fig. 4.11
Videofluoroscopic
swallow study
(anteroposterior view)

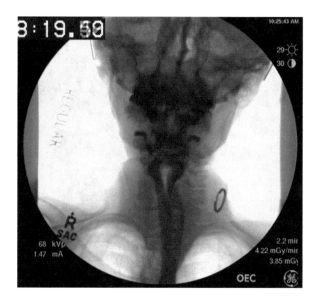

Fig. 4.12 Set-up of
fiberoptic endoscopic
evaluation of swallowing

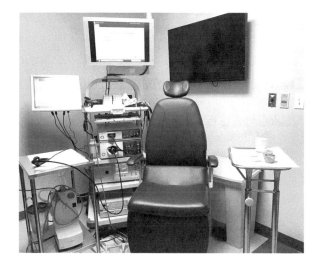

The structural integrity and mobility of the soft palate, base of tongue, oropharynx, larynx, and hypopharynx are visualized. In addition to the evaluation of the swallowing mechanism, the use of flexible endoscopy allows for appraisal of secretion management and possible laryngeal pathology [20]. With particular utility in patients who have undergone treatment for head and neck cancers, endoscopy affords thorough evaluation of post-surgical and post-radiation changes to the anatomy that may contribute to dysphagia. To evaluate the swallowing mechanism

Fig. 4.13 Visualization of vallecular residue during fiberoptic endoscopic evaluation of swallowing

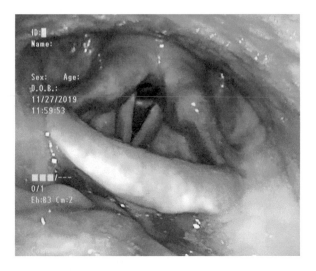

during FEES, various food and liquid consistencies can be dyed white or blue for improved visualization under endoscopy. Laryngeal penetration, aspiration, and pharyngeal residue can be observed (Fig. 4.13). In addition, the efficacy of compensatory strategies and maneuvers to improve swallowing safety and efficiency can be evaluated under visualization [22].

Treatment of Dysphagia in Head and Neck Cancers

Rehabilitation of dysphagia following the treatment of head and neck cancers is multifactorial. Treatment may focus on dietary modifications, use of compensatory strategies or maneuvers during swallowing, and exercises to improve swallow function.

Diet Allocation

Following oncologic intervention, patients may require changes to their diet to improve the safety and efficiency of swallowing. Depending on the severity of dysphagia, the functionality of the swallow may be impaired resulting in the need for changes in diet consistency, behavioral strategies, or alternate methods of nutrition and hydration to avoid nutritional deficiencies and pulmonary compromise [23]. Appropriate diet allocation can improve duration of meal times, nutritional status, and quality of life [24]. Examples of diet modifications include:

- Avoidance of solid consistencies due to impaired oral manipulation
- Thickened liquids for impaired airway protection

- Thin liquids if pharyngeal contractility is impaired
- Alternate methods of nutrition and hydration (e.g., nasogastric feeding tube or percutaneous endoscopic gastrostomy feeding tube)

Compensatory Strategies and Maneuvers

The use of compensatory strategies or postural maneuvers during swallowing may be needed to improve bolus flow or airway protection. In patients who have undergone surgical resection for head and neck cancers, appropriate postural changes have been shown to eliminate aspiration in 81% of patients [25]. The use of compensatory strategy or postural maneuver to improve impaired biomechanics should be evaluated under fluoroscopic visualization (VFSS) or endoscopic visualization (FEES) to determine its efficacy. Compensatory strategies, swallowing maneuvers, or postural changes to improve swallowing efficiency and safety may include:

Postural Changes

- *Chin tuck posture* (*chin-down posture or neck flexion*; Fig. 4.14): As the chin is posteriorly shifted, the tongue base and epiglottis more closely appose the posterior pharyngeal wall, while the vallecular space is widened. This posture may increase vallecular capacity and provide more time for swallow initiation, as well as improve extent and duration of laryngeal vestibule closure.

Fig. 4.14 Chin tuck maneuver

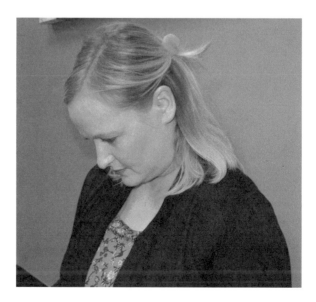

Fig. 4.15 Lateral head tilt

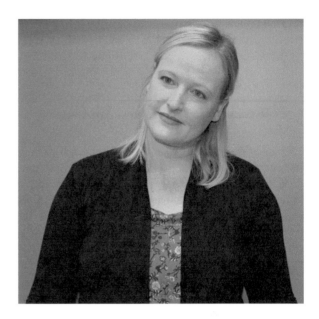

Fig. 4.16 Head rotation

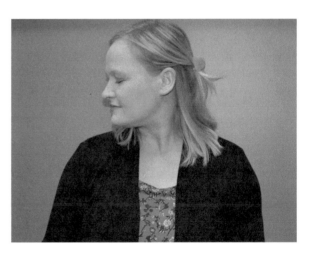

- *Lateral head tilt* (Fig. 4.15): Tilting the head laterally to the stronger side can improve pharyngeal clearance by diverting bolus flow from the weak side. By capitalizing on gravity, improved bolus flow can be achieved in the setting of unilateral oral and pharyngeal weakness.
- *Head rotation* (Fig. 4.16): A rotational head turn toward the weak side of the pharynx and larynx can divert a bolus away from the side of rotation. With the bolus lateralized from the weak side, improved bolus clearance can be achieved. This maneuver is also beneficial to promote airway closure in unilateral vocal fold immobility.

Compensatory Strategies

- *Effortful swallow*: The effortful swallow maneuver aims to increase tongue base retraction and pharyngeal pressure to improve bolus clearance through the pharynx and upper esophageal sphincter. Patients who experience pharyngeal residue may be asked to "squeeze hard" while they swallow to improve bolus clearance.
- *Supraglottic swallow maneuver*: The supraglottic swallow maneuver was designed to impose voluntary airway protection for patients who experience aspiration before or during the swallow. The patient is asked to hold their breath, swallow with a breath hold, and cough following the swallow to expel material that may have entered the laryngeal vestibule.
- *Super supraglottic swallow maneuver*: Designed to also improve airway protection similar to the supraglottic swallow, the super supraglottic maneuver provides further airway protection by engaging movement of the arytenoid cartilages to the petiole of the epiglottis and closure of the false vocal folds. The patient is asked to hold their breath, bear down, swallow, and cough after the swallow to expel material from the airway.
- *Mendelsohn maneuver*: The Mendelsohn maneuver aims to prolong laryngeal excursion and opening of the upper esophageal sphincter during swallowing. The patient is asked to hold their larynx in an elevated position using the muscles of the neck.

Swallowing Exercises

Changes to the swallowing musculature resulting in dysphagia following head and neck cancer treatment can occur because of muscle edema, fibrosis, and atrophy. Swallowing exercises aim to improve range of motion and strength. Weight-loaded exercises have shown to recover strength in weakened swallowing musculature. Prophylactic swallowing exercises, or swallowing exercises prescribed prior to the onset of dysfunction, have been shown to facilitate maintenance of oropharyngeal muscle function during radiation therapy [26].

Range of Motion and Strengthening Exercises

- Passive and active stretches for the jaw to improve interincisal opening of the mouth (Figs. 4.17 and 4.18)
- Tongue stretches and resistance exercises to increase lingual mobility and strength
- Effortful swallow to strengthen tongue base retraction and pharyngeal constriction

Fig. 4.17 Active jaw range of motion

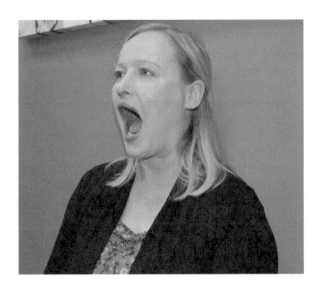

Fig. 4.18 Passive jaw range of motion

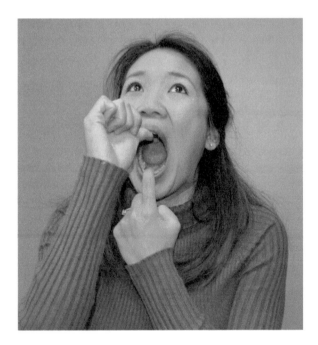

- Masako maneuver to increase base of tongue to posterior pharyngeal wall apposition
- Shaker exercise to improve duration and distention of upper esophageal sphincter opening
- Mendelsohn maneuver to promote laryngeal excursion and upper esophageal sphincter opening

Multidisciplinary Team

The treatment of head and neck cancers requires long-term surveillance from a variety of healthcare specialists. With the support of a multidisciplinary team, patients undergoing head and neck cancer treatment have a greater understanding of their diagnosis, the early and long-term impact of oncologic therapies, and the psychosocial and emotional manifestations of treatment.

The involvement of a multidisciplinary team begins at the initiation of care. From the time of diagnosis, a patient meets with members of the head and neck cancer team including the head and neck cancer surgeon, medical oncologist, radiation oncologist, dentist, speech-language pathologist, dietician, and nursing staff. Prior to the initiation of head and neck cancer treatment, these members are involved in treatment planning, identifying risk factors for treatment-related complications, and establishing psychosocial supports. During treatment, communication among the multidisciplinary team focuses on a patient's current status, progress throughout treatment, and need for treatment modifications to mitigate adverse outcomes. At the completion of head and neck cancer treatment, the multidisciplinary team is involved in disease surveillance, management of treatment-related side effects, and supportive care in quality-of-life issues [27].

With particular interest in dysphagia, the speech-language pathologist is an integral member of the head and neck cancer team. Speech-language pathologists provide assessment of swallowing function prior to surgical or medical interventions to identify existing dysphagia and risk factors for worsening of swallow function through treatment. In the pre-treatment phase, the speech-language pathologist is able to counsel a patient on the functional deficits that may result from oncologic treatment. Prophylactic swallowing exercises, compensatory strategies or maneuvers to improve swallow function, and dietary modifications may be provided in the early stages of oncologic treatment. During treatment, the speech-language pathologist provides ongoing assessment of swallowing function and recommendations for dietary modifications and compensatory strategies. Following oncologic treatment, the speech-language pathologist evaluates acute and long-term dysphagia and provides rehabilitation to improve functional outcomes.

Conclusion

Dysphagia remains a significant morbidity following head and neck cancer treatments. Impairments in swallowing function can occur along the continuum of treatment presenting in both the early and late stages of recovery. Continued advancements in surgical and medical interventions that aim to improve swallowing outcomes are promising. Speech-language pathologists are integral members of head and neck cancer treatment teams who provide specialized care to evaluate and diagnose dysphagia. With comprehensive diagnostics and early treatment interventions, preservation of swallowing function, limited alterations in diet, and maintenance of quality of life can be achieved.

References

1. Chaturvedi AK, Engels EA, Pfeiffer RM, Hernandez BY, Xiao W, Kim E, Biang B, Goodman MT, Sibug-Saber M, Cozen W, Liu L, Lynch CF, Wentzensen N, Jordan RC, Altekruse S, Anderson WF, Rosenberg RS, Gillison ML. Human papillomavirus and rising oropharyngeal cancer incidence in the United States. J Clin Oncol. 2011;29(32):4294–301.
2. Aylward A, Abdelaziz S, Hunt JP, Buchmann LO, Cannon RB, Rowe K, Snyder J, Wan Y, Deshmukj V, Newman M, Fraser A, Smith K, Herget K, Lloyd S, Hitchcock Y, Hashibe M, Monroe MM. Rates of dysphagia related diagnoses in long-term survivors of head and neck cancers. Otolaryngol Head Neck Surg. 2019;161(4):643–51. https://doi.org/10.1177/0194599819850154.
3. Iseli TA, Kulbersh BD, Iseli CE, Carroll WR, Rosenthal EL, Magnuson JS. Functional outcomes after transoral robotic surgery for head and neck cancer. Otolaryngol Head Neck Surg. 2009;141(2):166–71.
4. Hutcheson KA, Holsinger FC, Kupferman ME, Lewin JS. Functional outcomes after TORS for oropharyngeal cancer: a systematic review. Eur Arch Otorhinolaryngol. 2014;272(2):463–71.
5. Park YM, Kim WS, Byeon HK, Lee SY, Kim SH. Oncological and functional outcomes of transoral robotic surgery for oropharyngeal cancer. Br J Oral Maxillofac Surg. 2013;51(5):408–12.
6. Hirano M, Matsuoka H, Kuroiwa Y, Sato K, Tanaka S, Yoshida T. Dysphagia following various degrees of surgical resection for oral cancer. Ann Otol Rhinol Laryngol. 1992;101(2):138–41.
7. Lewin JS, Hutcheson KA, Barringer DA, May AH, Roberts DB, Holsinger FC, Diaz EM Jr. Functional analysis of swallowing outcomes after supracricoid partial laryngectomy. Head Neck. 2008;30(5):559–66.
8. Sullivan PA, Hartig GK. Dysphagia after total laryngectomy. Curr Opin Otolaryngol Head Neck Surg. 2001;9(3):139–46.
9. Maclean J, Cotton S, Perry A. Dysphagia following a total laryngectomy: the effect on quality of life, functioning, and psychological well-being. Dysphagia. 2009;24(3):314–21.
10. Kronenberger MB, Meyers AD. Dysphagia following head and neck cancer surgery. Dysphagia. 1994;9(4):236–44.
11. Rancati T, Schwarz M, Allen AM, Feng F, Popovtzer A, Mittal B, Eisbruch A. Radiation dose–volume effects in the larynx and pharynx. Int J Radiat Oncol Biol Phys. 2010;76(3):S64–9.
12. Platteaux N, Dirix P, Dejaeger E, Nuyts S. Dysphagia in head and neck cancer patients treated with chemoradiotherapy. Dysphagia. 2010;25(2):139–52.
13. Guchelaar HJ, Vermes A, Meerwaldt JH. Radiation-induced xerostomia: pathophysiology, clinical course and supportive treatment. Support Care Cancer. 1997;5(4):281–8.
14. Maria OM, Eliopoulos N, Muanza T. Radiation-induced oral mucositis. Front Oncol. 2017;7:89.
15. Deshpande TS, Blanchard P, Wang L, Foote RL, Zhang X, Frank SJ. Radiation-related alterations of taste function in patients with head and neck cancer: a systematic review. Curr Treat Options in Oncol. 2018;19(12):72.
16. Murphy, B. A., & Gilbert, J. (2009). Dysphagia in head and neck cancer patients treated with radiation: assessment, sequelae, and rehabilitation. In Seminars in radiation oncology (19, 1, pp. 35–42). Philadelphia: WB Saunders.
17. Sonies BC, Weiffenbach J, Atkinson JC, Brahim J, Macynski A, Fox PC. Clinical examination of motor and sensory functions of the adult oral cavity. Dysphagia. 1987;1(4):178–86.
18. Palmer JB, Kuhlemeier KV, Tippett DC, Lynch C. A protocol for the videofluorographic swallowing study. Dysphagia. 1993;8(3):209–14.
19. Rosenbek JC, Robbins JA, Roecker EB, Coyle JL, Wood JL. A penetration-aspiration scale. Dysphagia. 1996;11(2):93–8.
20. Eisenhuber E, Schima W, Schober E, Pokieser P, Stadler A, Scharitzer M, Oschatz E. Videofluoroscopic assessment of patients with dysphagia: pharyngeal retention is a predictive factor for aspiration. Am J Roentgenol. 2002;178(2):393–8.

21. Kendall KA, McKenzie S, Leonard RJ, Gonçalves MI, Walker A. Timing of events in normal swallowing: a videofluoroscopic study. Dysphagia. 2000;15(2):74–83.
22. Langmore SE, Kenneth SM, Olsen N. Fiberoptic endoscopic examination of swallowing safety: a new procedure. Dysphagia. 1988;2(4):216–9.
23. Wu CH, Ko JY, Hsiao TY, Hsu MM. Dysphagia after radiotherapy: endoscopic examination of swallowing in patients with nasopharyngeal carcinoma. Ann Otol Rhinol Laryngol. 2000;109(3):320–5.
24. Garcia JM, Chambers E IV. Managing dysphagia through diet modifications. Am J Nurs. 2010;110(11):26–33.
25. Logemann JA, et al. Effects of postural change on aspiration in head and neck surgical patients. Otolaryngol Head Neck Surg. 1994;110(2):222–7.
26. Carnaby-Mann G, et al. "Pharyngocise": randomized controlled trial of preventative exercises to maintain muscle structure and swallowing function during head-and-neck chemoradiotherapy. Int J Radiat Oncol Biol Phys. 2012;83(1):210–9.
27. Kelly SL, et al. Multidisciplinary clinic care improves adherence to best practice in head and neck cancer. Am J Otolaryngol. 2013;34(1):57–60.

Chapter 5
The Mutational Landscape of Head and Neck Squamous Cell Carcinoma: Opportunities for Detection and Monitoring Via Analysis of Circulating Tumor DNA

Kelechi Nwachuku, Daniel E. Johnson, and Jennifer R. Grandis

Introduction

HNSCC results, at least in part, from an accumulation of genetic alterations in onco-genic signaling pathways leading to aberrant growth and survival [3]. Our under-standing of the mutational landscape of HNSCC has been informed by a series of genomic studies carried out in the past decade. Elucidation of the key genetic altera-tions in HNSCC is likely to guide the use of targeted therapies aimed at altering the outcome of this lethal malignancy.

Even with an increased understanding of the genetic underpinnings of HNSCC, most cases of HNSCC are still diagnosed at an advanced stage, which impacts prog-nosis and survival [5]. Traditional screening methods rely on physical examination, which often requires access to experienced clinicians and specialized equipment. Understanding the mutational landscape of HNSCC is likely to inform the use of noninvasive techniques such as assessment of circulating tumor DNA (ctDNA) in the blood and/or saliva [5]. In HNSCC patients, both plasma and saliva contain detectable amounts of circulating DNA fragments encompassing tumor mutations; these fragments are detectable at the early stages of cancer, which may allow for early detection of HNSCC in high-risk individuals [5]. In addition, the use of non-invasive approaches that are sufficiently sensitive and specific for HNSCC may be used to monitor HNSCC patients following curative therapy [6]. This chapter will summarize our current understanding of the mutational landscape of HNSCC and

K. Nwachuku
School of Medicine, University of California at San Francisco, San Francisco, CA, USA

D. E. Johnson · J. R. Grandis (✉)
Department of Otolaryngology – Head and Neck Surgery, University of California at San Francisco, San Francisco, CA, USA
e-mail: Jennifer.Grandis@ucsf.edu

© Springer Nature Switzerland AG 2021
R. El Assal et al. (eds.), *Early Detection and Treatment of Head & Neck Cancers*, https://doi.org/10.1007/978-3-030-69852-2_5

will draw on that understanding to introduce ctDNA as a potential tool for use in the early detection and monitoring of HNSCC.

Mutational Landscape of HNSCC

The mutational landscape of HNSCC has been elucidated by a series of genomic sequencing studies [1, 7–9]. Mutations either confer a gain of function (e.g., driver mutations) or a loss of function, or have no apparent functional impact (known as silent mutations). In this chapter, we will restrict our discussion to gene mutations that are known to change the function of the protein encoded by the gene in question. The most common functional alterations include mutations in tumor suppressor genes such as *TP53*, *CDKN2A*, *NOTCH1*, and *PTEN* as well as oncogenic alterations (mutation or amplification) in *PIK3CA*, *CCND1*, *EGFR*, and *HRAS* (Table 5.1).

Deletion and/or mutation of *TP53* represent the most frequent somatic genomic alterations in HNSCC, occurring in 72% of HNSCC tumors [7]. HNSCC-associated *TP53* mutations alter p53 functional activity, including the sensing and repairing of DNA damage, as well as induction of apoptosis in response to extensive DNA damage. *TP53* mutations have been suggested to play an early role in HNSCC carcinogenesis [10]. Alterations in the tumor suppressor gene *CDKN2A* have similarly been implicated in HNSCC. *CDKN2A* encodes the cyclin-dependent kinase inhibitor p16/INK4A, which acts to block cell cycle progression from G1 to S phase [11]. *CDKN2A* can be downregulated or inactivated by various mechanisms in HNSCC, including hypomethylation of the promoter region, gene deletion, copy number loss, and mutation. The dysregulation of cyclin activity conferred by *CDKN2A* inactivation promotes tumorigenesis. Amplification of *CCND1* (encoding cyclin D1) leads to overexpression of this oncogene and augments the impact of *CDKN2A* loss of function in a significant subset of HNSCC patients [3]. Another proposed tumor suppressor gene frequently mutated in HNSCC is *NOTCH1*, which is mutated in 15% of tumors [9, 12]. The NOTCH1 protein is a transmembrane receptor that is known to play a variety of roles in cell growth and differentiation.

The *EGFR* gene has been implicated as a proto-oncogene in the development of HNSCC. *EGFR* encodes the epidermal growth factor receptor (EGFR), a cell surface member of the HER family of receptor tyrosine kinases. Upon activation through ligand binding, EGFR signals through the PI3K/AKT, RAS/RAF/MEK/ERK, and PLC/PKC pathways to promote cellular proliferation and survival, as well as invasion and metastasis [13]. EGFR is aberrantly overexpressed on the vast majority of HNSCC cells and tumors, often the result of *EGFR* gene amplification, and has been demonstrated as a key driver of oncogenesis in HNSCC [13].

Alterations in genes encoding intracellular signaling proteins downstream of EGFR have also been identified in HNSCC, particularly *PIK3CA* and *HRAS* [9].

Table 5.1 Genetic Alterations of Head and Neck Squamous Cell Carcinoma

Gene	Function	Predominating types of genetic alterations[a]	Frequency of genetic alterations in HNSCC (%)[b]	Functional impact of alterations
Genetic alterations predominant in HPV− tumors				
TP53 (*Tumor protein p53*)	Encodes the tumor suppressor protein p53	LOF, DEL	HPV+: 2% HPV−: 84%	Loss of tumor suppression
CDKN2A (*Cyclin-dependent kinase inhibitor 2A*)	Encodes the tumor suppressor proteins p16 (INK4A) and p14 (ARF)	LOF, DEL	HPV+: 0% HPV−: 57%	Loss of tumor suppression
NOTCH1 (*Notch homolog 1*)	Encodes the receptor protein Notch 1, involved Notch signaling pathway known to serve as a tumor suppressor in HNSCC	LOF	HPV+: 17% HPV−: 26%	Loss of tumor suppression
PTEN (*Phosphatase and tensin homolog*)	Encodes the tumor suppressor PTEN	DEL, LOF	HPV+: 6% HPV−: 12%	Loss of tumor suppression
CCND1 (*Cyclin D1*)	Encodes cyclin D1, which complexes with either CDK4 or CDK6	AMP	HPV+: 3% HPV−: 31%	Dysregulation of cell cycle contributing to tumorigenesis
EGFR (*Epidermal growth factor receptor*)	Encodes epidermal growth factor receptor which mediates cell proliferation and survival	AMP	HPV+: 6% HPV−: 15%	Promotes tumor cell proliferation and survival
HRAS (*HRas proto-oncogene, GTPase*)	Encodes H-Ras, a cell division regulator instructing growth and division	GOF	HPV+: 0% HPV−: 5%	Unfettered cell growth and division
FBXW7 (*F-box And WD repeat domain-containing 7*)	Encodes a component of a ubiquitin protein ligase complex	LOF	HPV+: 3% HPV−: 7%	Dysregulation of proteasome-mediated protein degradation of proteins including cyclin E
CASP8 (*Caspase 8*)	Encodes a central protease (caspase-8) in the extrinsic apoptosis pathway	LOF	HPV+: 3% HPV−: 11%	Loss of apoptosis and tumor suppression
FGFR1 (*Fibroblast growth factor receptor 1*)	Encodes fibroblast growth factor receptor 1 which mediates cellular migration, differentiation, proliferation, and survival	AMP	HPV+: 0% HPV−: 10%	Promotion of tumor survival and growth

(continued)

Table 5.1 (continued)

Gene	Function	Predominating types of genetic alterations[a]	Frequency of genetic alterations in HNSCC (%)[b]	Functional impact of alterations
TGFBR2 (Transforming growth factor beta receptor 2)	Encodes TGF-β receptor type 2	LOF	HPV+: 6% HPV−: 6%	Promotion of tumor growth and proliferation
FAT1 (FAT atypical cadherin 1)	Encodes the tumor suppressor protein FAT 1	LOF, DEL	HPV+: 3% HPV−: 32%	Loss of tumor suppression
AJUBA (Ajuba LIM protein)	A WNT pathway gene regulating mitosis, cell-cell adhesion, and gene transcription	LOF	HPV+: 0% HPV−: 7%	Dysregulation of Wnt/β-catenin signaling and cellular differentiation
NSD1 (Nuclear receptor–binding SET domain protein 1)	Encodes histone methyltransferase	LOF	HPV+: 8% HPV−: 12%	Alters chromatin structure, leading to changes in gene expression patterns
KMT2D (N-methyltransferase 2D)	Encodes histone methyltransferase	LOF	HPV+: 17% HPV−: 18%	Alters chromatin structure, leading to changes in gene expression patterns
FHIT (Fragile histidine triad diadenosine triphosphatase)	Encodes a P1-P3-bis(5′-adenosyl) triphosphate hydrolase involved in the metabolism of purines and tumor suppression	DEL	HPV+: 0% HPV−: 3%	Loss of tumor suppressor
CUL3 (Cullin-3)	Encodes cullin-3, anoxidative stress pathway protein	DEL	HPV+: 3% HPV−: 6%	Oxidative damage
KEAP1 (Kelch-like ECH-associated protein 1)	Encodes KEAP1, an oxidative stress pathway protein	LOF	HPV+: 0% HPV−: 5%	Oxidative damage
NFE2L2 (Nuclear factor, erythroid 2 Like 2)	Encodes NRF2, an oxidative stress pathway protein	AMP, GOF	HPV+: 0% HPV−: 14%	Oxidative damage
Genetic alterations predominant in HPV+ tumors				
PIK3CA (Phosphatidylinositol-4,5-bisphosphate 3-kinase catalytic subunit alpha)	Encodes p110 alpha protein, the catalytic subunit of enzyme PI3K involved in cell proliferation, migration and survival	AMP, GOF	HPV+: 56% HPV−: 34%	Promotes tumor cell proliferation and survival
HPVE6/7 (Human papillomavirus, E6 and E7)	Viral oncogenes encoding E6 and E7 that deactivate p53 and pRb, respectively	(Viral Oncogene)	HPV+: 100% HPV−: 0%	Loss of tumor suppression

Gene	Function	Mutation type	Frequency	Effect
RB1 (RB transcriptional corepressor 1)	Encodes RB tumor suppressor	LOF	HPV+: 6% HPV−: 4%	Loss of tumor suppression
BRCA1/2 (Breast cancer type 1 and 2 susceptibility protein)	Encode tumor suppressor proteins	LOF	HPV+: 3% HPV−: 3% (BRCA1) 4% (BRCA2)	Loss of tumor suppression
HLA-A/B (Major histocompatibility complex, class I, A and B)	Encode human leukocyte antigen (HLA) complexes helping body to distinguish self-antigen from foreign antigens	LOF	HPV+: 11% HPV−: 7%	May render immune system less capable of staving off cancer
ATM (ATM serine/threonine kinase)	Encodes DNA repair protein ATM	DEL	HPV+: 8% HPV−: 5%	DNA instability promoting carcinogenesis
TP63 (Tumor protein p63)	Regulates cell proliferation, differentiation, adhesion, and survival	AMP	HPV+: 28% HPV−: 19%	Contributes to cell invasion and migration
STAT1 (Signal transducer and activator of transcription 1)	Encodes the transcription factor STAT1 that mediates immune response to IFNs	AMP	HPV+: 6% HPV−: 5%	Possible loss of STAT1 mediated immune response promotes carcinogenesis
SOX2 (Sex-determining region Y-box 2)	Encodes transcription factor that maintains pluripotency in embryonic and neuro stem cells	AMP	HPV+: 28% HPV−: 21%	Promotion of tumor growth and proliferation
TRAF3 (TNF receptor–associated factor 3)	Mediates signal transduction from TNF receptor superfamily	LOF	HPV+: 22% HPV−: 1%	Likely loss of TRAF3-mediated immune response promotes carcinogenesis
CYLD (CYLD lysine 63 deubiquitinase)	Encodes a deubiquitinating enzyme that regulates NF-kB	LOF	HPV+: 11% HPV−: 3%	Dysregulation of apoptosis
DDX3X (DEAD-box helicase 3 X-linked)	Encodes the RNA helicase DDX3X	DEL	HPV+: 3% HPV−: 5%	Likely dysregulation of DNA translation and cell cycle[85]
E2F1 (E2F transcription factor 1)	Encodes the tumor suppressor protein E2F	AMP	HPV+: 19% HPV−: 2%	Loss of tumor suppression
JAK2 (Janus kinase 2)	Encodes the non-receptor tyrosine kinase JAK2, mediating cytokine receptor signaling	AMP	HPV+: 6% HPV−: 7%	Promotes tumor cell proliferation and survival

[a]LOF Loss of Function Mutation, DEL Deletion, AMP Amplification, GOF Gain of Function Mutation

[b]Frequency of mutations were taken from the analysis of the TCGA dataset which profiled 279 head and neck squamous cell carcinomas

PIK3CA encodes the p110α catalytic subunit of phosphoinositide 3-kinase (PI3K) which is important in cell proliferation, migration, and survival. *PIK3CA* has been shown to be both mutated and amplified in HNSCC and these alterations are associated with decreased survival of HNSCC patients [14, 15]. The PI3K signaling pathway is negatively regulated by phosphatase and tensin homolog (PTEN), a tumor suppressor. Mutations or epigenetic modifications of the *PTEN* gene resulting in loss of PTEN function or expression are common in HNSCC [16]. Activating mutations in *HRAS,* an oncogene, have been observed in 6% of HNSCC tumors [7]. However, activating mutations in *KRAS*, which have a high incidence in other cancers, are not found in HNSCC [7].

Several less-well-characterized genes have also been found to be frequently mutated in HNSCC, including *FBXW7, CASP8, FGF/FGFR, HLA-A/B, TGFBR2, FAT1, AJUBA, NSD1*, and *KMT2D* (Table 5.1). *FBXW7, or F-Box and WD Repeat Domain Containing 7*, is a tumor suppressor gene encoding a component of the ubiquitin protein ligase complex [14]. Interestingly, the complex containing FBXW7 is known to target NOTCH1 for proteolytic degradation. Mutations in FBXW7 abrogate this process. *CASP8* encodes a central protease (caspase-8) in the extrinsic apoptosis pathway and mutations in this gene occur in 9% of HNSCC tumors [7]. HNSCC-associated *CASP8* mutations have been shown to inhibit death receptor-mediated apoptosis and promote the activation of NF-κB, leading to augmentation of invasion, migration, and tumor growth [17, 18]. *CASP8* mutations have also been reported to co-occur with *HRAS* mutations in HNSCC tumors [19]. The fibroblast growth factor and receptor (FGF/FGFR) signaling pathway plays a key role in regulating cell functions such as migration, differentiation, proliferation, and suppression of apoptosis. Alteration of the *FGFR1* gene has been identified as a possible driver in a low-risk HNSCC patient (young, HPV-negative patient who did not smoke or drink). Notably, low-risk HNSCC patients are thought to have a distinct mutational landscape from high-risk patients [20]. Mutations in the immune surveillance/recognition pathway also occur in HNSCC, particularly in the *HLA-A/B* and *transforming growth factor beta receptor 2* (TGFBR2) genes, emphasizing the important role of the immune system in HNSCC carcinogenesis. Genes involved in the WNT signaling pathway, particularly *FAT1* and *AJUBA*, have also been implicated in HNSCC. *FAT1* (or *FAT atypical cadherin 1)* is a tumor suppressive gene that is altered in 29% of HNSCC tumors [7]. FAT1 protein normally acts to inhibit the nuclear localization of beta-catenin that is associated with WNT signaling. Mutations in FAT1 lead to hyperactive WNT signaling and promote tumorigenesis in HNSCC. AJUBA also acts as a negative regulator of WNT signaling, with HNSCC-associated mutations in this protein expected to increase oncogenic WNT signaling [21]. Other commonly mutated genes in HNSCC include *Nuclear receptor–binding SET domain protein* (NSD1*)* and *N-methyltransferase 2D* (KMT2D), which encode histone methyltransferases. Mutations in these genes confer alterations in chromatin structure, leading to changes in gene expression patterns that promote oncogenesis [22].

Comparison of Mutational Landscape of HPV-Positive and HPV-Negative HNSCC

The majority of HNSCC cases diagnosed in the United States and worldwide are tobacco-associated HPV-negative (HPV−) cancers. However, the incidence of HPV-driven (HPV+) HNSCC (particularly of the oropharynx) is rising, with increasing numbers of HPV+ HNSCC cases newly diagnosed each year throughout the world [23]. HPV+ HNSCC tumors typically exhibit better response to chemoradiation and HPV+ patients have a better overall prognosis. Notably, HPV+ and HPV− HNSCC exhibit differences in their mutational landscapes, which may provide important clues for understanding the better response and prognosis seen in HPV+ disease. Genetic alterations of *TP53* occur with a prevalence of 84% in HPV− HNSCC, but are rarely observed in HPV+ HNSCC [7]. Instead, loss of p53 expression in HPV+ HNSCC is driven by the HPV E6 oncoprotein, which promotes proteasomal degradation of the p53 protein. Similarly, the HPV E7 protein promotes proteasomal degradation and loss of the retinoblastoma (RB) protein. Of note, while HPV− HNSCC mutational signatures are characterized by nucleotide transitions of both purines (A↔G) and pyrimidines (C↔T), HPV+ HNSCC have a predominance of cytosine-to-thymidine (C > T) mutations at TpC sites [7, 24, 25]. This is due to viral induction of the apolipoprotein B mRNA editing enzyme, catalytic polypeptide-like (APOBEC) family of enzymes, which results in increased levels of cytosine deaminase-mediated mutagenesis [25]. Moreover, APOBEC has been implicated in producing the oncogenic E542K (c.1624G > A) and E545K (c.1633G > A) canonical mutations in *PIK3CA*. This is notable, as *PIK3CA* mutation appears to be more common in HPV+ HNSCC [26]. Although both HPV+ and HPV− HNSCC are driven by loss of p53 expression (via E6 or genetic deletion) or function (via mutation) and loss of RB expression (via E7) or function (via *CDKN2A* alterations), the mechanisms responsible are entirely distinct [23].

HPV+ HNSCC tumors have also been found to have enrichment of alterations in genes associated with DNA repair pathways (*BRCA1/2*, *ATM*, and Fanconi anemia genes); JAK/STAT signaling (*Janus Kinase 1/2* and *STAT1*); FGF signaling (*FGFR2*, *FGFR3* and *FGFR4*); as well as *PIK3CA*, *KRAS*, *E2F1*, *HLA-A/B*, *KMT2C*, *TRAF3*, *CYLD*, and *DDX3X* (Table 5.1) [27–29]. Deletion or truncation mutations of *TRAF3* are found in 22% of HPV+ tumors and truncating or missense mutations of *CYLD* are found in 11%. Mutations in these genes result in constitutive activation of the NF-κB signaling pathway [30]. Studies suggest that over half of all oropharyngeal squamous cell carcinomas currently diagnosed in the United States are HPV+, with epigenetic modifications distinct from HPV− oropharyngeal tumors, including viral and host methylation and chromatin modifications [31]. Increased alterations in the DNA damage response pathway in HPV+ HNSCCs has been suggested to account for the increased chemosensitivity and radiosensitivity of HPV+ cases along with the increased overall survival.

Although prior smaller studies of HPV+ tumors suggested an overall lower mutational burden compared to HPV− tumors, in actuality it is comparable (14.4 somatic exonic mutations in targeted cancer-associated genes compared to 15.2) confirmed by TCGA data analysis [27, 32]. In addition to differences in *TP53* alterations, HPV− tumors exhibit a higher prevalence of alterations in oxidative stress pathway genes (*KEAP1–CUL3–NFE2L2*), inactivation of *CDKN2A*, and amplification of *CCND1*, *genes encoding RTKs*, and the TERT promoter [2, 8, 10, 33]. HPV− tumors also have a high burden of focal EGFR amplifications which are not found in HPV+ tumors [2, 7, 27]. Of note, loss-of-function mutations of *FAT1* are uncommon in HPV+ HNSCC, but prevalent in HPV− HNSCC: 3% and 32% respectively [7, 34].

Alterations Associated with Early-Stage HNSCC

HNSCC is thought to arise through a progression of well-defined histopathological and clinical stages. Moreover, each stage is accompanied by specific genetic alterations (Fig. 5.1) [35]. This progression spans from benign hyperplasia, to dysplasia, to carcinoma in situ (CIS), and lastly, invasive carcinoma, that is, HNSCC. When stratified by HPV status, the genetic alterations in early-stage HNSCC tumors are different from those found in late-stage tumors. The earliest stage of HPV-associated tumors is characterized by HPV infection of crypt epithelium leading to expression of the viral oncogenes *E6* and *E7* [24]. The inactivation of p53 and RB by these oncogenes disrupts cell cycle regulation of the infected cells, which is considered to be the inception of HPV-induced carcinogenesis [36, 37]. The exact driver mutations that mediate HPV+ HNSCC remain largely unknown [38]. In fact, dysplastic lesions are seldom found in tonsils, where HPV-driven HNSCC most often develops [38]. Activation of the PI3K pathway by mutation and/or amplification of the *PIK3CA* oncogene is relatively common in HPV+ HNSCC, occurring in 50–60% of tumors [38]. HPV-infection is followed by aberrant differential of cells in the basal layer and gain of *E2F Transcription Factor 1* (*E2F1*) which often occurs with dysplasia [24]. CIS then follows and is associated with inactivating mutations or deletions of *TRAF3*, fragile histidine triad gene (*FHIT*), and *PTEN* [24, 36]. Lastly, aberrant cells invade through the basement membrane (cancer transformation), which is often accompanied by gain of *TP63*, *Sex Determining Region Y-Box 2* (*SOX2*), and *PIK3CA* [24, 36, 39].

Tobacco and alcohol use leads to DNA damage and genomic alterations that promote development of HPV− tumors (Fig. 5.1). The first stage in the progression to HNSCC is hyperplasia which often is accompanied by the loss of chromosome 9p21—the location of *CDKN2A* [24, 35]. Hyperplasia progresses to dysplasia which is often associated with loss of chromosomes 3p21 and 17p—the locations of the tumor suppressor genes *Ras association domain family member 1* (*RASSF1*) and *TP53*, respectively [35, 36]. Dysplasia then progresses to CIS, which is associated with losses of chromosomes 11q (containing *CCND1*), 13q (near the *Rb* locus), and

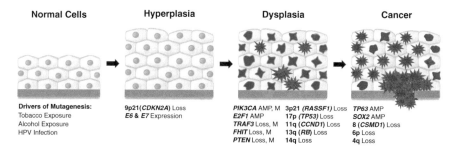

Fig. 5.1 Associated genetic alterations of the progressive states toward invasive HNSCC. Loci listed next to parenthesized genes contain those genes. The loci lacking specified genes are poorly defined microsatellite regions. AMP = Amplification, M = Mutation, and Loss = Genetic loss from deletion and/or epigenetic changes

14q (poorly defined microsatellites). CIS becomes HNSCC upon invasion through the basement membrane, an event that is associated with loss of chromosomes 8, 6p, and 4q [35]. Chromosome 8 contains the putative tumor suppressor gene *CUB And Sushi Multiple Domains 1* (*CSMD1*) and chromosomes 6p and 4q consist of poorly defined microsatellite regions including *TCTE, D6S265, D6S105* (chromosome 6p), *D8S262, D8S261, D8S273, D8S167*, and *D8S257* (chromosome 8), which are all lost at a high rate (approximately 40%) in invasive tumors [35, 36]. Other microsatellite regions lost at a high rate during tumorigenesis include *D3S1007, D3S1284, D3S1038, D3S1067* (chromosome 3p), *FABP2, D4S1613* (chromosome 4), *D9S736, IFN-α, D9S171* (chromosome 9p21), *JNT-2, D11S873, PYGM* (chromosome 11q13), *D13S133, D13S170* (chromosome 13q21), *D14S51, D14S81* (chromosome 14q), *TP53*, and *CHRNB-1* (chromosome 17p13) [35, 36]. Sidransky et al. tested a panel of 23 of these microsatellite markers in a DNA assay of saliva from HNSCC patients, comparing them to healthy controls, and detected microsatellite alterations in 86% of the HNSCC group (96% of the subset with microsatellite alterations found in their tumor) while no microsatellite alterations were detected in healthy controls [40]. This further establishes the association between these microsatellite markers and HNSCC while, similar to ctDNA, suggests an approach for detecting and monitoring HNSCC. Of note, studies are beginning to establish the roles of microRNAs (miRNAs) in HNSCC too [36, 41].

The role of HNSCC-associated mutations in causing tumor formation is still largely unknown, and a more complete understanding is hindered by the absence of studies sequencing premalignant lesions that progress to cancer. *TP53* has the most evidence for being a causative mutation to date in that it was discovered to be mutated in small p53-immunopositive focal patches in tumor-adjacent mucosal epithelium and dysplastic tissue leading to the hypothetical patch–field–tumor–metastasis progression model for HNSCC. This model suggests that *TP53* mutations in progenitor cells of the oral mucosa serve as a harbinger of subsequent oncogenic changes [36, 38, 42]. This hypothesis has been supported by data obtained in engineered mouse models [38, 43]. Studies have also shown that oral dysplastic epithelial lesions with aneuploidy have a high risk of malignant progression [44].

Circulating Tumor DNA (ctDNA) in HNSCC

Despite advancements in therapeutic interventions, the poor prognosis of HNSCC has remained stagnant over the last few decades, with 5-year survival rates of approximately 50% [5]. Implicated in this dilemma is diagnostic delay, associated with higher risk (30%) of advanced stage tumors and accompanying poorer prognosis [45]. Delays have the potential of being curtailed by noninvasive detection of novel biomarkers for monitoring at-risk individuals and/or suspicious lesions.

Cell-free DNA (cfDNA) are small fragments of nucleic acids that are shed from dying cells and are found in body fluids. (64) In individuals with cancer, a fraction of cfDNA becomes circulating tumor DNA (ctDNA), which harbors tumor-specific genetic and epigenetic alterations, including mutations and methylation patterns that can serve as diagnostic biomarkers in the management of HNSCC [41].

Tumor Detection

In HNSCC patients, tumor DNA is detectable not only in the blood, but also in saliva, given its close proximity to oral cavity and pharyngeal tumor sites (Fig. 5.2) [4]. The presence of ctDNA in HNSCC patients makes analysis of this DNA a particularly attractive diagnostic test. Moreover, the procurement of ctDNA is relatively noninvasive [46]. Circulating DNA can also be detected in early-stage disease and has demonstrated potential for detecting minimal residual disease—a limitation of many imaging-based methods (MRI, ultrasound, CT etc.) [46–48]. Furthermore, analysis of ctDNA has the potential of tracking dynamic tumor changes despite tumor heterogeneity, overcoming another major limitation of current detection methods, particularly those relying on tissue biopsies [49]. Studies have also correlated levels of ctDNA with the size and stage of tumors, further evincing its potential as a cancer detection and monitoring modality [50–55].

Because target nucleic acid levels can be very low in body fluids (e.g., 1 mutant DNA fragment/mL), highly sensitive techniques are necessary for mutational analysis of ctDNA [41, 51]. These techniques include "Tagged-amplicon deep Sequencing" (TAm-Seq), "beads, emulsions, amplification, and magnetics" (BEAMing), "Safe-Sequencing System" (Safe-SeqS), "Cancer Personalized Profiling by deep Sequencing" (CAPP-Seq), and PCR amplifications coupled with whole exome sequencing (WES) or next-generation sequencing (NGS) (Fig. 5.2) [41, 56].

Several studies have used these methods in investigating the utility of ctDNA in the detection of HNSCC [4]. Agrawal et al. queried the DNA from the saliva and/or plasma of 93 HNSCC patients, and identified the E7 gene in 30 patients (32%) [4]. In the remaining 63 patients (HPV− individuals), somatic mutations were evaluated in genes and gene regions commonly altered in HNSCC, including *PIK3CA*, *FBXW7*, *TP53*, *HRAS*, *CDKN2A*, and *NRAS*. In this study, multiplex PCR and

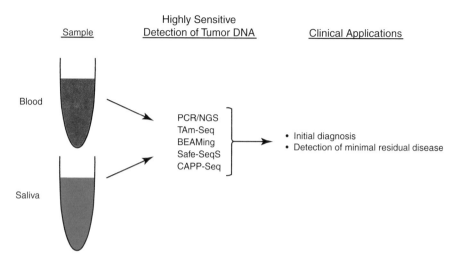

Fig. 5.2 Analysis of blood or saliva for diagnosis or detection of minimal residual disease

massively parallel sequencing was performed, identifying driver mutations in 58 out of the 63 samples. Whole Genome Sequencing was used to detect driver mutations in the remaining 5. In all, the most commonly mutated gene identified was *TP53*, a finding corroborated by other studies (86% of the 63 HPV− patients) [5]. Mutations were also identified in 12 of the 25 HPV+ patient samples. In the same study, when both saliva and plasma were tested in 47 patients, ctDNA was detected in 96%. When separated by tumor site in this same cohort, ctDNA was detected in 100% (*n* = 3), 100% (*n* = 7), 91% (*n* = 22), and 100% (*n* = 15) of tumors of the hypopharynx, larynx, oropharynx, and oral cavity, respectively. In comparing saliva and plasma testing, Agrawal et al. showed that saliva is preferentially enriched for ctDNA in cancers of the oral cavity with 100% of oral cancers being detected in the saliva compared to 47% to 70% in the saliva of patients with tumor located elsewhere in the upper aerodigestive tract [5]. Saliva was also shown to determine HPV status of primary tumor with a sensitivity and specificity of 92.9% and 100%, respectively [57]. Plasma had a similar sensitivity in determining tumor HPV status (96%) and was enriched with ctDNA in patients with tumors outside of the oral cavity with it being detectable in 86% to 100% of plasma samples compared to 80% in the plasma of patients with oral cavity cancers. Moreover, detection of ctDNA in plasma was found to be more sensitive for advanced-stage disease while detection in saliva was more sensitive for early-stage cancers. Of note, ctDNA levels alone were shown to have prognostic implications with reduced survival in HNSCC patients with advanced-stage disease.

These studies, along with large HNSCC genetic studies [7, 9, 12], suggest that a panel including *PIK3CA, NOTCH1, TP53, CDKN2A,* and *HPV16* DNA sequences would be able to detect >95% of invasive HNSCCs [4]. Further studies are needed in at-risk cohorts to determine the utility of this approach in detecting cancer prior to symptoms and findings on physical exam.

Tumor Monitoring

ctDNA analysis not only can be used for early tumor detection, but also for early relapse identification and monitoring of treatment response [4, 41]. There are a growing number of studies to determine the role of ctDNA in this setting [41]. One study investigated the presence of tumor DNA in the plasma or saliva of patients after surgical resection of their tumors [4]. Tumor DNA was found in three of nine patients studied post-op, prior to the development of recurrence. In contrast, no tumor DNA was detected in five patients who continued to show no evidence of disease for a median follow-up of 12 months [4]. This suggests that ctDNA may serve as an early identifier of relapse which could prompt earlier initiation of therapy.

In monitoring response to therapy via assessment of ctDNA, Binder et al. investigated the molecular mechanism of therapy-induced resistance to cetuximab by analyzing for mutant EGFR and RAS in the plasma of HNSCC patients [58]. They discovered that a large fraction (46%) of patients with progressive disease developed KRAS, HRAS, or NRAS mutations whereas no RAS mutations were detected in the nonprogressive subset of patients. This correlation was significant—RAS mutant clones with clinical resistance—(chi square $p = 0.032$) indicating that RAS mutations account for acquired resistance to EGFR-targeting therapy in a large proportion of HNSCC patients, despite the fact that RAS mutations are relatively rare in cetuximab-naïve primary tumors. This study illustrates the potential of analyzing ctDNA as an effective means to monitor therapy response and guide treatment decisions for optimized patient care. Studies on the use of ctDNA in tumor monitoring of HNSCC are currently limited, but are growing in number with increased awareness of the importance and promise of this approach.

Conclusions and Future Directions

The mutational landscape of HNSCC is an expanding body of knowledge that has the potential to guide disease detection and management. With roughly two-thirds of head and neck cancers presenting at advanced stages, the prognosis and survival of HNSCC remains poor. New approaches are needed for early HNSCC detection to improve outcomes. Circulating DNA has shown great promise as a noninvasively obtained biomarker in a number of HNSCC cohorts. Using the mutational signature of HNSCC to identify tumor DNA in body fluids has demonstrated the potential for detecting tumors at early stages and monitoring tumor relapse and response to treatment.

Even though great strides have been made in understanding the mutations that characterize HNSCC, identification of clear driver mutations has been limited by the paucity of mutational analysis studies of premalignant lesions, particularly in HPV+ HNSCC. In addition, with HNSCC arising from distinct anatomical sites of the aerodigestive tract (hypopharynx, larynx, oropharynx, and oral cavity) that potentially have distinct molecular features, the collective mutational landscape of HNSCC may not reveal the key mutations that give rise to tumor formation and progression across anatomic sites. Furthermore, most of the samples in the TCGA cohort and in many of the other sequencing studies were derived from the oral cavity, so that pharyngeal and laryngeal cancers are less well characterized genomically [24]. Studies to date of ctDNA as a biomarker in HNSCC management have also largely been restricted to cancers of the oral cavity and include a relatively small number of cases. Further investigation of ctDNA in larger HNSCC cohorts are needed to fully determine the value of this approach for early detection of both primary and recurrent disease.

Acknowledgments This work was supported by National Institutes of Health grants R01 DE024728 to DEJ and R01DE023685 and R35 CA231998 to JRG and the American Cancer Society.

References

1. Li H, et al. Genomic analysis of head and neck squamous cell carcinoma cell lines and human tumors: a rational approach to preclinical model selection. Mol Cancer Res. 2014; https://doi.org/10.1158/1541-7786.MCR-13-0396.
2. Van Waes C, Musbahi O. Genomics and advances towards precision medicine for head and neck squamous cell carcinoma. Laryngoscope Investig Otolaryngol. 2017;2:310–9.
3. Hoesli RC, et al. Genomic sequencing and precision medicine in head and neck cancers. Eur J Surg Oncol. 2017; https://doi.org/10.1016/j.ejso.2016.12.002.
4. Papadopoulos N, et al. Detection of somatic mutations and HPV in the saliva and plasma of patients with head and neck squamous cell carcinomas. Sci Transl Med. 2015;7:293ra104–293ra104.
5. Perdomo S, et al. Circulating tumor DNA detection in head and neck cancer: evaluation of two different detection approaches. Oncotarget. 2017;8:72621–32.
6. van Ginkel JH, Huibers MMH, van Es RJJ, de Bree R, Willems SM. Droplet digital PCR for detection and quantification of circulating tumor DNA in plasma of head and neck cancer patients. BMC Cancer. 2017;17:1–8.
7. Lawrence MS, et al. Comprehensive genomic characterization of head and neck squamous cell carcinomas. Nature. 2015;517:576–82.
8. Gaykalova DA, et al. Novel insight into mutational landscape of head and neck squamous cell carcinoma. PLoS One. 2014; https://doi.org/10.1371/journal.pone.0093102.
9. Stransky N, et al. The mutational landscape of head and neck squamous cell carcinoma. Science (80-). 2011;333:1157–60.
10. Morris LGT, et al. The molecular landscape of recurrent and metastatic head and neck cancers. JAMA Oncol. 2016;3:244.
11. Padhi S, et al. Role of CDKN2A/p16 expression in the prognostication of oral squamous cell carcinoma. Oral Oncol. 2017;73:27.
12. Agrawal N, et al. Exome sequencing of head and neck squamous cell carcinoma reveals inactivating mutations in NOTCH1. Science (80-). 2011; https://doi.org/10.1126/science.1206923.
13. Brand TM, Iida M, Wheeler D, L. Molecular mechanisms of resistance to the EGFR monoclonal antibody cetuximab. Cancer Biol Ther. 2011; https://doi.org/10.4161/cbt.11.9.15050.

14. Kommineni N, Jamil K, Pingali U, Addala L, Mur N. Association of PIK3CA gene mutations with head and neck squamous cell carcinomas. Neoplasma. 2015;62:72.
15. Hedberg ML, et al. Use of nonsteroidal anti-inflammatory drugs predicts improved patient survival for *PIK3CA*-altered head and neck cancer. J Exp Med. 2019;216:419 LP – 427.
16. Shao X, et al. Mutational analysis of the PTEN gene in head and neck squamous cell carcinoma. Int J Cancer. 1998; https://doi.org/10.1002/(SICI)1097-0215(19980831)77:5<684:: AID-IJC4>3.0.CO;2-R.
17. Li C, Egloff AM, Sen M, Grandis JR, Johnson DE. Caspase-8 mutations in head and neck cancer confer resistance to death receptor-mediated apoptosis and enhance migration, invasion, and tumor growth. Mol Oncol. 2014; https://doi.org/10.1016/j.molonc.2014.03.018.
18. Ando M, et al. Cancer-associated missense mutations of caspase-8 activate nuclear factor-κB signaling. Cancer Sci. 2013; https://doi.org/10.1111/cas.12191.
19. Pickering CR, et al. Integrative genomic characterization of oral squamous cell carcinoma identifies frequent somatic drivers. Cancer Discov. 2013; https://doi.org/10.1158/2159-8290. CD-12-0537.
20. Tillman BN, et al. Fibroblast growth factor family aberrations as a putative driver of head and neck squamous cell carcinoma in an epidemiologically low-risk patient as defined by targeted sequencing. Head Neck. 2016; https://doi.org/10.1002/hed.24292.
21. Haraguchi K, et al. Ajuba negatively regulates the Wnt signaling pathway by promoting GSK-3β-mediated phosphorylation of β-catenin. Oncogene. 2007;27:274.
22. Abba MC, et al. The head and neck cancer cell oncogenome: a platform for the development of precision molecular therapies. Oncotarget. 2015; https://doi.org/10.18632/oncotarget.2417.
23. Dok R, Nuyts S. HPV positive head and neck cancers: molecular pathogenesis and evolving treatment strategies. Cancers. 2016; https://doi.org/10.3390/cancers8040041.
24. Faraji, F. et al. The genome-wide molecular landscape of HPV-driven and HPV-negative head and neck squamous cell carcinoma293–325 (2018). doi:https://doi.org/10.1007/978-3-319-78762-6_11.
25. Hayes DN, Van Waes C, Seiwert TY. Genetic landscape of human papillomavirus-associated head and neck cancer and comparison to tobacco-related tumors. J Clin Oncol. 2015; https://doi.org/10.1200/JCO.2015.62.1086.
26. Henderson S, Chakravarthy A, Su X, Boshoff C, Fenton TR. APOBEC-mediated cytosine deamination links PIK3CA helical domain mutations to human papillomavirus-driven tumor development. Cell Rep. 2014; https://doi.org/10.1016/j.celrep.2014.05.012.
27. Seiwert TY, et al. Integrative and comparative genomic analysis of HPV-positive and HPV-negative head and neck squamous cell carcinomas. Clin Cancer Res. 2015; https://doi.org/10.1158/1078-0432.CCR-13-3310.
28. Shih JW, Tsai TY, Chao CH, Wu Lee YH. Candidate tumor suppressor DDX3 RNA helicase specifically represses cap-dependent translation by acting as an eIF4E inhibitory protein. Oncogene. 2008; https://doi.org/10.1038/sj.onc.1210687.
29. Zhang J, et al. Attenuated TRAF3 fosters activation of alternative NF-kB and reduced expression of antiviral interferon, TP53, and RB to promote HPV-positive head and neck cancers. Cancer Res. 2018; https://doi.org/10.1158/0008-5472.CAN-17-0642.
30. Hajek M, et al. TRAF3/CYLD mutations identify a distinct subset of human papillomavirus-associated head and neck squamous cell carcinoma. Cancer. 2017; https://doi.org/10.1002/ cncr.30570.
31. Harbison RA, et al. The mutational landscape of recurrent versus nonrecurrent human papillomavirus–related oropharyngeal cancer. JCI Insight. 2018; https://doi.org/10.1172/jci. insight.99327.
32. Hayes DN, Grandis JR, El-Naggar AK. The Cancer Genome Atlas: integrated analysis of genome alterations in squamous cell carcinoma of the head and neck. J Clin Oncol. 2013;31:6009.
33. Cho J, Johnson DE, Grandis JR. Therapeutic implications of the genetic landscape of head and neck cancer. Semin Radiat Oncol. 2018; https://doi.org/10.1016/j.semradonc.2017.08.005.

34. Kim KT, Kim BS, Kim JH. Association between FAT1 mutation and overall survival in patients with human papillomavirus-negative head and neck squamous cell carcinoma. Head Neck. 2016; https://doi.org/10.1002/hed.24372.

35. Califano J, et al. Genetic progression model for head and neck cancer: implications for field cancerization. Cancer Res. 1996;56:2488.

36. Leemans CR, Braakhuis BJM, Brakenhoff RH. The molecular biology of head and neck cancer. Nat Rev Cancer. 2011; https://doi.org/10.1038/nrc2982.

37. Zur Hausen H. Papillomaviruses and cancer: from basic studies to clinical. Papillomaviruses and cancer: from basic studies to clinical application. Nat Rev Cancer. 2002;2(5):342–50. https://doi.org/10.1038/nrc798.

38. Leemans CR, Snijders PJF, Brakenhoff RH. The molecular landscape of head and neck cancer. Nat Rev Cancer. 2018; https://doi.org/10.1038/nrc.2018.11.

39. Nekulova M, Holcakova J, Coates P, Vojtesek B. The role of P63 in cancer, stem cells and cancer stem cells. Cell Mol Biol Lett. 2011; https://doi.org/10.2478/s11658-011-0009-9.

40. Spafford MF, et al. Detection of head and neck squamous cell carcinoma among exfoliated oral mucosal cells by microsatellite analysis. Clin Cancer Res. 2001;7:607–12.

41. van Ginkel JH, Slieker FJB, de Bree R, van Es RJJ, Willems SM. Cell-free nucleic acids in body fluids as biomarkers for the prediction and early detection of recurrent head and neck cancer: a systematic review of the literature. Oral Oncol. 2017;75:8–15.

42. Wood HM, et al. The genomic road to invasion-examining the similarities and differences in the genomes of associated oral pre-cancer and cancer samples. Genome Med. 2017; https://doi.org/10.1186/s13073-017-0442-0.

43. Lim X, et al. Interfollicular epidermal stem cells self-renew via autocrine Wnt signaling. Science (80-.). 2013; https://doi.org/10.1126/science.1239730.

44. Torres-Rendon A, Stewart R, Craig GT, Wells M, Speight PM. DNA ploidy analysis by image cytometry helps to identify oral epithelial dysplasias with a high risk of malignant progression. Oral Oncol. 2009; https://doi.org/10.1016/j.oraloncology.2008.07.006.

45. Gómez I, Seoane J, Varela-Centelles P, Diz P, Takkouche B. Is diagnostic delay related to advanced-stage oral cancer? A meta-analysis. Eur J Oral Sci. 2009; https://doi.org/10.1111/j.1600-0722.2009.00672.x.

46. Han X, Wang J, Sun Y. Circulating tumor DNA as biomarkers for cancer detection. Genom Proteom Bioinform. 2017; https://doi.org/10.1016/j.gpb.2016.12.004.

47. Shaw JA, et al. Genomic analysis of circulating cell-free DNA infers breast cancer dormancy. Genome Res. 2012; https://doi.org/10.1101/gr.123497.111.

48. Chaudhuri AA, Binkley MS, Osmundson EC, Alizadeh AA, Diehn M. Predicting radiotherapy responses and treatment outcomes through analysis of circulating tumor DNA. Semin Radiat Oncol. 2015; https://doi.org/10.1016/j.semradonc.2015.05.001.

49. Ignatiadis M, Lee M, Jeffrey SS. Circulating tumor cells and circulating tumor DNA: challenges and opportunities on the path to clinical utility. Clin Cancer Res. 2015; https://doi.org/10.1158/1078-0432.CCR-14-1190.

50. Forshew T, et al. Noninvasive identification and monitoring of cancer mutations by targeted deep sequencing of plasma DNA. Sci Transl Med. 2012; https://doi.org/10.1126/scitranslmed.3003726.

51. Bettegowda C, et al. Detection of circulating tumor DNA in early- and late-stage human malignancies. Sci Transl Med. 2014; https://doi.org/10.1126/scitranslmed.3007094.

52. Diehl F, et al. Circulating mutant DNA to assess tumor dynamics. Nat Med. 2008; https://doi.org/10.1038/nm.1789.

53. Newman AM, et al. An ultrasensitive method for quantitating circulating tumor DNA with broad patient coverage. Nat Med. 2014; https://doi.org/10.1038/nm.3519.

54. Sausen M, et al. Clinical implications of genomic alterations in the tumour and circulation of pancreatic cancer patients. Nat Commun. 2015; https://doi.org/10.1038/ncomms8686.

55. Beaver JA, et al. Detection of cancer DNA in plasma of patients with early-stage breast cancer. Clin Cancer Res. 2014; https://doi.org/10.1158/1078-0432.CCR-13-2933.

56. Heitzer E, Ulz P, Geigl JB. Circulating tumor DNA as a liquid biopsy for cancer. Clin Chem. 2015; https://doi.org/10.1373/clinchem.2014.222679.
57. Chai RC, et al. A pilot study to compare the detection of HPV-16 biomarkers in salivary oral rinses with tumour p16INK4a expression in head and neck squamous cell carcinoma patients. BMC Cancer. 2016; https://doi.org/10.1186/s12885-016-2217-1.
58. Braig F, et al. Liquid biopsy monitoring uncovers acquired RAS-mediated resistance to cetuximab in a substantial proportion of patients with head and neck squamous cell carcinoma. Oncotarget. 2016; https://doi.org/10.18632/oncotarget.8943.

Chapter 6
Circulating Biomarkers in Head and Neck Cancer

Taichiro Nonaka and David T. W. Wong

Introduction

Head and neck cancer was ranked as the seventh common cancer in the world with estimated 880,000 new cases and 450,000 deaths in 2018 [1]. Squamous cell carcinoma (SCC) is the most predominant histological type that mainly occurs along the oropharyngeal mucosa. The overall survival rate has remained unchanged for decades despite the improved surgery and treatment options. Currently, available screening techniques, such as imaging and protein biomarkers, are not sufficient to detect the presence of head and neck cancers in their early stages. Tissue biopsy is the standard diagnostic method, but it does not provide information about the heterogeneity and evolution of tumors [2]. Liquid biopsy is a highly desirable method for cancer detection since it can provide real-time information in a minimally invasive manner [3]. Circulating tumor DNA (ctDNA), circulating tumor cells (CTCs), and exosomal miRNAs are emerging biomarkers that can be applied to cancer detection, treatment planning, and response monitoring [4]. Of note, ctDNA and exosomal miRNAs are present in multiple body fluids, including saliva, and are very promising biomarkers for cancer [5]. In this chapter, we summarize the current array of circulating biomarkers (ctDNA, CTCs, and exosomal miRNAs) and their potential clinical applications in early detection and treatment of head and neck cancer.

T. Nonaka (✉) · D. T. W. Wong (✉)
Center for Oral/Head and Neck Oncology Research, School of Dentistry, University of California, Los Angeles, Los Angeles, CA, USA

Division of Oral Biology and Medicine, School of Dentistry, University of California, Los Angeles, Los Angeles, CA, USA
e-mail: tnonaka@ucla.edu; dtww@ucla.edu

© Springer Nature Switzerland AG 2021
R. El Assal et al. (eds.), *Early Detection and Treatment of Head & Neck Cancers*, https://doi.org/10.1007/978-3-030-69852-2_6

Circulating Tumor DNA and Circulating Tumor Cells

Early Detection

ctDNA refers to a cell-free DNA that is derived from cancer cells circulating freely in blood. Patients with cancer have higher concentrations of ctDNA than healthy individuals [6]. ctDNA mainly originates from apoptotic or necrotic tumor cells and contains the mutations present in the tumor (Fig. 6.1). In 1994, Vasioukhin et al. and Sorenson et al. first demonstrated the presence of tumor-specific RAS mutations in plasma cell-free DNA [7, 8]. Several other studies have demonstrated a high concordance of mutational profiles between plasma ctDNA and matched tumor samples in lung cancer [9], breast cancer [10, 11], and colorectal cancer [12, 13].

A recent proof-of-principle study has shown that ctDNA is a promising biomarker for the presence of head and neck cancer [14]. In a cohort of 93 patients with head and neck squamous cell carcinoma (HNSCC) including 20 cases of early-stage cancer, plasma and saliva samples were screened for somatic mutations (*TP53*, *PIK3CA*, *NOTCH1*, *FBXW7*, *CDKN2A*, *NRAS*, and *HRAS*) and human papillomaviruses (HPV16 and 18) (Table 6.1). Plasma ctDNA was shown to be a more sensitive biomarker than salivary ctDNA for oropharynx, hypopharynx, and larynx cancer (plasma ctDNA: 86–100% vs. salivary ctDNA: 47–70%). However, salivary ctDNA showed better sensitivity than plasma ctDNA (100% vs. 80%) in oral cancer, indicating that oral cancer–derived DNA is more readily detected in saliva due to the close proximity of the tumor to saliva. Importantly, when both plasma and saliva were tested in combination, the overall ctDNA detection rate was 96%, irrespective of tumor location or stage. These findings indicated that in order to obtain highly sensitive results, a combination of appropriate body fluids should be tested, depending on the type of tumor present. *TP53* was the most frequently detected ctDNA in the plasma of patients with oral cancer (85%), and this was also the case for tumors of other anatomical sites (oropharynx 100%, hypopharynx 100%, and larynx 86%). HPV16 DNA was detected somewhat less frequently compared to the high prevalence rates of *TP53* ctDNA, likely because *TP53* mutations and HPV positivity are mutually exclusive [15]. The Cancer Genome Atlas Network showed high *TP53* mutation rate (86%) in 243 HPV-negative samples, while only one out of 36 HPV-positive cases (2.8%) had a nonsynonymous *TP53* mutation, which is consistent with this data [16].

For cancers with a viral etiology such as nasopharyngeal carcinoma, detection of the cancer-associated viral DNA may provide a good strategy for identifying individuals with early-stage disease. Chan et al. screened asymptomatic volunteers for plasma Epstein–Barr virus (EBV) DNA and found 69 of the 1318 participants (5.2%) had viral DNA, among whom three individuals were diagnosed with nasopharyngeal carcinoma [17]. They further confirmed this result in a prospective cohort with a total of 20,174 participants, demonstrating that 34 of 309 participants (11%) with persistent EBV-positive results developed nasopharyngeal carcinoma [18]. Population screening of viral DNA in plasma is a promising approach to detect early-stage cancer.

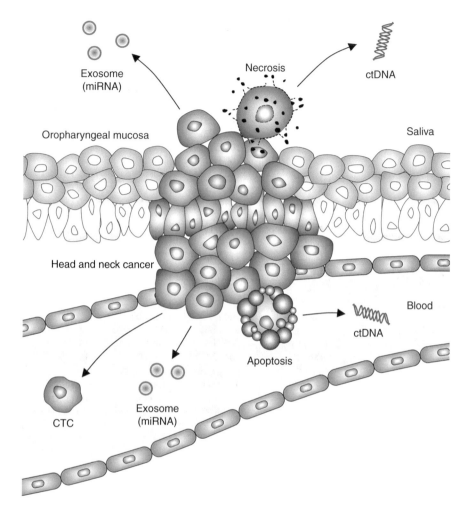

Fig. 6.1 Circulating biomarkers in head and neck cancer. Circulating tumor DNA (ctDNA), circulating tumor cells (CTCs), and exosomal miRNAs are complementary biomarkers present in plasma and/or saliva. Apoptotic tumor cells release ctDNA into blood, whereas necrotic tumor cells shed ctDNA into saliva. Tumor cells release exosomal miRNAs into blood and saliva. Primary tumor and metastatic lesions release CTCs into blood. (Reprinted with permission from [3]. Copyright 2018, SAGE Publications)

Some primary and metastatic tumors release subsets of CTCs into the blood (Fig. 6.1). CTCs are capable of providing whole cellular information, and increased CTC levels exhibit diagnostic features. CTCs have been tested in numerous studies for diagnosis of primary tumors and metastatic relapse [19]. Nichols et al. and He et al. reported that CTCs were detected in 6 of 15 (40.0%) and 3 of 9 (33.3%) patients diagnosed with head and neck cancer [20, 21]. Buglione together with his team reported that CTCs are more commonly found in the advanced stages than in the early stages [22]. Moreover, Jatana et al. and Gröbe et al. reported that an

Table 6.1 Summary of saliva and plasma ctDNA biomarker profiles identified in head and neck squamous cell carcinoma

			% of positivity (no. detected/no. examined)		
		ctDNA	Saliva	Plasma	Saliva or plasma[a]
Site	Oral cavity	*TP53*	100 (36/36)	85 (11/13)	100 (13/13)
		PIK3CA	100 (2/2)	50 (1/2)	100 (2/2)
		NOTCH1	100 (3/3)	NA	NA
		CDKN2A	100 (2/2)	NA	NA
		Translocation	100 (2/2)	NA	NA
		HPV16 DNA	100 (1/1)	NA	NA
		(Total)	100 (46/46)	80 (12/15)	100 (15/15)
	Oropharynx	*TP53*	80 (4/5)	100 (1/1)	100 (1/1)
		PIK3CA	25 (2/8)[b]	100 (5/5)	100 (5/5)
		FBXW7	67 (2/3)	100 (3/3)	100 (3/3)
		HPV16 DNA	41 (7/17)	92 (11/12)	92 (11/12)
		NRAS	0 (0/1)	0 (0/1)	0 (0/1)
		(Total)	47 (16/34)[b]	91 (20/22)	91 (20/22)
	Larynx	*TP53*	70 (7/10)	86 (6/7)	100 (7/7)
	Hypopharynx	*TP53*	67 (2/3)	100 (3/3)	100 (3/3)
Stage	Early (I + II)	*TP53*	100 (16/16)	75 (6/8)	100 (8/8)
		HPV16 DNA	100 (2/2)	100 (1/1)	100 (1/1)
		PIK3CA	100 (1/1)	0 (0/1)	100 (1/1)
		NOTCH1	100 (1/1)	NA	NA
		(Total)	100 (20/20)	70 (7/10)	100 (10/10)
	Late (III + IV)	*TP53*	87 (33/38)	94 (15/16)	100 (16/16)
		PIK3CA	33 (3/9)[b]	100 (6/6)	100 (6/6)
		FBXW7	67 (2/3)	100 (3/3)	100 (3/3)
		HPV16 DNA	38 (6/16)	91 (10/11)	91 (10/11)
		NOTCH1	100 (2/2)	NA	NA
		CDKN2A	100 (2/2)	NA	NA
		Translocation	100 (2/2)	NA	NA
		NRAS	0 (0/1)	0 (0/1)	0 (0/1)
		(Total)	70 (51/73)[b]	92 (34/37)	95 (35/37)
HPV	HPV16	HPV16 DNA	40 (12/30)	86 (18/21)	86 (18/21)
Overall			76 (71/93)[b]	87 (41/47)	96 (45/47)

Reprinted with permission from [3]. Copyright 2018, SAGE Publications

All biomarker data and detection rates were extracted from the results of the safe-sequencing system (Safe-SeqS) and digital polymerase chain reaction published by Wang et al. (2015)

NA not applicable

[a]Detection rates in "saliva or plasma" were calculated only if patients' data from both saliva and plasma were available

[b]One patient with PIK3CA-negative but human papillomavirus (HPV)–positive saliva was counted in the total number

increased number of CTCs is correlated with worse prognosis, and the presence of CTCs is correlated with locoregional relapse [23, 24]. However, CTCs seem to be much less sensitive than ctDNA for early detection of cancer. Bettegowda et al. reported that no CTCs were detected in early-stage bladder, breast, and colorectal cancers, whereas ctDNA was detected in 81% of these cancers [11]. These findings suggest that the presence of CTCs symbolizes a late stage and represents a prognostic marker but not an early diagnostic marker (Fig. 6.2a).

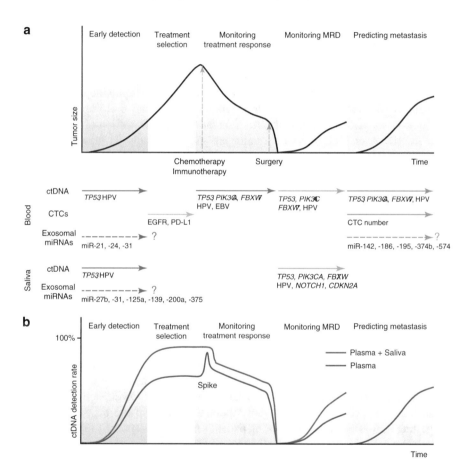

Fig. 6.2 Potential clinical applications of circulating biomarkers in the treatment of head and neck cancer. (**a**) Schematic time course of disease management and tumor size in patient with head and neck cancer undergoing chemotherapy (or immunotherapy) and surgery. Plasma ctDNA analysis allows early detection, monitoring of treatment response, monitoring of minimal residual disease (MRD), and prediction of metastasis. CTC analysis can assist the selection of targeted therapies. Exosomal miRNAs currently offer limited insight into clinical applications. Salivary ctDNA analysis can provide complementary information. (**b**) Use of plasma and salivary ctDNA in combination allows for higher sensitivity in detection of cancer than the use of plasma ctDNA alone. A spike in ctDNA level reflects transient tumor cell death by systemic therapy. (Reprinted with permission from [3]. Copyright 2018, SAGE Publications)

Treatment Selection

CTCs can be used to test the presence of drug targets. Cetuximab, a monoclonal antibody targeting the extracellular domain of the epidermal growth factor receptor (EGFR), has been approved for the treatment of advanced HNSCC [25, 26]. Measuring cell-surface expression of EGFR on CTCs provides critical information for planning anti-EGFR treatment (Fig. 6.2a). This is consistent with the finding that Cetuximab treatment was more effective in reducing EGFR-positive CTCs than conventional chemotherapy in HNSCC [27].

EGFR downstream signaling molecules participate in the resistance of HNSCC to Cetuximab. It is particularly important to screen RAS mutations before Cetuximab treatment because tumors harboring activating RAS do not respond to EGFR-targeted therapy. Braig et al. investigated plasma ctDNA in a liquid biopsy cohort of 20 patients with HNSCC treated with Cetuximab and found 6 out of 20 patients (30%) acquired KRAS, NRAS, or HRAS mutations [28]. Detection of RAS mutations in ctDNA or CTCs may help tailor anti-EGFR therapy, as these mutations correlate significantly with treatment efficacy and disease progression. More importantly, mutational loads should be monitored during the therapy so the loss of cetuximab response can be reliably predicted. Thus, CTCs may be used for mutational monitoring to guide treatment decisions.

In the tumor microenvironment, tumor cells can express programmed cell death ligand 1 (PD-L1) that downregulates effector T-cell activity, thereby protecting tumors from immune attack [29]. Detection of CTCs expressing PD-L1 on their surface can be predictive of the response to anti-PD-L1 immunotherapy (Fig. 6.2a) [30]. In breast cancer, Mazel et al. reported that PD-L1-expressing CTCs were detected in 11 out of 16 (68.8%) patients, suggesting its usefulness in treatment planning [31]. PD-L1 expression on CTCs was also reported in other tumor types, such as lung [32], bladder [33], prostate, and colorectal cancers [34], and was significantly associated with poor survival. In head and neck cancer, Strati et al. found PD-L1 expression in $CD45^-EpCAM^+$ CTCs in 24 of 94 patients (25.5%) before treatment, 8 of 34 (23.5%) after chemotherapy, and 12 of 54 (22.2%) at the end of treatment [35]. Oliveira-Costa et al. investigated PD-L1 expression in OSCC-derived $CD45^-$ cytokeratin(CK)$^+$ CTCs and found transcriptional and protein expression of PD-L1, suggesting its usefulness for monitoring patient's treatment response [36]. Moreover, Kulasinghe et al. isolated $CD45^-EpCAM^+CK^+$ CTCs from a patient with laryngeal cancer and detected high expression of PD-L1 by immunocytochemistry [37].

Despite evidence of the benefits in treatment selection, detecting CTCs is challenging due to their extremely low numbers. It is estimated that only one to two CTCs are present per 7.5 mL of blood, making them difficult to study [21]. Currently, the only Food and Drug Administration (FDA)–approved platform for isolating CTCs is CellSearch [38]. CellSearch is a standardized, semiautomated system that enables positive selection of CTCs based on the expression of the epithelial marker EpCAM. Testing of therapeutic targets on a small population of CTCs in patients with HNSCC is currently under investigation, but its clinical utility has not yet been established.

Monitoring Treatment Response

ctDNA is advantageous in real-time monitoring of the treatment response compared to imaging [39]. ctDNA is a more sensitive biomarker than CTCs or other cancer antigens, such as 15-3 (CA15-3), for predicting treatment response (Fig. 6.2a) [40]. Earlier therapeutic interventions can be enabled through the detection of differential early dynamics of mutations, which predict treatment response in the context of systemic therapy.

The median half-life of plasma EBV DNA was 3.99 days (range, 1.85–28.29 days) as shown by a study examining the clearance of EBV during chemotherapy in naso-pharyngeal carcinoma [41]. Another research reported that the half-life of plasma ctDNA (*APC*, *KRAS*, *TP53*, and *PIK3CA*) in colorectal cancer was 114 min after surgery, suggesting that ctDNA is the most preferable biomarker when monitoring fast changes in the size of the tumor due to its rapid dynamics [12]. The above studies indicate that tumor dynamics in cancer patients undergoing chemotherapy or surgery can be reliably monitored by ctDNA measurement (Fig. 6.2a). Currently, a clinical trial to evaluate ctDNA as a biomarker for treatment response in HNSCC is ongoing and the results are awaited (ClinicalTrials.gov Identifier: NCT03540563).

Monitoring Minimal Residual Disease

Previous studies have shown that ctDNA levels can be used for monitoring minimal residual disease (MRD) after surgery [42]. In principle, detection of ctDNA may be the best method for measuring MRD since the PCR-based approach, with a sensitive readout, is the most effective detection modality (Fig. 6.2a). Diehl et al. were able to detect mutations as low as 0.01% in cell-free DNA in patients with colorectal cancer, and those with MRD relapsed within 1 year after surgery [12]. In a prospective cohort of 230 patients with colorectal cancer, relapse-free survival was 90% for the ctDNA-negative group and 0% for the ctDNA-positive group after surgery [43]. Another study was performed on 55 patients with breast cancer, demonstrating that postoperative ctDNA detection accurately predicted poor relapse-free survival [44]. It is yet to be confirmed whether identifying MRD-positive patients could improve the situation of patients with cancer, but placing patients into groups of high or low risk on the basis of ctDNA levels will allow the earliest therapeutic intervention.

Predicting Metastasis

The idea of using ctDNA as a surrogate marker is based on the evidence that it shares common mutational profiles with primary and secondary tumors [11, 40]. To back up the above statement, many studies have reported that ctDNA is a sensitive biomarker for detecting metastasis, reflecting the tumor burden in many cancers, including head and neck cancer [11, 40, 45].

The prognostic value of CTC enumeration has also been demonstrated in various tumor types via large clinical trials [46–48]. There is growing evidence that detection of CTCs correlates with poor survival in patients with head and neck cancer [23, 24, 49, 50]. Additionally, CTC number was correlated with a higher incidence of regional metastasis in head and neck cancer [51]. However, these studies were unable to provide threshold CTC values correlating with poor prognosis, as CTC numbers are highly variable among individuals. Although the clinical value of CTC analysis remains controversial, there is evidence indicating that CTC numbers after surgery or systemic therapy can predict treatment outcomes and metastasis (Fig. 6.2a) [52].

The low numbers of CTCs make their detection challenging. CellSearch method selects for tumor cells expressing EpCAM; therefore, downregulation of EpCAM during the epithelial–mesenchymal transition may make CTCs undetectable. Actually, only one-third of CTCs are found to be EpCAM-positive in patients with metastatic breast cancer [53]. This limitation might be overcome by combining different technologies and using additional markers. With this in mind, we propose that the combined use of ctDNA and CTCs may be an ideal strategy to assess the risk for metastasis in head and neck cancer.

Circulating Exosomal miRNAs

Exosomes are nanoscale extracellular vesicles of endocytic origin that carry diverse cellular constituents (e.g., DNA, RNA, and proteins) and play a vital role in exchanging molecular information between cells [54]. Given their contents, exosomes could potentially be exploited as cancer biomarkers. Among the constituents found in exosomes, miRNAs are the most relevant markers for cancer diagnosis since they regulate both oncogenes and tumor suppressor genes [55]. A certain set of exosomal miRNAs forms cancer biomarkers because of the correlation between miRNA profiles in plasma and tumors [56, 57]. This has led to the exploration of the use of the miRNA signature as a diagnostic tool in various cancers [58–60], including head and neck cancer. A study carried out by Summerer et al. showed that high numbers of circulating miR-142, miR-186, miR-195, miR-374b, and miR-574 represent prognostic biomarkers for head and neck cancer [61]. Similarly, elevated levels of miR-21 and miR-24 were detected in plasma from patients with head and neck cancer [62, 63]. Moreover, amplified miR-31 was detected in the plasma of patients with head and neck cancer, and was reduced after tumor resection, suggesting its origin is from the tumor [63]. Downregulation of tumor-suppressive miR-486 was highly associated with OSCC recurrence, suggesting miR-486 could act as a biomarker to monitor OSCC recurrence after surgery [64]. These findings provide considerable evidence that exosomal miRNAs can be used as a valuable tool in the diagnosis of cancer (Fig. 6.2a).

The miRNA database, miRandola, offers a large catalogue of extracellular, non-coding RNAs found in a variety of diseases and currently consists of 1002 miRNAs with 3283 entries (http://mirandola.iit.cnr.it/) [65]. Despite being extensively investigated, the reliability of exosomal miRNA is hampered by heterogeneous results, likely due to inconsistent methods among the studies [66]. Additionally, it is not confirmed whether immune cells make a strong contribution to circulating miRNA levels. Systemic or local inflammation may perturb miRNA expression and its reproducibility, even within the same individual [67]. From this, there is no consensus about the diagnostic performance of exosomal miRNAs in head and neck cancer, and more studies are needed to further characterize exosomal miRNAs. Validation in large clinical trials with standardized protocols is required to substantiate the value of exosomal miRNAs in a clinical setting.

Salivary Diagnostics

In the past decade, saliva researchers have come up with salivary diagnostics to detect oral and systemic diseases [68]. A certain amount of salivary constituents are derived from physiological interactions with blood, as shown by proteomic studies, indicating that 20–30% of the salivary proteome reflects that of plasma [69, 70]. The above relationship between blood and saliva reveals an additional resource for diagnosing systemic diseases. Saliva has unique advantages over other body fluids for clinical diagnosis. Saliva can be collected noninvasively without patient discomfort. Saliva does not coagulate, hence it is much easier to handle and process than blood. Given a wide variety of constituents and close physiological interactions with blood, saliva can be regarded as a mirror of oral and systemic health, rendering it an attractive biofluid for disease diagnosis.

Salivary ctDNA

Genomic analysis shows that about 70% of salivary cell-free DNA originates from the host while the other 30% originates from microorganisms [71]. Salivary ctDNA has been revealed to be a more sensitive biomarker than the plasma ctDNA for early-stage oral cancer (Table 6.1). A proof-of-principle study demonstrated *TP53* ctDNA detection in saliva of patients with early-stage oral cancer with 100% sensitivity [14]. Even in patients with cancers at other sites (oropharynx, hypopharynx, and larynx), *TP53* ctDNA was found in the saliva of 67% to 80% of these patient groups, making it a promising biomarker for detecting head and neck cancer (Fig. 6.2a).

Qureishi et al. examined the accuracy of PCR-based HPV DNA detection in saliva from patients with oropharyngeal squamous cell carcinoma (OPSCC) and found acceptable diagnostic accuracy, with a positive predictive value of 96% [72]. The sensitivity and specificity of saliva testing when compared to the reference p16 immunohistochemistry (IHC) on surgical biopsies were 72% and 90%, respectively. In a prospective study, Martin-Gomez et al. confirmed oral rinse as a reliable and noninvasive source of HPV DNA in patients with OPSCC [73]. Among 171 cases, the concordance rate between oral rinse and tumor specimens was 74% for HPV16. Other HPV types (e.g., HPV 18, 31, 33, and 35) showed even higher concordance rates (>94%), demonstrating the feasibility of HPV detection in saliva (Fig. 6.2a).

Another possible implication of oral HPV detection is in the monitoring of disease after treatment for HPV-positive OPSCC. In a retrospective study, Ahn et al. demonstrated that positive post-treatment saliva HPV status was associated with higher risk of recurrence (hazard ratio, 10.7; 95% CI, 2.36–48.50) ($P = 0.002$) [74]. Rettig et al. showed similar results that evaluated the predictive value of HPV DNA in saliva [75]. In the prospective cohort of 124 HPV-positive OPSCC, HPV DNA was present in 54% of oral rinse samples from patients prior to treatment but was seen in only 5% following treatment. Importantly, 5 of 6 patients (83%) with persistent HPV DNA in oral rinse developed recurrent disease, implicating saliva as a possible surveillance tool. Saliva is enriched with tumor- or HPV-specific DNA originating from tumor cells in the oropharyngeal cavity, and analyzing both plasma and saliva maximizes the effectiveness for screening head and neck cancer (Fig. 6.2b).

Salivary miRNA

Circulating cell-free miRNAs turned out to be unexpectedly stable in saliva [76]. The endogenous miRNAs in saliva degrade at a slower rate compared to exogenous miRNAs. Profiling of salivary miRNAs showed they are packed in exosomes which make them resistant to destruction by RNases [77, 78]. Some studies have shown that salivary miRNAs can serve as potential biomarkers for head and neck cancer. Park et al. reported that miR-125a and miR-200a were significantly less abundant in saliva from patients with oral cancer than in healthy individuals [76]. Similarly, the expression of miR-139 and miR-375 were decreased in saliva collected from patients with oral cancer compared to their expression in healthy controls [79, 80]. Additionally, increased expression of miR-27b and miR-31 was observed in saliva from patients with oral cancer [81, 82]. Importantly, expression levels of miR-139 and miR-31 reverted to baseline after excision of the lesions, suggesting their potential use as prognostic biomarkers [79, 81]. Although certain sets of salivary miRNAs may serve as putative biomarkers for head and neck cancer, further research is required to validate these findings and to elucidate the molecular mechanisms involved.

Salivary Exosomes

Salivary exosomes are nanoscale extracellular vesicles (EVs) secreted from salivary gland and/or oral epithelial cells. They are enclosed by a phospholipid bilayer, containing a unique protein cargo that reflects the cells of origin (Fig. 6.3). Commonly detected proteins include tetraspanins, heat shock proteins, water channel, major histocompatibility complexes, Rab GTPases, and ESCRT [83, 84]. Other proteins found in exosomes include signaling, cytoskeletal, metabolic, and carrier proteins. Comprehensive analyses on mammalian EVs have generated extensive catalogues of constituents (proteins, nucleic acids, and lipids) found in different types of EVs isolated from cells, tissue, or body fluids, including saliva. The databases are publicly available at Vesiclepedia (http://www.microvesicles.org) [85] and ExoCarta (http://www.exocarta.org) [86].

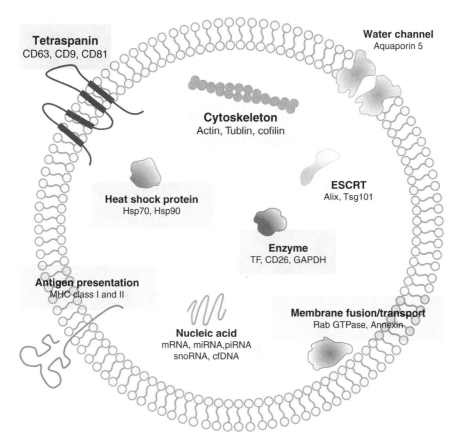

Fig. 6.3 Structure and content of a salivary exosome. The exosome is surrounded by a phospholipid bilayer. Membrane protein markers in most salivary exosomes include tetraspanin, water channel, and major histocompatibility complex (MHC) class I. The intravesicular contents include nucleic acids (RNA and DNA) and various cytosolic proteins, such as enzymes, heat shock proteins, cytoskeleton, endosomal sorting complex required for transport (ESCRT)–associated proteins, and membrane fusion/transport–associated proteins from the parental cells of origin. (Reprinted with permission from [68]. Copyright 2017, Elsevier Inc.)

The nanostructure of tumor-derived exosomes adds another layer of complexity to the characterization of exosomes [87]. Nanostructural analysis using atomic force microscopy (AFM) and field emission scanning electron microscopy (FESEM) revealed trilobed structures of salivary exosomes in healthy donors, indicating their elastic mechanical properties [88, 89]. Salivary exosomes have a spherical morphology when stresses are not applied while they have a heterogeneous surface due to the embedded proteins in a dense lipid membrane. Characterization of salivary exosomes at the single-vesicle level revealed irregular morphologies and aggregations in patients with oral cancer [90]. The study also revealed an increased size of salivary exosomes in oral cancer (98.3 ± 4.6 nm) compared to those in healthy individuals (67.4 ± 2.9 nm) ($p < 0.05$). These morphological aberrations indicate that some amount of salivary exosomes consist of tumor-derived exosomes that were directly released into saliva. Additionally, high-resolution AFM identified multivesicular bodies (MVBs) in oral cancer saliva (Fig. 6.4) [90]. The presence of membrane ruptures in MVBs indicates the sites for exosome release as well as filamentous extension of nucleic acids. The images from the above studies demonstrate salivary exosomes as potential indicators of oral cancer.

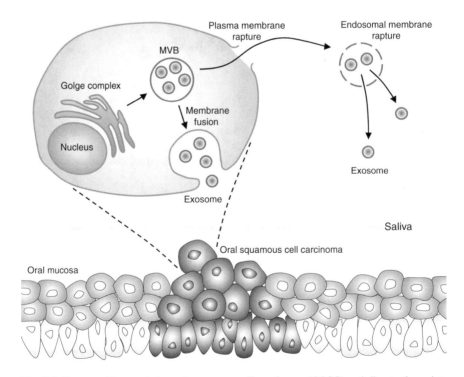

Fig. 6.4 Exosome biogenesis in oral squamous cell carcinoma (OSCC) and direct release into saliva. Exosomes are generated via the trans-Golgi network and accumulated in multivesicular body (MVB). Exosomes are released into saliva by two different mechanisms: constitutive release via membrane fusion or aberrant release via membrane rupture. (Reprinted with permission from [68]. Copyright 2017, Elsevier Inc.)

Conclusions and Future Perspectives

An increasing amount of evidence suggests the clinical utility of circulating bio-markers in patient stratification and monitoring of disease status. ctDNA that is actively released in plasma and saliva is preferred for the early detection of head and neck cancer, whereas CTCs from metastatic lesions can be used to predict poor prognosis. CTC analysis for the expression of surface molecules (e.g., EGFR, PD-L1) can provide critical information necessary for planning immunotherapy. Other circulating biomarkers such as exosomal miRNAs can provide additional lay-ers of information; thus, targeting multiple types of biomarkers that have indepen-dent mechanisms of release may increase the specificity and sensitivity of cancer diagnosis.

A key question concerning the circulating biomarkers (ctDNA, CTCs, and exo-somal miRNAs) is the extent to which they are representative of the whole tumor. In this regard, biomarkers should be assessed in terms of inclusivity of all tumor fea-tures. CTCs are unable to represent a heterogeneous tumor and this compromises their clinical relevance, despite being considered to have full cellular information. Exosomes are supposed to represent a large portion of the tumor, since they are believed to have originated from the whole tumor, reflecting the heterogeneous characteristic of the tumor. However, exosomal miRNAs are selectively assembled through the trans-Golgi network and can only represent a portion of the cellular miRNAs. Further studies with large patient cohorts using standardized protocols are required to determine whether each approach, individually as well as in combina-tion, can improve overall survival.

Simultaneous analysis of the circulating biomarkers in multiple body fluids is an ideal strategy to provide complementary information and represents a critical mile-stone toward the implementation of liquid biopsies in personalized medicine. Utilizing saliva is noninvasive and informative; thus, salivary diagnostics may fulfill the ambitions of precision medicine initiatives.

Saliva-exosomics is a term to describe next-generation salivaomics that studies salivary exosomes through the use of the advanced "omics" technologies to better delineate their specific functions and biomarkers [68]. In patients with cancer, saliva contains a unique set of the exosomes that originate from cancerous lesions (Fig. 6.5). This may be due to the processing and selection of cancer-derived exo-somes in the salivary glands. However, the amount and content of salivary exo-somes vary greatly, even in patients who have the same type of tumor and stage; thus there is a need for more in-depth understanding of salivary exosomes to estab-lish biomarkers and develop new therapeutic approaches.

Routine isolation and analysis of circulating biomarkers in the clinical setting is challenging. Establishing simple, rapid, and affordable technologies to analyze cir-culating biomarkers is essential for point-of-care application. Current technologies (e.g., ddPCR, next-generation sequencing) have faced drawbacks, such as high cost, long processing time, and complicated data manipulation. We have developed a novel saliva liquid biopsy technology termed electric field–induced release and

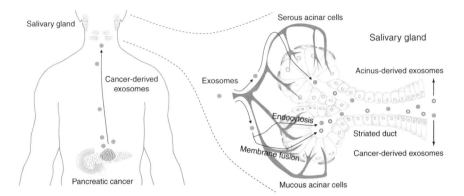

Fig. 6.5 Schematic representation of the exosome-mediated transfer of cancer-derived products from distal tumor to salivary gland tissue. Cancer-derived exosomes enter the circulation and reach the salivary glands. Exosome uptake at salivary gland acinar cells occurs via endocytosis or membrane fusion. Two different salivary exosomes are released into saliva. Cancer-derived exosomes are released through endocytosis followed by exocytosis at the opposite luminal membrane, while acinus-derived exosomes are released through fusion of MVBs with the plasma membrane. Both types of salivary exosomes carry cargos that include cancer-derived products. (Reprinted with permission from [68]. Copyright 2017, Elsevier Inc.)

measurement (EFIRM), which can detect minute amounts of ctDNA and RNA directly, only requiring 40 μL of saliva [91–93]. Combining this electrochemical sensing technology and other outstanding components (e.g., rapid biomarker isolation techniques) is desirable for efficient detection of circulating biomarkers, facilitating the development of point-of-care devices for routine clinical use.

Acknowledgments The work was supported by National Institutes of Health grants UH2/UH3 CA206126, U01 CA233370, and U01 DE017790 to D.T.W.W.; DE027759 and DE029272 to T.N.

Conflicts of Interest D.T.W.W. is a consultant to Liquid Diagnostics, GlaxoSmithKline, Wrigley, and Colgate-Palmolive.

References

1. Bray F, Ferlay J, Soerjomataram I, Siegel RL, Torre LA, Jemal A. Global cancer statistics 2018: GLOBOCAN estimates of incidence and mortality worldwide for 36 cancers in 185 countries. CA Cancer J Clin. 2018;68:394–424.
2. Gerlinger M, Rowan AJ, Horswell S, Math M, Larkin J, Endesfelder D, Gronroos E, Martinez P, Matthews N, Stewart A, Tarpey P, Varela I, Phillimore B, Begum S, McDonald NQ, Butler A, Jones D, Raine K, Latimer C, Santos CR, Nohadani M, Eklund AC, Spencer-Dene B, Clark G, Pickering L, Stamp G, Gore M, Szallasi Z, Downward J, Futreal PA, Swanton C. Intratumor heterogeneity and branched evolution revealed by multiregion sequencing. N Engl J Med. 2012;366:883–92.

3. Nonaka T, Wong DTW. Liquid biopsy in head and neck cancer: promises and challenges. J Dent Res. 2018;97:701–8.
4. Siravegna G, Marsoni S, Siena S, Bardelli A. Integrating liquid biopsies into the management of cancer. Nat Rev Clin Oncol. 2017;14:531–48.
5. Weber JA, Baxter DH, Zhang S, Huang DY, Huang KH, Lee MJ, Galas DJ, Wang K. The microRNA spectrum in 12 body fluids. Clin Chem. 2010;56:1733–41.
6. Leon SA, Shapiro B, Sklaroff DM, Yaros MJ. Free DNA in the serum of cancer patients and the effect of therapy. Cancer Res. 1977;37:646–50.
7. Sorenson GD, Pribish DM, Valone FH, Memoli VA, Bzik DJ, Yao SL. Soluble normal and mutated DNA sequences from single-copy genes in human blood. Cancer Epidemiol Biomark Prev. 1994;3:67–71.
8. Vasioukhin V, Anker P, Maurice P, Lyautey J, Lederrey C, Stroun M. Point mutations of the N-ras gene in the blood plasma DNA of patients with myelodysplastic syndrome or acute myelogenous leukaemia. Br J Haematol. 1994;86:774–9.
9. Newman AM, Bratman SV, To J, Wynne JF, Eclov NC, Modlin LA, Liu CL, Neal JW, Wakelee HA, Merritt RE, Shrager JB, Loo BW Jr, Alizadeh AA, Diehn M. An ultrasensitive method for quantitating circulating tumor DNA with broad patient coverage. Nat Med. 2014;20:548–54.
10. Beaver JA, Jelovac D, Balukrishna S, Cochran R, Croessmann S, Zabransky DJ, Wong HY, Toro PV, Cidado J, Blair BG, Chu D, Burns T, Higgins MJ, Stearns V, Jacobs L, Habibi M, Lange J, Hurley PJ, Lauring J, VanDenBerg D, Kessler J, Jeter S, Samuels ML, Maar D, Cope L, Cimino-Mathews A, Argani P, Wolff AC, Park BH. Detection of cancer DNA in plasma of patients with early-stage breast cancer. Clin Cancer Res. 2014;20:2643–50.
11. Bettegowda C, Sausen M, Leary RJ, Kinde I, Wang Y, Agrawal N, Bartlett BR, Wang H, Luber B, Alani RM, Antonarakis ES, Azad NS, Bardelli A, Brem H, Cameron JL, Lee CC, Fecher LA, Gallia GL, Gibbs P, Le D, Giuntoli RL, Goggins M, Hogarty MD, Holdhoff M, Hong SM, Jiao Y, Juhl HH, Kim JJ, Siravegna G, Laheru DA, Lauricella C, Lim M, Lipson EJ, Marie SK, Netto GJ, Oliner KS, Olivi A, Olsson L, Riggins GJ, Sartore-Bianchi A, Schmidt K, Shihl M, Oba-Shinjo SM, Siena S, Theodorescu D, Tie J, Harkins TT, Veronese S, Wang TL, Weingart JD, Wolfgang CL, Wood LD, Xing D, Hruban RH, Wu J, Allen PJ, Schmidt CM, Choti MA, Velculescu VE, Kinzler KW, Vogelstein B, Papadopoulos N, Diaz LA Jr. Detection of circulating tumor DNA in early- and late-stage human malignancies. Sci Transl Med. 2014;6:224ra24.
12. Diehl F, Schmidt K, Choti MA, Romans K, Goodman S, Li M, Thornton K, Agrawal N, Sokoll L, Szabo SA, Kinzler KW, Vogelstein B, Diaz LA Jr. Circulating mutant DNA to assess tumor dynamics. Nat Med. 2008;14:985–90.
13. Thierry AR, Mouliere F, El Messaoudi S, Mollevi C, Lopez-Crapez E, Rolet F, Gillet B, Gongora C, Dechelotte P, Robert B, Del Rio M, Lamy PJ, Bibeau F, Nouaille M, Loriot V, Jarrousse AS, Molina F, Mathonnet M, Pezet D, Ychou M. Clinical validation of the detection of KRAS and BRAF mutations from circulating tumor DNA. Nat Med. 2014;20:430–5.
14. Wang Y, Springer S, Mulvey CL, Silliman N, Schaefer J, Sausen M, James N, Rettig EM, Guo T, Pickering CR, Bishop JA, Chung CH, Califano JA, Eisele DW, Fakhry C, Gourin CG, Ha PK, Kang H, Kiess A, Koch WM, Myers JN, Quon H, Richmon JD, Sidransky D, Tufano RP, Westra WH, Bettegowda C, Diaz LA Jr, Papadopoulos N, Kinzler KW, Vogelstein B, Agrawal N. Detection of somatic mutations and HPV in the saliva and plasma of patients with head and neck squamous cell carcinomas. Sci Transl Med. 2015;7:293ra104.
15. Leemans CR, Braakhuis BJ, Brakenhoff RH. The molecular biology of head and neck cancer. Nat Rev Cancer. 2011;11:9–22.
16. The Cancer Genome Atlas Network. Comprehensive genomic characterization of head and neck squamous cell carcinomas. Nature. 2015;517:576–82.
17. Chan KC, Hung EC, Woo JK, Chan PK, Leung SF, Lai FP, Cheng AS, Yeung SW, Chan YW, Tsui TK, Kwok JS, King AD, Chan AT, van Hasselt AC, Lo YM. Early detection of nasopharyngeal carcinoma by plasma Epstein-Barr virus DNA analysis in a surveillance program. Cancer. 2013;119:1838–44.
18. Chan KCA, Woo JKS, King A, Zee BCY, Lam WKJ, Chan SL, Chu SWI, Mak C, Tse IOL, Leung SYM, Chan G, Hui EP, Ma BBY, Chiu RWK, Leung SF, van Hasselt AC, Chan ATC,

Lo YMD. Analysis of plasma Epstein-Barr virus DNA to screen for nasopharyngeal cancer. N Engl J Med. 2017;377:513–22.

19. Alix-Panabieres C, Pantel K. Clinical applications of circulating tumor cells and circulating tumor DNA as liquid biopsy. Cancer Discov. 2016;6:479–91.

20. He S, Li P, Long T, Zhang N, Fang J, Yu Z. Detection of circulating tumour cells with the CellSearch system in patients with advanced-stage head and neck cancer: preliminary results. J Laryngol Otol. 2013;127:788–93.

21. Nichols AC, Lowes LE, Szeto CC, Basmaji J, Dhaliwal S, Chapeskie C, Todorovic B, Read N, Venkatesan V, Hammond A, Palma DA, Winquist E, Ernst S, Fung K, Franklin JH, Yoo J, Koropatnick J, Mymryk JS, Barrett JW, Allan AL. Detection of circulating tumor cells in advanced head and neck cancer using the CellSearch system. Head Neck. 2012;34:1440–4.

22. Buglione M, Grisanti S, Almici C, Mangoni M, Polli C, Consoli F, Verardi R, Costa L, Paiar F, Pasinetti N, Bolzoni A, Marini M, Simoncini E, Nicolai P, Biti G, Magrini SM. Circulating tumour cells in locally advanced head and neck cancer: preliminary report about their possible role in predicting response to non-surgical treatment and survival. Eur J Cancer. 2012;48:3019–26.

23. Grobe A, Blessmann M, Hanken H, Friedrich RE, Schon G, Wikner J, Effenberger KE, Kluwe L, Heiland M, Pantel K, Riethdorf S. Prognostic relevance of circulating tumor cells in blood and disseminated tumor cells in bone marrow of patients with squamous cell carcinoma of the oral cavity. Clin Cancer Res. 2014;20:425–33.

24. Jatana KR, Lang JC, Chalmers JJ. Identification of circulating tumor cells: a prognostic marker in squamous cell carcinoma of the head and neck? Future Oncol. 2011;7:481–4.

25. Bonner JA, Harari PM, Giralt J, Azarnia N, Shin DM, Cohen RB, Jones CU, Sur R, Raben D, Jassem J, Ove R, Kies MS, Baselga J, Youssoufian H, Amellal N, Rowinsky EK, Ang KK. Radiotherapy plus cetuximab for squamous-cell carcinoma of the head and neck. N Engl J Med. 2006;354:567–78.

26. Vermorken JB, Mesia R, Rivera F, Remenar E, Kawecki A, Rottey S, Erfan J, Zabolotnyy D, Kienzer HR, Cupissol D, Peyrade F, Benasso M, Vynnychenko I, De Raucourt D, Bokemeyer C, Schueler A, Amellal N, Hitt R. Platinum-based chemotherapy plus cetuximab in head and neck cancer. N Engl J Med. 2008;359:1116–27.

27. Tinhofer I, Hristozova T, Stromberger C, Keilhoiz U, Budach V. Monitoring of circulating tumor cells and their expression of EGFR/phospho-EGFR during combined radiotherapy regimens in locally advanced squamous cell carcinoma of the head and neck. Int J Radiat Oncol Biol Phys. 2012;83:e685–90.

28. Braig F, Voigtlaender M, Schieferdecker A, Busch CJ, Laban S, Grob T, Kriegs M, Knecht R, Bokemeyer C, Binder M. Liquid biopsy monitoring uncovers acquired RAS-mediated resistance to cetuximab in a substantial proportion of patients with head and neck squamous cell carcinoma. Oncotarget. 2016;7:42988–95.

29. Baumeister SH, Freeman GJ, Dranoff G, Sharpe AH. Coinhibitory pathways in immunotherapy for Cancer. Annu Rev Immunol. 2016;34:539–73.

30. Butt AQ, Mills KH. Immunosuppressive networks and checkpoints controlling antitumor immunity and their blockade in the development of cancer immunotherapeutics and vaccines. Oncogene. 2014;33:4623–31.

31. Mazel M, Jacot W, Pantel K, Bartkowiak K, Topart D, Cayrefourcq L, Rossille D, Maudelonde T, Fest T, Alix-Panabieres C. Frequent expression of PD-L1 on circulating breast cancer cells. Mol Oncol. 2015;9:1773–82.

32. Boffa DJ, Graf RP, Salazar MC, Hoag J, Lu D, Krupa R, Louw J, Dugan L, Wang Y, Landers M, Suraneni M, Greene SB, Magana M, Makani S, Bazhenova L, Dittamore RV, Nieva J. Cellular expression of PD-L1 in the peripheral blood of lung cancer patients is associated with worse survival. Cancer Epidemiol Biomark Prev. 2017;26:1139–45.

33. Anantharaman A, Friedlander T, Lu D, Krupa R, Premasekharan G, Hough J, Edwards M, Paz R, Lindquist K, Graf R, Jendrisak A, Louw J, Dugan L, Baird S, Wang Y, Dittamore R, Paris PL. Programmed death-ligand 1 (PD-L1) characterization of circulating tumor cells (CTCs) in muscle invasive and metastatic bladder cancer patients. BMC Cancer. 2016;16:744.

34. Satelli A, Batth IS, Brownlee Z, Rojas C, Meng QH, Kopetz S, Li S. Potential role of nuclear PD-L1 expression in cell-surface vimentin positive circulating tumor cells as a prognostic marker in cancer patients. Sci Rep. 2016;6:28910.
35. Strati A, Koutsodontis G, Papaxoinis G, Angelidis I, Zavridou M, Economopoulou P, Kotsantis I, Avgeris M, Mazel M, Perisanidis C, Sasaki C, Alix-Panabieres C, Lianidou E, Psyrri A. Prognostic significance of PD-L1 expression on circulating tumor cells in patients with head and neck squamous cell carcinoma. Ann Oncol. 2017;28:1923–33.
36. Oliveira-Costa JP, de Carvalho AF, da Silveira da GG, Amaya P, Wu Y, Park KJ, Gigliola MP, Lustberg M, Buim ME, Ferreira EN, Kowalski LP, Chalmers JJ, Soares FA, Carraro DM, Ribeiro-Silva A. Gene expression patterns through oral squamous cell carcinoma development: PD-L1 expression in primary tumor and circulating tumor cells. Oncotarget. 2015;6:20902–20.
37. Kulasinghe A, Perry C, Kenny L, Warkiani ME, Nelson C, Punyadeera C. PD-L1 expressing circulating tumour cells in head and neck cancers. BMC Cancer. 2017;17:333.
38. Riethdorf S, Fritsche H, Muller V, Rau T, Schindlbeck C, Rack B, Janni W, Coith C, Beck K, Janicke F, Jackson S, Gornet T, Cristofanilli M, Pantel K. Detection of circulating tumor cells in peripheral blood of patients with metastatic breast cancer: a validation study of the CellSearch system. Clin Cancer Res. 2007;13:920–8.
39. Haber DA, Velculescu VE. Blood-based analyses of cancer: circulating tumor cells and circulating tumor DNA. Cancer Discov. 2014;4:650–61.
40. Dawson SJ, Tsui DW, Murtaza M, Biggs H, Rueda OM, Chin SF, Dunning MJ, Gale D, Forshew T, Mahler-Araujo B, Rajan S, Humphray S, Becq J, Halsall D, Wallis M, Bentley D, Caldas C, Rosenfeld N. Analysis of circulating tumor DNA to monitor metastatic breast cancer. N Engl J Med. 2013;368:1199–209.
41. Wang WY, Twu CW, Chen HH, Jan JS, Jiang RS, Chao JY, Liang KL, Chen KW, Wu CT, Lin JC. Plasma EBV DNA clearance rate as a novel prognostic marker for metastatic/recurrent nasopharyngeal carcinoma. Clin Cancer Res. 2010;16:1016–24.
42. Reinert T, Scholer LV, Thomsen R, Tobiasen H, Vang S, Nordentoft I, Lamy P, Kannerup AS, Mortensen FV, Stribolt K, Hamilton-Dutoit S, Nielsen HJ, Laurberg S, Pallisgaard N, Pedersen JS, Orntoft TF, Andersen CL. Analysis of circulating tumour DNA to monitor disease burden following colorectal cancer surgery. Gut. 2016;65:625–34.
43. Tie J, Wang Y, Tomasetti C, Li L, Springer S, Kinde I, Silliman N, Tacey M, Wong HL, Christie M, Kosmider S, Skinner I, Wong R, Steel M, Tran B, Desai J, Jones I, Haydon A, Hayes T, Price TJ, Strausberg RL, Diaz LA Jr, Papadopoulos N, Kinzler KW, Vogelstein B, Gibbs P. Circulating tumor DNA analysis detects minimal residual disease and predicts recurrence in patients with stage II colon cancer. Sci Transl Med. 2016;8:346ra92.
44. Garcia-Murillas I, Schiavon G, Weigelt B, Ng C, Hrebien S, Cutts RJ, Cheang M, Osin P, Nerurkar A, Kozarewa I, Garrido JA, Dowsett M, Reis-Filho JS, Smith IE, Turner NC. Mutation tracking in circulating tumor DNA predicts relapse in early breast cancer. Sci Transl Med. 2015;7:302ra133.
45. Lebofsky R, Decraene C, Bernard V, Kamal M, Blin A, Leroy Q, Rio Frio T, Pierron G, Callens C, Bieche I, Saliou A, Madic J, Rouleau E, Bidard FC, Lantz O, Stern MH, Le Tourneau C, Pierga JY. Circulating tumor DNA as a non-invasive substitute to metastasis biopsy for tumor genotyping and personalized medicine in a prospective trial across all tumor types. Mol Oncol. 2015;9:783–90.
46. Groot Koerkamp B, Rahbari NN, Buchler MW, Koch M, Weitz J. Circulating tumor cells and prognosis of patients with resectable colorectal liver metastases or widespread metastatic colorectal cancer: a meta-analysis. Ann Surg Oncol. 2013;20:2156–65.
47. Ma X, Xiao Z, Li X, Wang F, Zhang J, Zhou R, Wang J, Liu L. Prognostic role of circulating tumor cells and disseminated tumor cells in patients with prostate cancer: a systematic review and meta-analysis. Tumour Biol. 2014;35:5551–60.
48. Wang S, Zheng G, Cheng B, Chen F, Wang Z, Chen Y, Wang Y, Xiong B. Circulating tumor cells (CTCs) detected by RT-PCR and its prognostic role in gastric cancer: a meta-analysis of published literature. PLoS One. 2014;9:e99259.

49. Jatana KR, Balasubramanian P, Lang JC, Yang L, Jatana CA, White E, Agrawal A, Ozer E, Schuller DE, Teknos TN, Chalmers JJ. Significance of circulating tumor cells in patients with squamous cell carcinoma of the head and neck: initial results. Arch Otolaryngol Head Neck Surg. 2010;136:1274–9.
50. Kulasinghe A, Perry C, Jovanovic L, Nelson C, Punyadeera C. Circulating tumour cells in metastatic head and neck cancers. Int J Cancer. 2015;136:2515–23.
51. Hristozova T, Konschak R, Stromberger C, Fusi A, Liu Z, Weichert W, Stenzinger A, Budach V, Keilholz U, Tinhofer I. The presence of circulating tumor cells (CTCs) correlates with lymph node metastasis in nonresectable squamous cell carcinoma of the head and neck region (SCCHN). Ann Oncol. 2011;22:1878–85.
52. Toss A, Mu Z, Fernandez S. Cristofanilli M. CTC enumeration and characterization: moving toward personalized medicine. Ann Transl Med. 2014;2:108.
53. de Albuquerque A, Kaul S, Breier G, Krabisch P, Fersis N. Multimarker analysis of circulating tumor cells in peripheral blood of metastatic breast cancer patients: a step forward in personalized medicine. Breast Care (Basel). 2012;7:7–12.
54. Simons M, Raposo G. Exosomes--vesicular carriers for intercellular communication. Curr Opin Cell Biol. 2009;21:575–81.
55. Chen X, Liang H, Zhang J, Zen K, Zhang CY. Secreted microRNAs: a new form of intercellular communication. Trends Cell Biol. 2012;22:125–32.
56. Mitchell PS, Parkin RK, Kroh EM, Fritz BR, Wyman SK, Pogosova-Agadjanyan EL, Peterson A, Noteboom J, O'Briant KC, Allen A, Lin DW, Urban N, Drescher CW, Knudsen BS, Stirewalt DL, Gentleman R, Vessella RL, Nelson PS, Martin DB, Tewari M. Circulating microRNAs as stable blood-based markers for cancer detection. Proc Natl Acad Sci U S A. 2008;105:10513–8.
57. Rosenfeld N, Aharonov R, Meiri E, Rosenwald S, Spector Y, Zepeniuk M, Benjamin H, Shabes N, Tabak S, Levy A, Lebanony D, Goren Y, Silberschein E, Targan N, Ben-Ari A, Gilad S, Sion-Vardy N, Tobar A, Feinmesser M, Kharenko O, Nativ O, Nass D, Perelman M, Yosepovich A, Shalmon B, Polak-Charcon S, Fridman E, Avniel A, Bentwich I, Bentwich Z, Cohen D, Chajut A, Barshack I. MicroRNAs accurately identify cancer tissue origin. Nat Biotechnol. 2008;26:462–9.
58. Rabinowits G, Gercel-Taylor C, Day JM, Taylor DD, Kloecker GH. Exosomal microRNA: a diagnostic marker for lung cancer. Clin Lung Cancer. 2009;10:42–6.
59. Skog J, Wurdinger T, van Rijn S, Meijer DH, Gainche L, Sena-Esteves M, Curry WT Jr, Carter BS, Krichevsky AM, Breakefield XO. Glioblastoma microvesicles transport RNA and proteins that promote tumour growth and provide diagnostic biomarkers. Nat Cell Biol. 2008;10:1470–6.
60. Taylor DD, Gercel-Taylor C. MicroRNA signatures of tumor-derived exosomes as diagnostic biomarkers of ovarian cancer. Gynecol Oncol. 2008;110:13–21.
61. Summerer I, Unger K, Braselmann H, Schuettrumpf L, Maihoefer C, Baumeister P, Kirchner T, Niyazi M, Sage E, Specht HM, Multhoff G, Moertl S, Belka C, Zitzelsberger H. Circulating microRNAs as prognostic therapy biomarkers in head and neck cancer patients. Br J Cancer. 2015;113:76–82.
62. Hsu CM, Lin PM, Wang YM, Chen ZJ, Lin SF, Yang MY. Circulating miRNA is a novel marker for head and neck squamous cell carcinoma. Tumour Biol. 2012;33:1933–42.
63. Liu CJ, Kao SY, Tu HF, Tsai MM, Chang KW, Lin SC. Increase of microRNA miR-31 level in plasma could be a potential marker of oral cancer. Oral Dis. 2010;16:360–4.
64. Yan Y, Wang X, Veno MT, Bakholdt V, Sorensen JA, Krogdahl A, Sun Z, Gao S, Kjems J. Circulating miRNAs as biomarkers for oral squamous cell carcinoma recurrence in operated patients. Oncotarget. 2017;8:8206–14.
65. Russo F, Di Bella S, Vannini F, Berti G, Scoyni F, Cook HV, Santos A, Nigita G, Bonnici V, Lagana A, Geraci F, Pulvirenti A, Giugno R, De Masi F, Belling K, Jensen LJ, Brunak S, Pellegrini M, Ferro A. miRandola 2017: a curated knowledge base of non-invasive biomarkers. Nucleic Acids Res. 2018;46:D354–D9.

66. Ono S, Lam S, Nagahara M, Hoon DS. Circulating microRNA biomarkers as liquid biopsy for cancer patients: Pros and Cons of current assays. J Clin Med. 2015;4:1890–907.
67. Pritchard CC, Kroh E, Wood B, Arroyo JD, Dougherty KJ, Miyaji MM, Tait JF, Tewari M. Blood cell origin of circulating microRNAs: a cautionary note for cancer biomarker studies. Cancer Prev Res (Phila). 2012;5:492–7.
68. Nonaka T, Wong DTW. Saliva-Exosomics in cancer: molecular characterization of cancer-derived exosomes in saliva. Enzyme. 2017;42:125–51.
69. Bandhakavi S, Stone MD, Onsongo G, Van Riper SK. Griffin TJ. A dynamic range compression and three-dimensional peptide fractionation analysis platform expands proteome coverage and the diagnostic potential of whole saliva. J Proteome Res. 2009;8:5590–600.
70. Yan W, Apweiler R, Balgley BM, Boontheung P, Bundy JL, Cargile BJ, Cole S, Fang X, Gonzalez-Begne M, Griffin TJ, Hagen F, Hu S, Wolinsky LE, Lee CS, Malamud D, Melvin JE, Menon R, Mueller M, Qiao R, Rhodus NL, Sevinsky JR, States D, Stephenson JL, Than S, Yates JR, Yu W, Xie H, Xie Y, Omenn GS, Loo JA, Wong DT. Systematic comparison of the human saliva and plasma proteomes. Proteomics Clin Appl. 2009;3:116–34.
71. Rylander-Rudqvist T, Hakansson N, Tybring G, Wolk A. Quality and quantity of saliva DNA obtained from the self-administered oragene method--a pilot study on the cohort of Swedish men. Cancer Epidemiol Biomark Prev. 2006;15:1742–5.
72. Qureishi A, Ali M, Fraser L, Shah KA, Moller H, Winter S. Saliva testing for human papilloma virus in oropharyngeal squamous cell carcinoma: a diagnostic accuracy study. Clin Otolaryngol. 2018;43:151–7.
73. Martin-Gomez L, Giuliano AR, Fulp WJ, Caudell J, Echevarria M, Sirak B, Abrahamsen M, Isaacs-Soriano KA, Hernandez-Prera JC, Wenig BM, Vorwald K, McMullen CP, Wadsworth JT, Slebos RJ, Chung CH. Human papillomavirus genotype detection in oral gargle samples among men with newly diagnosed oropharyngeal squamous cell carcinoma. JAMA Otolaryngol Head Neck Surg. 2019;145:460.
74. Ahn SM, Chan JY, Zhang Z, Wang H, Khan Z, Bishop JA, Westra W, Koch WM, Califano JA. Saliva and plasma quantitative polymerase chain reaction-based detection and surveillance of human papillomavirus-related head and neck cancer. JAMA Otolaryngol Head Neck Surg. 2014;140:846–54.
75. Rettig EM, Wentz A, Posner MR, Gross ND, Haddad RI, Gillison ML, Fakhry C, Quon H, Sikora AG, Stott WJ, Lorch JH, Gourin CG, Guo Y, Xiao W, Miles BA, Richmon JD, Andersen PE, Misiukiewicz KJ, Chung CH, Gerber JE, Rajan SD, D'Souza G. Prognostic implication of persistent human papillomavirus type 16 DNA detection in oral rinses for human papillomavirus-related oropharyngeal carcinoma. JAMA Oncol. 2015;1:907–15.
76. Park NJ, Zhou H, Elashoff D, Henson BS, Kastratovic DA, Abemayor E, Wong DT. Salivary microRNA: discovery, characterization, and clinical utility for oral cancer detection. Clin Cancer Res. 2009;15:5473–7.
77. Gallo A, Tandon M, Alevizos I, Illei GG. The majority of microRNAs detectable in serum and saliva is concentrated in exosomes. PLoS One. 2012;7:e30679.
78. Michael A, Bajracharya SD, Yuen PS, Zhou H, Star RA, Illei GG, Alevizos I. Exosomes from human saliva as a source of microRNA biomarkers. Oral Dis. 2010;16:34–8.
79. Duz MB, Karatas OF, Guzel E, Turgut NF, Yilmaz M, Creighton CJ, Ozen M. Identification of miR-139-5p as a saliva biomarker for tongue squamous cell carcinoma: a pilot study. Cell Oncol (Dordr). 2016;39:187–93.
80. Wiklund ED, Gao S, Hulf T, Sibbritt T, Nair S, Costea DE, Villadsen SB, Bakholdt V, Bramsen JB, Sorensen JA, Krogdahl A, Clark SJ, Kjems J. MicroRNA alterations and associated aberrant DNA methylation patterns across multiple sample types in oral squamous cell carcinoma. PLoS One. 2011;6:e27840.
81. Liu CJ, Lin SC, Yang CC, Cheng HW, Chang KW. Exploiting salivary miR-31 as a clinical biomarker of oral squamous cell carcinoma. Head Neck. 2012;34:219–24.
82. Momen-Heravi F, Trachtenberg AJ, Kuo WP, Cheng YS. Genomewide study of salivary microRNAs for detection of oral cancer. J Dent Res. 2014;93:86S–93S.

83. Gonzalez-Begne M, Lu B, Han X, Hagen FK, Hand AR, Melvin JE, Yates JR. Proteomic analysis of human parotid gland exosomes by multidimensional protein identification technology (MudPIT). J Proteome Res. 2009;8:1304–14.

84. Ogawa Y, Miura Y, Harazono A, Kanai-Azuma M, Akimoto Y, Kawakami H, Yamaguchi T, Toda T, Endo T, Tsubuki M, Yanoshita R. Proteomic analysis of two types of exosomes in human whole saliva. Biol Pharm Bull. 2011;34:13–23.

85. Kalra H, Simpson RJ, Ji H, Aikawa E, Altevogt P, Askenase P, Bond VC, Borras FE, Breakefield X, Budnik V, Buzas E, Camussi G, Clayton A, Cocucci E, Falcon-Perez JM, Gabrielsson S, Gho YS, Gupta D, Harsha HC, Hendrix A, Hill AF, Inal JM, Jenster G, Kramer-Albers EM, Lim SK, Llorente A, Lotvall J, Marcilla A, Mincheva-Nilsson L, Nazarenko I, Nieuwland R, Nolte-'t Hoen EN, Pandey A, Patel T, Piper MG, Pluchino S, Prasad TS, Rajendran L, Raposo G, Record M, Reid GE, Sanchez-Madrid F, Schiffelers RM, Siljander P, Stensballe A, Stoorvogel W, Taylor D, Thery C, Valadi H, van Balkom BW, Vazquez J, Vidal M, Wauben MH, Yanez-Mo M, Zoeller M, Mathivanan S. Vesiclepedia: a compendium for extracellular vesicles with continuous community annotation. PLoS Biol. 2012;10:e1001450.

86. Simpson RJ, Kalra H, Mathivanan S. ExoCarta as a resource for exosomal research. J Extracell Vesicles. 2012:1.

87. Cheng J, Nonaka T, Wong DTW. Salivary exosomes as nanocarriers for cancer biomarker delivery. Materials (Basel). 2019;12:654.

88. Palanisamy V, Sharma S, Deshpande A, Zhou H, Gimzewski J, Wong DT. Nanostructural and transcriptomic analyses of human saliva derived exosomes. PLoS One. 2010;5:e8577.

89. Sharma S, Rasool HI, Palanisamy V, Mathisen C, Schmidt M, Wong DT, Gimzewski JK. Structural-mechanical characterization of nanoparticle exosomes in human saliva, using correlative AFM, FESEM, and force spectroscopy. ACS Nano. 2010;4:1921–6.

90. Sharma S, Gillespie BM, Palanisamy V, Gimzewski JK. Quantitative nanostructural and single-molecule force spectroscopy biomolecular analysis of human-saliva-derived exosomes. Langmuir. 2011;27:14394–400.

91. Pu D, Liang H, Wei F, Akin D, Feng Z, Yan Q, Li Y, Zhen Y, Xu L, Dong G, Wan H, Dong J, Qiu X, Qin C, Zhu D, Wang X, Sun T, Zhang W, Li C, Tang X, Qiao Y, Wong DT, Zhou Q. Evaluation of a novel saliva-based epidermal growth factor receptor mutation detection for lung cancer: a pilot study. Thorac Cancer. 2016;7:428–36.

92. Tu M, Wei F, Yang J, Wong D. Detection of exosomal biomarker by electric field-induced release and measurement (EFIRM). J Vis Exp. 2015:52439.

93. Wei F, Lin CC, Joon A, Feng Z, Troche G, Lira ME, Chia D, Mao M, Ho CL, Su WC, Wong DT. Noninvasive saliva-based EGFR gene mutation detection in patients with lung cancer. Am J Respir Crit Care Med. 2014;190:1117–26.

Chapter 7
Proinflammatory Signaling Pathways and Genomic Signatures in Head and Neck Cancers

Zhong Chen, Ramya Viswanathan, Ethan L. Morgan, Jun Jeon, and Carter Van Waes

Introduction

Deregulation of inflammatory and immune responses has been observed and recognized as important in the pathogenesis and therapeutic resistance of cancer, including head and neck cancers (HNCs). Among HNCs, head and neck squamous cell carcinomas (HNSCCs) account for ~90% of these cancers histologically and have been most broadly studied. Subsets of HNSCCs and other HNCs aberrantly express a repertoire of cytokines, chemokines, and soluble factors that promote tumor cell growth, survival, migration, as well as inflammatory and angiogenic responses in the tumor microenvironment (TME) that enhance tumorigenesis. Among these, interleukin-1 (IL-1) expressed by tumor cells and tumor necrosis factor (TNF) expressed in the TME by immune and other cells induce the activation of NF-κB, a family of transcription factors that regulate the expression of additional cytokines and other mediators of the malignant phenotype and deregulated immune responses. Dissection of signaling pathways and genomic alterations in HNSCCs and other HNCs reveals that many of these converge upon NF-κB and other transcription factors that regulate multiple genes and features of the malignant phenotype, identifying pathways of interest. Protein ubiquitination and the proteasome play a key role in regulating NF-κB, and are among targets of genomic or other alterations, and thus may be potential therapeutic targets. The Cancer Genome Atlas (TCGA) and genomic characterization of libraries of cell lines and patient-derived xenograft models have identified several key, recurrent alterations affecting these pathways that can enable mechanistic and preclinical studies to identify new therapeutic

Z. Chen (✉) · R. Viswanathan · E. L. Morgan · J. Jeon · C. Van Waes (✉)
Tumor Biology Section, Head and Neck Surgery Branch, National Institute on Deafness and Other Communication Disorders, National Institutes of Health, Bethesda, MD, USA
e-mail: chenz@nidcd.nih.gov; vanwaesc@nidcd.nih.gov

© Springer Nature Switzerland AG 2021
R. El Assal et al. (eds.), *Early Detection and Treatment of Head & Neck Cancers*, https://doi.org/10.1007/978-3-030-69852-2_7

targets. Functional genomics using RNAi, CRISPR, and drug libraries can be integrated with these findings to identify drivers and mediators that represent key targets for therapy. In this chapter, we have summarized the discovery history and current advances in understanding HNSCC, focusing on proinflammatory signaling pathways and genomic signatures. The topics include (1) the networks of proinflammatory cytokines, chemokines, and growth factors, focusing on their roles in HNSCC pathogenesis, co-expression patterns, clinical correlates, and therapeutic potential; (2) NF-κB signaling and the crosstalk with other pathways and related current biomarker identification and drug development; (3) regulation of inflammatory signaling by ubiquitination, the association with genomic alterations and transcriptomic expression, and recent developments in drug discovery; and (4) genomic signatures and transcriptomic landscapes of proinflammatory and other signaling molecules, including overview of HNSCC TCGA and Pan TCGA projects, high-throughput characterization of human cell lines, and genome-wide gene perturbation and functional analyses. Advances in cutting-edge experimental technologies, such as high-throughput sequencing, single-cell partition, and multiplex staining and imaging, plus big data collection, computation pipelines, and bioinformatics proficiency have empowered us to precisely understand and construct the molecular atlas of HNSCC in an unprecedented magnitude and depth. The comprehensive characterization of cancers has significantly influenced how we classify HNSCC into molecular subtypes and changed our clinical practice for patient diagnosis, prognosis, and therapy.

Networks of Proinflammatory Cytokines, Chemokines, and Growth Factors

Malignant and stromal cells secrete cytokines, chemokines, and other soluble factors that play a critical role in the promotion of cell growth, survival, inflammation, migration, angiogenesis, therapeutic resistance, and other complex interactions in the TME [1–4] (Fig. 7.1). These factors contribute to the phenotype of HNC through proinflammatory signaling within its local and the systemic environment. This section summarizes the role of these factors in HNC development, prognosis, and response to treatments, which may help investigators elucidate potential targets that may synergize with existing targeted and immune-based therapies.

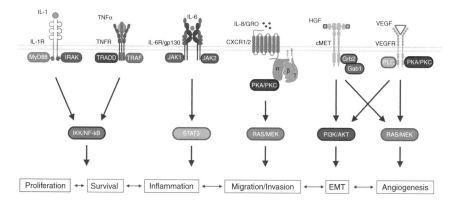

Fig. 7.1 Networks of proinflammatory cytokines, chemokines, and growth factors in HNSCC. The proinflammatory and proangiogenic cytokines, chemokines, and growth factors are produced by cancer, inflammatory, or stromal cells in the tumor microenvironment. Their receptors are structured with distinct extracellular domains for ligand binding and intracellular domains that mediate signal transduction. Interleukin-1a or interleukin-b binds to interleukin-1 receptor (IL-1R1) extracellular immunoglobulin domains and transduces intracellular signaling via MyD88 and IRAK to activate IKK and NF-kB pathway. TNFα binds to the trimeric TNF receptor (TNFR) and mediates signaling via the receptor's death domain (DD) through TRADD and TRAFs. Multimeric structure of IL-6 receptor (IL-6R) is comprised of IL-6R chains complexed with gp130, which mediates signaling through JAK1/2 and activates the STAT3 pathway. IL-8 or GRO binds to CXCR1/2, which are seven-transmembrane G protein-coupled receptors (Gα, β, γ), that mediate signaling through protein kinase A and protein kinase C (PKA/C) to activate RAS/MEK pathways. Binding of HGF to c-MET elicits downstream signaling mediated by adaptor proteins, Gab1 and Grb2, to activate PI3K/AKT and RAS/MEK pathways. The binding of VEGF to VEGFR leads to formation of receptor dimer and then activates the phospholipases C (PLC) and PKA/C, which mediate signaling through RAS/MEK and PI3K/AKT pathways. The activation of these signaling pathways collectively promotes oncogenesis of HNSCC, through enhanced cell proliferation, survival, inflammation, migration, invasion, EMT, and angiogenesis. (Figure was created using BioRender.com.)

Role of Interleukins, Chemokines, and Growth Factors in HNC Pathogenesis

Soluble factors that can transmit inflammatory signals include a variety of different classes of signaling molecules, which are small proteins secreted and used by immune, stromal, and epithelial cells in the TME to regulate immune and inflammatory responses. As the receptors for the same signaling molecule may be located in various compartments of TME, understanding their parallel and overlapping downstream effects in both the tumor and immune cell populations may have important implications for multi-targeting of therapy. Notable families of inflammatory and growth mediators are cytokines called interleukins (IL) and members of tumor necrosis factor (TNF), chemokine, and growth factor receptor tyrosine kinase families (Fig. 7.1). In the TME, these factors, pathways, and mediators play key roles in the balance between cancer pathogenesis and eradication, through the promotion of cancer cell proliferation, survival, migration, inflammation and anti-tumor immunity, and angiogenesis [5].

The IL-1 family is a key regulator of cancer immunity and inflammation that can directly or indirectly promote tumor inflammatory responses, metastasis, and angiogenesis. The role of IL-1α/β and their interaction via the type 1 IL-1 receptor (IL-1R) have been extensively studied in cancer [6]. IL-1 signaling is initiated through the recruitment of both the IL-1R accessory protein and the adaptor protein MyD88 to the receptor complex, which results in signal transduction downstream through proinflammatory effector pathways such as the inhibitor-kappaB (IκB) kinase (IKK) and nuclear factor kappaB (NF-κB) pathway [7]. IL-1R present in endothelial cells have also been shown to trigger NF-κB-independent pathway molecules such as the MYD88-ARNO-ARF6 cascade to disrupt vascular stability in inflammatory disease models, which may also have important implications for tumorigenesis [8]. IL-1 may be expressed by HNSCC cells and immune cells recruited to the TME. Our early work demonstrated that IL-1-IL1R-IKK-NF-κB signaling axis is aberrantly active and contributes to tumorigenesis and metastasis in two murine SCC models [9–12], and this was consistent with increased levels in patient serum and tumor specimens [13–17]. TNFα and TNF-related apoptosis-inducing ligand (TRAIL) are another family of cytokines that can be induced in response to stress or radiation therapy, or produced by T lymphocytes and can promote either cancer cell survival or cell death. TNF binds TNF family receptors that can alternatively induce IKK-NF-κB and prosurvival genes, or caspase-mediated cell death, in different contexts [18]. We demonstrated that response elements for NF-κB and other transcriptional cofactors downstream of IL-1 and TNF are prevalent and regulate the expression of several proinflammatory and angiogenic cytokines, including IL-6, IL-8, IL-8 ortholog growth-regulated oncogene-α (GROα), granulocyte-macrophage colony-stimulating factor (GM-CSF), and vascular endothelial growth factor (VEGF) in human HNSCC cell lines. Many of these cytokines and growth factors have been studied for their involvement in cancer. Biologically, IL-6 is able to initiate its activities through the various downstream pathways [19–21], and it has been implicated in promoting proliferation, EMT, and tumor-promoting inflammatory responses [11, 20, 21].

Several cytokines subclassified as chemokines have been associated with increased malignant features [22]. Their downstream mechanisms and contribution to HNSCC phenotypes have been elucidated for factors such as GROα and IL-8 [23, 24]. GROα, or CXCL1, mainly asserts its effect through the G protein-coupled receptor CXCR2, which mediates tumor survival and spread through pathways such as PI3K/AKT/mTOR, RAS/RAF/MEK/ERK, and NF-κB [10, 24–27]. IL-8, or CXCL8, is an interleukin that binds to both CXCR1 and CXCR2, and evidence suggests that IL-8 expression is not only increased in HNSCC but also influenced by other factors such as IL-1α, epithelial growth factor receptor (EGFR) antagonists, and hepatocyte growth factor (HGF) [17, 25, 26, 28]. Mechanistically, the effect of IL-8 is dependent on CXCR1/2-mediated NOD1/RIP2 and NF-κB signaling pathway to certain degree [23].

Factors that are primarily known for their role in stimulating growth and angiogenesis, such as VEGF, HGF, and GM-CSF, have also been observed in various HNSCC cell lines and models [9, 12, 14, 25, 26, 28–30]. VEGF is one of the most prominent angiogenic factors known to contribute to tumor growth [31]. HNSCC cells express VEGF receptors (VEGFR) 1, 2, and 3, which all have their own VEGF family ligand preference and affinity, as well as activate different downstream signaling pathways that ultimately contribute to angiogenesis and vasculogenesis [32, 33]. HGF is a growth factor that regulates many normal physiological processes such as tissue growth, remodeling, migration, regeneration, and differentiation. The activated form of HGF binds the receptor mesenchymal epithelial transition factor (c-Met) on the cell surface to activate various intracellular signaling cascades such as Src, MAPK, and PI3K to increase cell survival and motility [34]. c-MET is over-expressed in many HNSCC cases, and rarely, mutations in its kinetic domains can increase metastatic potential, interfere with response to radiation treatment, and worsen recurrence [35]. GM-CSF is a growth factor secreted in response to immune activation and inflammatory signals, and while it has been traditionally associated with regulating immune cell activity, evidence suggests it is also secreted by non-immune cells in the TME to promote cancer pathogenesis [36]. GM-CSF acts through CD116 (also called GM-CSF receptor, GMCSFR), which is closely linked to JAK2 activation, and downstream activation of STAT5 and MAPK to regulate cell proliferation [37, 38]. Increased expression of GM-CSF and its receptor is noted in various human HNSCC tumor cell lines [39], and GM-CSF has been shown to stimulate proliferation and migration of tumor cells in in vitro and in vivo model of HNSCC [40].

Co-expression of Proinflammatory Factors as Clinical Correlates

Many of the proinflammatory mediators of HNSCC have been shown to be modulated together, which has important clinical implications for estimating disease prognosis and response to treatment. Early studies on patient serum as well as various human HNSCC cell lines and tumor specimens showed increased expression of key proinflammatory molecules such as IL-1α, IL-6, IL-8, GROα, GM-CSF, and VEGF [14, 15], which have been replicated in multiple different laboratories [41–44]. Thus, certain proinflammatory molecules are expressed and modulated together, and the prognostic value in longitudinally analyzing the markers together as a panel was assessed.

Certain distinct patterns of proinflammatory factors were related to different stages of HNSCC. In cell lines and a mouse model, the malignant stages of HNSCC correlated with shift in the inflammatory cytokine profile from that of premalignant lesions [45, 46]. Interestingly, saliva samples of patients with premalignant oral lesions showed increased levels of TNFα and IL-6 [47]. Lastly, metastatic or recurrent lesions in an in vitro study showed increased expression of IL-6, IL-6R, TGF-β, and VEGF compared to that of nonmetastatic cells or normal keratinocytes, and proinflammatory TNFα was only secreted by stage IV, metastatic, or recurrence-derived cell lines [48]. Correspondingly, resistance of HNSCC to TNFα occurs through activation of NF-κB and prosurvival genes of the BCL-2 and inhibitor of apoptosis protein (IAP) families [49, 50] and inactivation of the TP53/TP63/TP73 family of tumor suppressors [51, 52].

Clinically, analysis of mean serum concentration of IL-6, IL-8, HGF, VEGF, and GROα in HNSCC patients showed that they were increased compared to matched controls [53]. The subsequent 3-year prospective serum study of HNSCC patients with stage III/IV oropharyngeal SCC receiving chemoradiation therapy showed that increasing levels of IL-6, IL-8, VEGF, HGF, and/or GROα predicted decreased cause-specific survival while higher baseline VEGF was correlated with increased survival [13]. More recently, it was shown that patients with newly diagnosed, curable HNSCC who were undergoing chemoradiotherapy exhibited significant increase in levels of IL-1β, IL-6, and IL-10 at 7 weeks after treatment compared to that of before treatment [54].

Cytokine- and Chemokine-Based Therapies and Their Potentials

Many proinflammatory factors discussed thus far are intricately related to the pathogenesis of HNSCC, and several strategies have been explored to inhibit the oncogenic pathways and responses that these factors often elicit in HNSCC. IL-1 signaling plays a role in tumor cell resistance to EGFR inhibitor erlotinib in HNSCC cells [55]. However, IL-1 has also been shown to increase natural killer (NK) and T cell-mediated cytotoxicity [56, 57], which are mechanisms by which cetuximab facilitates anti-tumor activity [58]. Thus, the opposing roles of IL-1 in cancer cloud the rationale for targeting IL-1 for therapy. A recent study by Espinosa-Cotton et al. demonstrated that recombinant IL-1α induced T cell-dependent anti-tumor activity in immunocompetent mice, and increased serum IL-1α level was associated with favorable progression-free survival (PFS) in recurrent/metastatic (R/M) HNSCC patients treated with cetuximab-based therapy [59]. This suggested the potential for combining IL-1 with immune-based therapy such as anti-PD1 immune checkpoint therapy, which has yet to be fully investigated.

It has been established that IL-6 expression is increased in many conditions driven by inflammation and enhances STAT3 (signal transducers and activators of transcription 3) activation to further increase HNSCC survival and therapy resistance though IL-6-mediated positive feedback loops [21, 60–62]. Further, tumor-infiltrating immune cells have been shown to downmodulate anti-tumor immunity through effects of STAT3 activation in tumor and immune cells [63–66]. These findings underscore the potential of targeting the IL-6/STAT3 pathway in

HNSCC. The safety and tolerability of targeting the IL-6/JAK/STAT3 pathway in humans have been well established in various inflammatory conditions, and their use in the treatment of solid tumors, including HNSCC, is undergoing active pre-clinical and clinical investigations [67]. Specifically, AZD9150, a STAT3 antisense oligonucleotide, has demonstrated safe and effective activity in a phase I trial for advanced staged lymphoma and non-small-cell lung cancer with stable disease or partial response rate in 44% of studied patients. Notably, a preclinical study has shown that the decoy oligonucleotide to the STAT3 response element in the FOS promoter suppressed HNSCC tumor growth through inhibiting STAT3 binding to DNA [68], and this study was later moved into phase 0, where it showed a decrease in STAT3-dependent gene expression in HNSCC tumors without significant toxic effects on patients [69]. Lastly, the benefit of combining immune checkpoint thera-pies (ICTs) with IL6/JAK/STAT3 pathway inhibitors has been investigated for vari-ous types of cancers [70–72], including HNSCC (NCT02646748). The currently ongoing phase 1b/2 (SCORES) study of durvalumab (anti-PD-L1) with AZD9150 or AZD5069 (anti-CXCR2) for advanced solid tumors and R/M HNSCC has been showing enhanced activity in the durvalumab plus AZD9150 combination group compared to other combination or monotherapy groups [73].

Recently, there has been an increased interest in chemokine-targeted therapies that aim to improve the efficacy of ICTs, as expression of chemokines such as IL-8, which can recruit myeloid-derived suppressor cells (MDSCs), has been correlated with poor response to ICTs [74, 75]. A large-scale retrospective analysis of 1344 patients with advanced cancers, including squamous cell cancers, revealed that high levels of IL-8 in plasma and tumor neutrophil infiltration were associated with decreased efficacy of ICT-based therapies, including nivolumab (anti-PD1) and/or ipilimumab (anti-CTLA4), everolimus (mTOR inhibitor), or docetaxel, in four dif-ferent phase 3 clinical trials [74]. Single-cell RNA sequencing of immune cells shows that high IL-8 expression in myeloid cells was associated with downregula-tion of antigen-presentation machinery, which is critical for T cell-based tumor cytotoxicity [76]. Previously, MDSCs have been shown to inhibit T cell function in TME and by reducing MDSC recruitment through blockade of CXCR1/2 using SX-682 enhanced both NK-cell and T cell-based immunotherapeutic efficacy in murine oral cancer mice models [77, 78].

In summary, proinflammatory cytokines, growth factors, and chemokines have been shown to assert both direct and indirect effects on the pathogenesis of HNC. A select panel of these markers has been shown to be potentially useful in determining HNC surveillance with respect to growth, metastasis, prognosis, and response to therapy. Mechanistic elucidation of how these factors influence the oncogenic sig-naling pathways has allowed for combination therapies that were able to synergize with each other, and factors that enhance immune-based cytotoxicity or reduce immunosuppression show promising potential for complementing ICTs for treat-ment of HNSCC.

NF-κB Pathway and Crosstalk with Other Signaling in Head and Neck Cancers

NF-κB (nuclear factor kappa-light-chain-enhancer of activated B cells) is a family of proteins that regulates diverse cellular processes such as cell growth, apoptosis, inflammatory, and immune responses [79] and plays a critical role in the tumorigenesis of a variety of cancer types, including head and neck, lung, breast, prostate, colon, gastrointestinal, liver, pancreatic, and hematopoietic malignancies [80–85]. This family comprises five subunits with a conserved REL homology domain (RHD) in their N terminus – RELA (p65), RELB, c-REL, NF-κB1 (p105/p50), and NF-κB2 (p100/p52) [79]. The RHD binds to DNA through the N terminus and interacts with the inhibitors of κB (IκB) through the C-terminus. The RHD is also critical for dimer formation between the NF-κB members such as RELA/p50, RELB/p52, c-REL/p50, RELA/RELA, and RELA/c-REL [86, 87]. RELA, c-REL, and RELB are synthesized as mature proteins, while p50 and p52 are synthesized as part of their precursor protein complexes p105 and p100, respectively. The C-termini of p105 and p100 contain IκB-like ankyrin repeats which are phosphorylated, ubiquitinated, and partially degraded by the proteasome, thereby releasing the processed units, p50 and p52, respectively [87, 88]. In addition, RELA, c-REL, and RELB contain a transactivation domain (TAD) that transactivates their target genes, while p50 and p52, which lack these TADs, rely on their interactions with other proteins to suppress or activate transcription [89].

Classical and Alternative NF-κB Signaling Pathways

In the absence of any stimulus, NF-κB dimers remain in the cytoplasm with the nuclear localization signal (NLS) sequestered by the inhibitors of κBs (IκB), and their activation is mediated by the inhibitor of κB kinases (IKK) through the classical and alternative signaling pathways [79, 89, 90] (Fig. 7.2). The classical pathway is activated when signals such as proinflammatory cytokines (e.g., TNFα or IL1) or bacterial cell wall lipopolysaccharides (LPS) bind to TNF receptors (TNFRs) or Toll-like receptors (TLRs). This leads to the stimulation of IKKβ, which is present in a complex with IKKα and the regulatory protein IKKγ (also known as NEMO). This complex phosphorylates IκB, which targets IκB to ubiquitination and degradation by the proteasome [91], thereby exposing the NLS of RELA/p50 or c-REL/p50 heterodimer and leading to its nuclear translocation and activation of target genes (Fig. 7.2). In addition, IKKβ along with other kinases phosphorylates RELA at Serine 536, while protein kinase A phosphorylates RELA at Serine 276 [92]. These phosphorylation events have been shown to be important for NF-κB signaling, and their aberrant activations are prevalent in malignant tissues of HNSCC patients [93, 94]. Metastatic cell lines were associated with increased constitutive and TNFα-inducible activation of NF-κB and proinflammatory cytokines, and these were

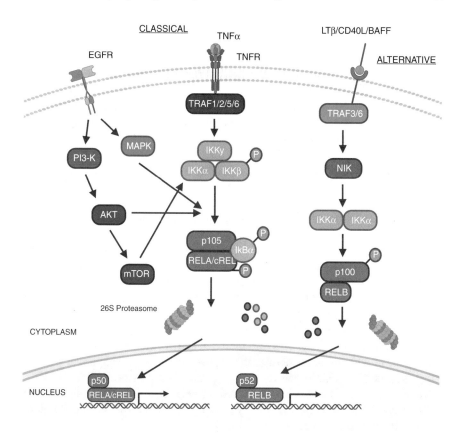

Fig. 7.2 Classical and alternative NF-κB signaling pathway. NF-κB proteins are shown in red. The classical pathway (shown in the middle) is induced when signals such as TNFα bind to its receptor TNFR and is mediated by TRAF1/2/5/6. This leads to the phosphorylation of IKKβ, which is in complex with IKKα and the regulatory protein IKKγ (shown in green), which phosphorylates IκB and targets it for ubiquitination and degradation by the 26S proteasome. Degradation of IκB and partial processing of p105 by the proteasome to create p50 lead to the nuclear translocation of RELA/p50 or c-REL/p50 dimers and activation of their target genes. In the alternative pathway (shown on the right), binding of LTβ/CD40L/BAFF to their respective receptors leads to the activation of NIK by signaling through TRAF3/6 and activation of IKKα/IKKα complex. This leads to the phosphorylation and partial processing of p100 to yield p52 which then, along with RELB, translocate into the nucleus and regulate their target genes. Other pathways that crosstalk with the NF-κB signaling pathway include, but not limited to, the EGFR pathway and MAPK pathway (shown on the left). (Figure was created using BioRender.com.)

dependent on an intact IκBα [9, 16, 49, 95]. Gene profiling from squamous cell carcinomas established in syngeneic mice revealed that early response genes that are differentially expressed in the metastatic cells are related to NF-κB [96]. When NF-κB was inactivated using a dominant negative IκBα mutant and the changes in gene expression with transformation and progression of murine SCC were studied using a cDNA microarray, NF-κB was found to regulate the expression of >60% of the genes that were differentially expressed in metastatic cells. This also inhibited the malignant phenotypic characteristics such as increased proliferation, migration, cell survival, angiogenesis, and tumor progression suggesting that NF-κB is a key mediator of malignant SCC [97].

The alternative NF-κB pathway is modulated by distinct TNF family cytokines and other factors such as CD40, BAFF, and lymphotoxin-β (LTβ) through TNFR-associated factors (TRAF) 3/6 and NF-κB-inducing kinase (NIK) (Fig. 7.2). TRAF3 negatively regulates the alternative NF-κB pathway by binding to NIK resulting in constitutive ubiquitin-mediated proteasomal degradation keeping NIK steady-state levels low in unstimulated cells [78]. Conversely, when ligand is bound, TRAF3 is ubiquitinated and degraded by the proteasome, and NIK accumulates [78]. This leads to the activation of the IKKα/IKKα complex which mediates the processing of p100 to p52 through phosphorylation, ubiquitination, and degradation [87], thereby causing nuclear translocation of RELB/p52 complex and transactivation. In addition, the HNSCC TCGA project identified *TRAF3* deletion in HPV+ tumors [98], and we showed an increase in the expression and activity of the alternative NF-κB pathway components including RELB/p52 in TRAF3-deficient HPV+ tumors and cell lines. Inversely, overexpressing TRAF3 in HPV+ cell lines with low levels of endogenous TRAF3 resulted in inhibition of RELB/p52 expression, localization, and NF-κB reporter activity. This also inhibited cell growth, migration, and colony formation, in addition to increasing the expression of tumor suppressor proteins suggesting that TRAF3, in general, acts as a tumor suppressor in HPV+ HNSCC cells [99]. Loss of TRAF3 also attenuated its other role in antiviral signaling in HPV+ HNSCC and may be one way by which progression from episomal to integrated HPV infection can be enhanced [100].

In order to address the observation that HPV+ tumors have a better prognosis and to understand the role of NF-κB subunits in the tumorigenesis of oral cancers, Mishra et al. studied the DNA binding activity and expression pattern of different subunits of NF-κB and correlated it to the presence of HPV infection. Tissues collected from normal, precancerous, and oral cancer patients showed that NF-κB was constitutively activated and NF-κB members were upregulated in oral cancer tissues. Expression of the NF-κB subunits increased with the severity of the lesions with p50 showing the highest DNA binding activity [101]. Similar results were obtained by Gupta et al. in a spectrum of tongue cancer tissues and cell lines; they showed that p50 and c-REL were associated with increased severity of the lesions in both HPV+ and HPV− tumors, while RELA in HPV+ TSCCs was associated with well-differentiated tumors with better prognosis [102]. We demonstrated that classical pathway component c-REL has a distinct role from RELA in HNSCC. When induced by TNFα, c-REL binds TP53 family member ΔNTP63, and displaces TP73, to abrogate its tumor suppressor function [52].

Crosstalk of NF-κB Pathway with Other Signaling Pathways

The delicate balance of NF-κB signaling pathway also depends on other interacting pathways such as the EGFR-mediated PI3K/Akt/mTOR pathway that is frequently deregulated in HNSCC [103] (Fig. 7.2). This pathway is activated by several ligands, including epidermal growth factor (EGF) and transforming growth factor-α (TGF-α), which lead to the activation of the class I phosphoinositide 3-kinases (PI3K), Akt, and mammalian target of rapamycin (mTOR) [104]. Akt, its substrate GSK and mTOR, can form a complex to affect the phosphorylation of the IKKα, which as part of the IKK complex leads to phosphorylation of IκB and activation of the classical pathway and prosurvival genes [105–108] (Fig. 7.2). In HNSCC, a malignant phenotype is often associated with activated EGFR and NF-κB pathway. Our previous study revealed that overexpression of both IKKα and IKKβ contributes to the increased expression and activation of components of the EGFR pathway along with NF-κB pathway, suggesting that inhibiting both the pathways may result in better suppression of NF-κB pathway activation and proliferation of HNSCC cells [109].

Mitogen-activated protein kinases (MAPK), a family of serine/threonine kinases, can also activate the NF-κB pathway by activating IKK [84] (Fig. 7.2). In a kinase-mediated phosphorylation cascade, MAPK kinase kinases (MAP 3K) activate a MAPK kinase (MKK), which further activates a MAP kinase (MAPK) [84]. IKK proteins are activated by a MAP 3K called TGFβ-activated kinase 1 (TAK1), which further leads to activation of the NF-κB pathway [110]. TNFα and IL-1 induce NF-κB activation through another MAP 3K, MEKK3. MAP kinases also regulate the group of transcription factors in activator protein-1 (AP-1) family, which consists of subfamilies that include Jun (c-Jun, JunB, and JunD) and Fos (c-Fos, FosB, Fra1, and Fra2) [111], which form dimers and regulate several key processes such as cell growth, differentiation, and apoptosis [112]. The high DNA binding activity and differential expression of the members of AP-1, particularly c-Fos, c-Jun, and JunB, have been noted in various carcinomas, including oral carcinomas [113, 114]. c-Fos/JunD dimers were found in oral cancer tissues, while its precancerous counterparts predominantly contained JunD homodimers [114]. Also, interesting was that a higher expression and DNA binding activity of AP-1 were noted in tongue tumor tissues and cancer cell lines when c-Fos partnered with Fos-related antigen 2 (Fra-2) while c-Jun joined the complex in poorly differentiated and HPV(−) carcinomas [115].

CK2 (casein kinase 2 or II) is another protein kinase that shows high expression in HNSCC patients and is linked to severity of the disease and its prognosis [116, 117]. CK2 phosphorylates IKKβ and contributes to aberrant NF-κB activation [118]. Furthermore, knockdown of a specific subunit of CK2 (CK2α) differentially regulated NF-κB signaling pathway and downstream molecules and proapoptotic genes such as *TP53* and *TP63* and contributed to the malignant phenotype in HNSCC cells [119]. CK2 inhibitor CX-4945 inhibited prosurvival mediators including the NF-κB pathway and BCL-xL expression and enhanced the expression of proapoptotic TP53 and p21 reporter activities in human HNSCC cells lines and xenograft models, although it had only modest anti-tumor activity in xenografts. When MEK inhibitor PD-0325901 (PD-901) was added, there was a better response in the xenograft experiments suggesting that the MEK-ERK-AP-1 pathway offers some resistance to CK2 inhibitors and MEK inhibitor PD-901 was active in HNSCC cells resistant to CX-4945 [120].

Current Biomarkers and Drug Development Related to NF-κB Pathways

The transcriptome and proteome of human HNSCC and murine syngeneic SCC showed that 60% of the genes differentially expressed were related to the NF-κB pathway and manipulation of such genes resulted in altered tumorigenesis, suggesting that NF-κB and its related pathways could be potential biomarkers in the prognosis of HNSCC [121]. Constitutive activation of NF-κB is seen in the majority of HNSCCs, and increased nuclear localization of phosphorylated RELA is observed in patients with malignant HNSCC. Therefore, intensity of nuclear phosphorylated RELA could be a proteomic biomarker to predict the risk of malignant HNSCC and survival of the patients [121]. Elevated proinflammatory cytokines and their genes modulated by NF-κB cell lines and tumors of HNSCC patients may also be used as biomarkers in prognosis of malignancy of HNSCC [13].

As activation of NF-κB is dependent on IKK-mediated phosphorylation, ubiquitination, and proteasomal degradation of IkBs, proteasome and IKK inhibitors were studied. While proteasome inhibitors were found to be most active in lymphomas and myeloma, in combination with other therapies, they induced only partial antitumor activity or even had antagonistic effects with EGFR inhibitors in HNSCC and other cancers [122]. In a study of HNSCC patients treated with proteasome inhibitor, Allen et al. performed immunohistochemistry (IHC) staining of the different NF-κB subunits, which included phosphorylated RELA (pRELA), and pERK1/2 and pSTAT3 on tissues obtained from HNSCC patients and matched non-cancerous epithelial tissues. The cancer tissues had an increased NF-κB staining, including pRELA, compared to the matched non-malignant tissue where it was restricted to the basal layer. This pattern corresponded to nuclear Ki67 staining, which is a marker for cell proliferation. Furthermore, when the presence and localization of the proteins were compared in pre-treatment tumor biopsies, 100% of the biopsies showed nuclear co-staining for all the five NF-κB proteins, including pRELA, RELB as well as pSTAT3, and pERK1/2. Only NF-κB and RELA but not RELB subunits or STAT3 were inhibited by proteasome inhibitor in some tumors. These results support the conclusion that nuclear activation of NF-κB is increased in HNSCC tissues and that proteasome inhibitors showed limited effect on alternative NF-κB and other prosurvival pathways [123]. In a larger study, Gaykalova et al. performed IHC on 100 HNSCC and 13 controls and found that HPV− tumors had an increased overall staining of STAT3 and NF-κB compared to HPV+ tumors. In particular, nuclear activation of STAT3 and NF-κB was also higher in HPV− tumors compared to HPV+ tumors, suggesting that HPV− HNSCC is characterized by coactivated NF-κB and STAT3 pathways. This result also correlated with the signatures of transcription factors (TF) obtained by gene expression analysis, which showed that HPV+ and HPV− HNSCCs differed significantly in their TF signatures with increased expression of direct targets of STATs, NF-κB, and AP-1 in HPV− tumors [124]. Overall, proteasome and especially IKK inhibitors were found to have limited activity and narrow therapeutic windows due to immune and hematologic toxicity, suggesting targeting driver oncogenes and the pathways that converge on NF-κB may provide more specific targets for therapy in HNSCC.

One such pathway that presented as a therapeutic option is the PI3K/mTOR pathway [103]. Altered expression or mutations of the catalytic subunit of PI3K (*PI3KCA*) are common in HNSCC [98]. PI3K-AKT signaling has been implicated in NF-κB transactivation through IKK as noted above, as well as phosphorylation of RELA and c-REL subunits, and co-factor CBP/p300 [125]. The latter cofactor may inversely regulate transactivation of prosurvival transcription factor NF-kB or TP53 tumor suppressor [126]. HNSCC displaying differences in activated PI3K-AKT, mutant *TP53*, or TGFβ receptors (*TGFβR*) showed differences in sensitivity to PI3K/mTOR-targeted agents. The PI3K/mTOR inhibitor PF-04691502 (PF-502) inhibited prosurvival signaling and enhanced the expression of TP53 in HNSCC with a low expression of TP53, but not those overexpressing mutant *TP53/TGFβR2*. This also increased apoptosis and, therefore, had significant therapeutic effect alone and when combined with radiation. This suggested that the action of PI3K/mTOR inhibitor PF502 on PI3K-Akt pathway is modified by the nature of *TP53*, and these regulatory aspects should be taken into consideration in future clinical trials of PI3K-mTOR inhibitors [127].

Following this, the ATP-competitive dual PI3K/mTOR inhibitor, PF-05212384, was tested in preclinical HNSCC models for its ability to radiosensitize HNSCC cells in vitro and in mouse model. PF-05212384 (PF-384) effectively inhibited PI3K and mTOR, resulting in significant radiosensitization of tumor cells grown in vitro when compared to normal human fibroblasts. This was also reflected in the delay in γH2AX foci resolution, which is an indicator of DNA damage, and 24-hour exposure resulted in cell cycle block in the cells exposed to PF-05212384. Following this, PF-384 delayed the regrowth of UM-SCC1 xenograft tumors in nude mice suggesting that PI3K/mTOR pathway might be a good candidate axis for sensitizing HNSCC cells to radiation and that PF-384 might be a potential radiosensitizer for HNSCC [128]. However, HNSCCs usually have other pathways like MEK/ERK/ AP-1 coactivated along with mTOR pathway, and these might make the treatments resistant. Therefore, PF-384 was tested on a panel of HNSCC cell lines with different *PIK3CA* expression and mutation status, and it showed variable activity with different HNSCC cell lines. Although PF-384 was effective in inhibiting the direct targets of PI3K/mTOR, its action on coactivated ERK was insufficient to cause inhibition of tumor growth in mice suggesting that other pathways such as MEK/ ERK contribute to the resistance against PF-384. When a MEK inhibitor PD-0325901 (PD-901) was added to the treatment, it enhanced the anti-tumor effect of PF-384 [129].

In a window of opportunity trial, the classic allosteric inhibitor of PI3K-mTOR pathway, rapamycin, was put to the test on patients with advanced HNSCC for 21 days. The results showed that 14 of the 16 patients treated with rapamycin had clinical reduction in the size of their tumors. Also, four of the patients (25%) met RECIST criteria for a 30% reduction, which included one complete response, suggesting that inhibition of the mTOR pathway presents itself as an attractive therapeutic target in HNSCC [130]. Another upstream regulator of the mTOR pathway, EGFR, has also been targeted in HNSCC therapy. Cetuximab is an EGFR antibody that is approved therapy for HNSCC patients although it is extremely expensive and its overall impact on survival is modest [131]. Two small molecule inhibitors of EGFR tyrosine kinase, gefitinib and erlotinib, which were also approved by the Food and Drug Administration (FDA) have been used to inhibit EGFR signaling. In a pilot dose escalation study using gefitinib combined with weekly paclitaxel and radiation therapy, inhibition of EGFR and downstream signaling by gefitinib was seen only in one out of the seven tumors studied. The addition of gefitinib to paclitaxel and radiation therapy did not improve the response of locally advanced HNSCC over paclitaxel and radiation therapy alone [132]. Following this, a panel of HNSCC cell lines and tumors were treated with gefitinib, and the proteomic responses of EGFR and downstream signaling molecules were analyzed pre- and post-treatment. Gefitinib sensitivity was directly correlated to inhibition of phosphorylated Akt (p-AKT) and phosphorylated STAT-3 (p-STAT3) in tumor from only one patient, suggesting that p-AKT and p-STAT3 could potentially serve as biomarkers for predicting sensitivity to therapeutics targeting the rare HNSCC in which EGFR drives tumorigenesis [133].

Soleimani et al. summarized the current NF-κB inhibitors that inhibit colorectal cancer based on their function and how they affected NF-κB activity. Inhibitors such as curcumin, which also showed clinical activity against HNSCC, work by suppressing NF-κB activation and thereby inhibiting proliferation [83]. A clinical trial in patients with preneoplastic oral lesions showed slightly higher clinical response with curcumin than placebo [134], but the solubility and bioavailability of curcumin are limited. Other inhibitors that have clinical activity against colorectal cancer mediate their inhibition through regulation of apoptosis, inflammation, metastasis, drug resistance, and radio-resistance. However, they seem to have some common themes such as abrogation or decreased NF-κB signaling and inactivation of NF-κB subunits or inhibition of phosphorylation of NF-κB signaling pathway components [83].

In summary, NF-κB signaling pathway is a key pathway that is aberrantly activated in the majority of HNSCCs. As discussed above, its various players cannot only be used as biomarkers in predicting the severity of the disease and survival of the patients, they can also be thought of as potential therapeutic candidates. However, the NF-κB signaling pathway crosstalks with several other pathways and therefore inhibiting the players of the pathway without getting a compensatory response from other pathways remain a challenge. Combination of chemotherapeutics targeting the NF-κB and related pathways along with radiation seems the more effective therapeutic option in preclinical models.

Regulation of Inflammatory Signaling by Ubiquitination and Proteasome

As one of the hallmarks of cancer, chronic inflammation is an important driver of malignancy [135]. Therefore, to prevent chronic inflammation that might lead to malignant transformation, inflammatory signaling is tightly regulated to ensure that only an appropriate response to inflammatory stimuli is mounted. A key regulator of many signaling pathways is protein ubiquitination, which plays a pivotal role in the activation and termination of many signaling pathways. As such, defects in the ubiquitin system can result in the aberrant activation or the failure to terminate inflammatory signaling, leading to a chronic inflammatory state [136, 137]. Here, we will discuss how the ubiquitin system regulates inflammatory signaling and how this system could be a potential therapeutic target in HNSCC.

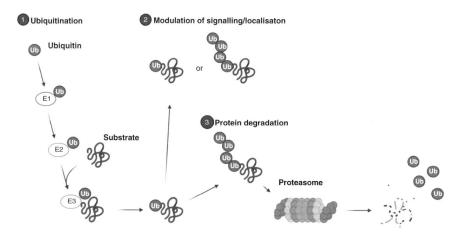

Fig. 7.3 The ubiquitin enzymatic cascade and the ubiquitin-proteasome system (USP). (1) A simplified diagram of the ubiquitin enzymatic cascade. Addition of ubiquitin to protein substrates can have several consequences, including (2) the modulation of signal transduction or protein localization or (3) proteasomal degradation. (Figure was created using BioRender.com)

The Ubiquitin System

Ubiquitin is a small, highly conserved, ubiquitously expressed protein found in all eukaryotic species, from yeast to humans [136, 137]. Ubiquitin regulates a wide range of cellular functions, from protein degradation to the modulation of signal transduction, which is achieved through the conjugation of ubiquitin to protein substrates through a stepwise, enzymatic cascade [136–138]. This process requires three classes of enzyme: E1 ubiquitin-activating enzymes, E2 ubiquitin-conjugating enzymes, and E3 ubiquitin ligases (Fig. 7.3). The human genome encodes for 8 E1 proteins (only 2 E1 proteins are involved in ubiquitination), around 50 E2 proteins, and over 700 E3 proteins, demonstrating the complexity of the ubiquitin system [136]. E3 ligases catalyze the transfer of ubiquitin to a protein substrate; therefore, E3 ligases add specificity to the ubiquitin system [137]. In addition, ubiquitin can be removed by deubiquitinating enzymes (DUBs), of which there have been around 100 characterized, in 7 distinct families [138]. Ubiquitin contains 76 amino acids, including 7 lysine residues – at amino acid position 6 (K6), K11, K27, K33, K48, and K63; the C-terminus of ubiquitin can be conjugated to any of these seven lysines on another ubiquitin, forming polyubiquitin chains of different linkages [137]. Additionally, ubiquitin can be directly attached to the N-terminal methionine of another ubiquitin to form linear polyubiquitin chains [137]. Polyubiquitin chains can either be linear or branched; in addition to the type of lysine linkage, this can result in a distinct biological function. For example, K11- and K48-polyubiquitin chains are predominantly associated with targeting proteins for degradation, whereas K63-polyubiquitin chains form linkers between signaling proteins that are associated with the propagation of extracellular signals into downstream functions, such as transcriptional activation [136].

Ubiquitin-Mediated Regulation of Inflammatory Signaling

Ubiquitination is a critical regulator of inflammatory signaling, including the NF-κB, STAT3, and AP-1 pathways, which may be activated by ligand-receptor interactions [139] and are aberrantly activated in HNSCC. Upon cytokine-receptor engagement of TNFα to TNFR1, a complex of TRADD, TRAF2, RIP1, and cIAP1/2 is recruited to the receptor. This induces K63-polyubiquitination on RIP1 by UBC13, an E2 protein, and cIAP1/2, which are E3 ligases [140]; this polyubiquitin chain serves as a binding platform for the regulatory proteins TAB1 and TAB2 through their ubiquitin binding domains (UBDs) [141]. This leads to the recruitment, autophosphorylation, and activation of TAK1 [142]. TAK1 phosphorylates IKKα, which subsequently induces IκBα phosphorylation at serine 32 and 36, resulting in its K48-polyubiquitination, proteasomal degradation, and subsequent NF-κB activation [143]. Ubiquitination of IκBα is mediated by the E3 ligase Skp1-Cullin1-F-box protein (SCF)$^{β-TrCP}$ – the β-TrCP subunit adds specificity to the E3 ligase. The degradation of IκBα results in the release of the NF-κB subunits RELA, revealing their nuclear localization sequences and promoting NF-κB transactivation [143]. Furthermore, activated TAK1 can also induce the MAPK signaling pathway; TAK1 phosphorylates MKK6 in an ubiquitin-dependent manner, resulting in JNK/p38 activation [142]. In addition to TNFα, other cytokines can also induce proinflammatory signaling which require ubiquitination. IL-1α/β can activate NF-κB and JNK/p38 signaling via the E3 ligase TRAF6 [144], and other cytokines, such as IL-6 and TNFα, can induce STAT3 activation, either directly or indirectly [145].

The trimeric IKK complex comprised of IKKγ (NEMO), IKKα, and IKKβ can bind to K63-polyubiquitin chains on RIP1, bringing these components into the proximity of TAK1, and allowing phosphorylation and activation of the IKK complex [141]. In addition to the K63-polyubiquitination-mediated activation of NF-κB, linear ubiquitination is required for NF-κB activation [146, 147]. Linear polyubiquitination is mediated by the E3 ligase linear ubiquitin chain assembly complex (LUBAC) [146]. LUBAC-mediated ubiquitination is required for the classical NF-κB pathway and potentially JNK-mediated AP-1 activity [147]. Furthermore, LUBAC binds to and ubiquitinates NEMO, and these functions are essential for NF-κB activation.

In contrast, deubiquitinating enzymes (DUBs) can also modulate inflammatory signaling, primarily resulting in the termination of signaling and preventing chronic inflammation [148]. A20 [also known as TNF alpha-induced protein 3 (TNFAIP3)], a member of the ovarian tumor (OTU) family of deubiquitinases, has well-defined role in inflammatory signaling. Unusually, A20 can also function as an E3 ligase [149]. A20 can terminate inflammatory signaling via three main mechanisms: (i) the DUB function of A20 removes K63-polyubiquitin chains form RIP1 and NEMO; (ii) the E3 ligase function K48-polyubiquitinates RIP and UBC13, promoting their proteasomal degradation; and (iii) A20 disrupts the interaction of TRAF2/5 and cIAP1/2 with UBC13, preventing their ability to function as E3 ligases [150]. Another well-characterized DUB involved in inflammatory signaling is CYLD, a member of the USP family of DUBs [151]. CYLD removes K63-polyubiquitin chains form RIP1, TRAF2, TRAF6, and NEMO, as well as removes M1-linear polyubiquitination from RIP1 [152]. Thus, both A20 and CYLD negatively regulate NF-κB and AP-1 signaling. Other DUBs can also modulate inflammatory signaling: Cezanne (OTUD7B), an OTU family member, and USP21, a USP family member, can remove K63-linked polyubiquitin chains from RIP1 [153, 154]. Conversely, the OTU family member OTUB1 can stabilize both cIAP1/2 and UBC13, resulting in enhanced inflammatory signaling [155, 156]. Additionally, USP11 has been shown to deubiquitinate and stabilize IκBα, promoting NF-κB nuclear translocation [157].

The Ubiquitin System in HNSCC: Genomic and Transcriptomic Expression Data

Copy-Number Alteration and mRNA Expression

Several genome-wide studies have been published that examine the genomic and transcriptomic alterations in HNSCC [98, 158]. Several of these have focused on inflammatory signaling pathways, including NF-κB [99, 100]. Interestingly, these studies have highlighted the prevalence of alterations in the ubiquitin system in HNSCC (reviewed in [159]). In coding the HNSCC TCGA dataset, frequent amplifications and overexpression of *BIRC2/3* (on chromosome 11q22), encoding the E3 ligases cIAP1/2, were observed [98]. cIAP1/2 are critical mediators of TNFα signaling, promoting K63-mediated polyubiquitination of RIP1 and K48-mediated polyubiquitination and subsequent proteasomal degradation of TRAF3. A key finding of TCGA study demonstrated that the *TRAF3* gene, located on chromosome 14q32.32, was commonly deleted, and occasionally mutated, in HPV+ HNSCC [98]. TRAF3 is an E3 ligase that functions as a negative regulator of both classical and alternative NF-κB [160]. Further studies demonstrated that these mutants or the loss of TRAF3 resulted in enhanced NF-κB signaling and promoted HPV+ HNSCC [99, 100, 160].

Somatic Mutations

Mutational analysis identified that the SCF family E3 ligase FBXW7 (SCF[FBXW7]) is one of the most commonly mutated genes in HNSCC [161]; this E3 ligase promotes the degradation of the AP-1 component c-Jun and NF-κB2, thereby inhibiting both AP-1 and NF-κB signaling [162, 163]. The most prevalent *FXBW7* mutations are so-called "hot-spot" mutations (R505 > R479 > R465) in the substrate binding domain; these mutations inhibit the interaction between SCF[FBXW7] and its substrates, resulting in their stabilization [164]. Therefore, these mutations may promote both AP-1 and NF-κB signaling in HNSCC. Other common mutations identified in HNSCC are in *CUL3* and *KEAP1*, an E3 ligase and a CUL3-specific adapter protein, respectively. The CUL3-KEAP1 complex targets IKKβ for proteasomal degradation, inhibiting NF-κB signaling [165]. Mutations, or loss, of either *CUL3* or *KEAP1* can thus result in increased inflammatory signaling through NF-κB. Additionally, it has been demonstrated in non-tumorigenic RPE cells that *CUL3* inactivation in combination with *TP53* inactivation results in an oncogenic phenotype driven by NF-κB and AP-1 signaling [166]. Interestingly, mutations in *CUL3* significantly co-occur with mutations in *TP53* in HNSCC [98], suggesting that the CUL3-KEAP1 E3 ligase may function in concert with deleted, mutated, or degraded TP53 in HNSCC to promote inflammatory signaling. In addition, the deubiquitinase *CYLD* is also commonly mutated in HPV+ HNSCC, and this phenotype promotes NF-κB signaling [100].

Targeting the Ubiquitin System in HNSCC

The abovementioned studies have identified several ubiquitin system components that are deregulated in HNSCC and may be attractive therapeutic targets. In the past 20 years, targeting the ubiquitin system has gained a lot of traction as a potential target for cancer therapies [167]. Currently, several avenues have been approached; as enzymes that contain a well-defined active site, targeting of E3 ligases and DUBs with small molecule inhibitors has a lot of potential. However, inhibition of the proteasome has been the most successful strategy so far, with several inhibitors currently approved by the FDA [168].

Proteasome Inhibitors

One of the first components of the ubiquitin system that was targeted for inhibition was the proteasome, resulting in the accumulation of tumor suppressors, such as TP53 and p27. Additionally, proteasome inhibition significantly inhibits the inflammatory response; IκBα accumulation results in the inhibition of NF-κB signaling and the subsequent release of proinflammatory cytokines [168]. Thus, proteasome inhibition can have multiple effects that inhibit cell proliferation and promote apoptosis.

Proteasome inhibitors have been trialed in many cancers, including multiple myeloma (MM) and many different lymphomas [168]. Bortezomib is a reversible inhibitor that binds to the catalytic site of the proteasome and is currently FDA approved for the treatment of MM and mantle cell lymphoma (MCL). Subsequent studies have shown that the efficacy of Bortezomib in MM and MCL is likely due to multiple mechanisms, including the inhibition of proliferation, induction of apoptosis, and the inhibition of NF-κB-dependent cytokine secretion [169]. A problem with Bortezomib is the intrinsic resistance observed in many patients [169]. Therefore, the second generation of proteasome inhibitors was developed to overcome these issues. Carfilzomib is an irreversible inhibitor of the proteasome and is currently FDA approved for MM patients who would have previously received treatment, potentially with Bortezomib [170].

Proteasome inhibitors have been tested as a potential therapeutic option to inhibit NF-κB signaling in HNSCC. Early studies showed that Bortezomib treatment inhibited NF-κB signaling in both mouse and human squamous cell carcinomas [123]. However, despite inhibition of NF-κB, other inflammatory pathways were unaffected (AP-1 and STAT3), and the responses were variable [171, 172]. While further combination studies with Bortezomib combined with histone deacetylase (HDAC) inhibitors or cisplatin greatly enhanced the induction of apoptosis and anti-tumor responses, toxicities were also increased [173]. Therefore, proteasome inhibition has the potential to inhibit inflammatory signaling in HNSCC, and combination therapy with Bortezomib, or next-generation proteasome inhibitors such as carfilzomib, deserves further investigation.

IAP Antagonists

Another target of the ubiquitin system that has gained attention in recent years is the E3 ligases cIAP1/2. As mentioned previously, the cIAP1/2 are often amplified or overexpressed in HNSCC [174, 175]. The dual function of these proteins is critical for their potential as a therapeutic target in cancer; inhibition of cIAPs results in the inhibition of downstream inflammatory signaling and the induction of apoptosis though the extrinsic pathway [175].

Compounds targeting cIAPs (IAP antagonists) are mimicked after the natural IAP antagonist, second mitochondria-derived activator of caspase (SMAC) – thus, they are also called SMAC mimetics. Upon mitochondrial release, SMAC is cleaved and dimerizes. The N-terminal domain of SMAC contains a four-amino-acid sequence (AVPI; ala, val, pro, ile) which binds to the BIR3 and BIR2 domain of IAPs [175]. IAP antagonists mimic this sequence, allowing binding to IAPs. Upon binding, cIAP1/2 undergo a conformation change, autoubiquitination, and proteasomal degradation [175]. In addition, SMAC mimetics target XIAP, thereby allowing caspase activation and apoptotic cell death to occur [176]. The IAP antagonists developed thus far are monovalent or bivalent, based on how many BIR domains the IAP antagonist can bind to. The mechanism of action of IAP antagonists is primarily the induction of TNFα-dependent apoptosis; despite inhibition of classical NF-κB signaling, cIAP depletion results in the stabilization of NIK, thereby driving alternate NF-κB signaling [176]. This results in the autocrine production of TNFα and the induction of apoptosis. In agreement with this, IAP antagonist-induced apoptosis is enhanced by the addition of death ligands, such as TNFα and TRAIL [177, 178].

There are currently several IAP antagonists in clinical trials: four monovalent (Debio-1143, GDC-0917, LCL-161, and GDC-0152), two bivalent (birinapant and HGS-1029), and one that is not based on the AVPI peptide (ASTX-660). All these inhibitors are in early phase clinical trials for solid cancers [179]. Additionally, birinapant and HGS-1029 are being tested in lymphoma [180]. So far, clinical efficacy has been shown in phase I trials in ovarian cancer and melanoma [181, 182]. Additionally, combination therapies with standard chemotherapies (cisplatin, paclitaxel), radiation therapy, or immune checkpoint inhibitors are currently being tested [183, 184] (Fig. 7.4).

In HNSCC, several IAP antagonists have been shown to have benefits in vitro and sensitize HNSCC cancer cells to standard chemotherapeutics, TNFα and TRAIL [177, 183]. In addition, birinapant, Debio-143, and LCL161 sensitize HNSCC cells to radiation therapy [177, 184, 185]. Interestingly, HNSCC cell lines containing *FADD* amplifications demonstrate increased sensitivity to IAP antagonists and were more sensitive to combination therapy with radiation, resulting in

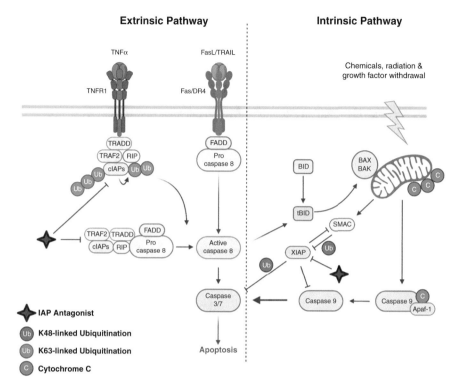

Fig. 7.4 Extrinsic and intrinsic apoptosis pathways. The extrinsic apoptosis pathway is induced by the ligand binding (TNF, FASL, or TRAIL) to cell death receptors (TNFR, FAS, or DR4, respectively). The death domain of TNFR1 recruits TNF receptor-associated death domain (TRADD) protein, an adaptor molecule that allows binding of TRAF2 and c-IAP1 and c-IAP2 to the receptor complex. c-IAP1/2 induce K63-linked RIP1 ubiquitination and subsequent downstream signaling through NF-κB and AP-1. In the absence of cIAPs, RIP1 cannot be ubiquitinated and instead forms a cytosolic complex with the adaptor molecule Fas-associated via death domain (FADD) and caspase 8, leading to the induction of apoptosis via caspase 3/7 activation. As cIAP-mediated ubiquitination of RIP1 prevents the formation of these death-inducing complexes, SMAC mimetics can be used to drive cell death by causing degrading c-IAPs. The intrinsic pathway of apoptosis can be triggered by cytotoxic insults and involves the release of cytochrome c and SMAC from the mitochondria into the cytosol. Caspase 8-induced cleavage of BH3-interacting death domain agonist (BID) to truncated BID (tBID) can also cause mitochondrial permeabilization. Cytochrome c is released to the cytosol, which leads to the activation of caspase-9 and later caspase-3 and caspase-7; released cytochrome c binds apoptosis protease-activating factor (Apaf1) and induces formation of the apoptosome, activating caspase 9, inducing apoptosis via caspase 3/7 activation. Additionally, SMAC is released from mitochondria and can directly inhibit XIAP, another IAP protein. SMAC mimetics can therefore inhibit XIAP to promote apoptosis. (Figure was created using BioRender.com.)

enhanced TNFα-dependent apoptosis [177]. Furthermore, some IAP antagonists were more effective in HPV+ HNSCC [185]. Finally, recent studies using the IAP antagonist ASTX660 have showed promise in HNSCC, promoting TNFα- and TRAIL-induced cell death in HNSCC cell lines and radiation-induced immunogenic death in preclinical models [186, 187]. These data suggest that IAP antagonists may be most effective when the underlying genetics, or HPV status, of a tumor are known, making them an attractive target in personalized medicine.

In summary, it is becoming clear that inhibition of inflammatory signaling via the ubiquitin system is an attractive therapeutic target in HNSCC. The use of proteasome inhibitors and IAP antagonists offers the ability to target several oncogenic pathways at once, including the inhibition of proliferation and the induction of apoptosis.

Genomic Signatures and Transcriptomic Landscapes of Proinflammatory and Other Signaling Molecules

Cancer is a complex genetic disease, derived from uncontrolled proliferative cells with accumulated genomic alterations and functional defects. The most prominent genetic alteration is the somatic mutation, which can be acquired by phenotypically normal cells through the lineage of mitotic divisions [188]. The intrinsic mechanisms of mutation include inherent genetic defects, replicational errors, and/or deficiency for DNA repair during the cell division [188]. The extrinsic mechanisms of mutation are mediated through the effects of exogenous mutagens, such as carcinogens from tobacco smoke and alcohol, and infection with oncogenic viruses, such as human papillomaviruses (HPV). These are among the potent inducers and promoters that can increase somatic mutation rates and induce genomic instability and chromosomal alterations [189], especially in HNSCC and SCC from the lung, esophageal, cervix, and bladder [190]. The accumulations of these genetic alterations during the growth of cancer cells over years or decades can lead to the development of heterogeneous genomic alterations, which are difficult to be characterized, classified, and utilized for patient diagnosis and prognosis in the clinics, particularly when medical practice is only based on traditional pathological and histological methods. To address these problems and understand the most comprehensive molecular portraits of human cancers, The Cancer Genome Atlas (TCGA) and other large collaborative projects have been established, which performed multiplexed in-depth investigations of the major cancer types using cutting-edge genome characterization technologies and large integrated datasets.

Table 7.1 Open datasets and resources of cancer tissues and cell lines with genomic and proteomic information and sensitivity to genetic and small molecule perturbations

Project name (Abbreviation)	Leading institutes	Description	Total samples HNSCC samples	Website	Reference
Cancer tissues					
The Cancer Genome Atlas (*TCGA*)	NCI/NHGRI/NIH	A landmark cancer genomics program which molecularly characterized over 20,000 primary cancer and matched normal samples spanning 33 cancer types and generated over 2.5 petabytes of genomic, epigenomic, transcriptomic, and proteomic data	>11,000 cancer cases >530 HNSCC cases	http://cancergenome.nih.gov/ https://gdc.cancer.gov https://www.cbioportal.org	Hutter and Zenklusen [191] Cancer Genome Atlas Network [98]
TCGA Pan-Cancer Atlas *PanCanAtlas*	NCI/NHGRI/NIH	Uniquely comprehensive, in-depth, and interconnected analyses across 33 cancer types with a collection of 27 papers divided into three main categories: cell-of-origin patterns, oncogenic processes, and signaling pathways. Each category is anchored by a flagship paper providing a summary of the core findings for that topic	>11,000 cancer cases >530 HNSCC cases	https://gdc.cancer.gov/about-data/publications/pancanatlas https://www.cell.com/pb-assets/consortium/pancanceratlas/pancani3/index.html https://www.cbioportal.org	Hoadley et al. [199] Ding et al. [200] Sanchez-Vega et al. [201] Campbell et al. [190]
Normal tissues					
Genotype-Tissue Expression (*GTEx*)	NCI/NHGRI/NHLBI NIDA/NIMH/NINDS	A comprehensive resource to study tissue-specific gene expression and regulation. Samples were collected from adult organ and tissue donors or surgical donors of 54 non-diseased tissue sites. Primary molecular assays include whole genome-seq, whole exome-seq, and RNA-seq and provide open access to data including gene expression, quantitative trait loci (eQTLs), and histology images	~1000 deceased adults	https://gtexportal.org/home/	GTEx Consortium, *Nature*, 2017[193]

(continued)

Table 7.1 (continued)

Project name (Abbreviation)	Leading institutes	Description	Total samples HNSCC samples	Website	Reference
Cancer cell lines					
Cancer Cell Line Encyclopedia (CCLE)	Broad Institute & Novartis Institutes for Biomedical Research	A detailed genetic and pharmacologic characterization of a large panel of human cancer models, to develop integrated analyses that link distinct pharmacologic vulnerabilities to genomic and proteomic patterns	1775 cell lines 71 HNSCC lines	https://portals. broadinstitute.org/ccle https://depmap.org/ portal/ccle/	Ghandi et al. [205] Barretina, et al. [204]
RNAi/shRNA/CRISPR					
Deep RNAi Interrogation of Viability Effects in cancer (DRIVE)	Novartis Institutes for Biomedical Research	Large-scale RNAi screen in which viability effects of mRNA knockdown were assessed for 7837 genes using an average of 20 shRNAs per gene	398 cancer cell lines 10 HNSCC cell lines	https://oncologynibr. shinyapps.io/drive/	McDonald, et al. [209]
Project Achilles	Broad Institute	Systematically identifies and catalogs gene essentiality across hundreds of genomically characterized cancer cell lines using genome-scale lentiviral-based pooled shRNA or CRISPR-Cas9 libraries to knockout individual genes and identify those affecting cell survival	>700 cancer cell lines >40 HNSCC cell lines	https://depmap.org/ portal/achilles/	Behan et al. [210]
The Cancer Dependency Map (DepMap)	Broad Institute & Sanger Institute	Integrated datasets to profile hundreds of cancer cell lines for genomic information and sensitivity to genetic and small molecule perturbations to define a landscape of genetic targets for therapeutics	1775 cell lines 71 HNSCC cell lines	https://depmap.org/ portal/	Tscherniak et al., *Cell*, 2017 [194]

Drug screening

Name	Institution	Description	Scale	URL	Reference
Profiling Relative Inhibition Simultaneously in Mixtures (PRISM)	Broad Institute & Harvard University	A powerful approach to rapidly screen thousands of drugs across hundreds of human cancer models on an unprecedented scale to identify predictive biomarkers of sensitivity and new lineages for treatment	>500 cancer cell lines 27 HNSCC lines	https://depmap.org/portal/prism/	Yu et al. [213] Corsello et al. [211] Corsello et al. [212]
Genomics of Drug Sensitivity in Cancer (GDSC)	Wellcome Sanger Institute & Mass General Hospital	Screening large panels of characterized human cancer cell lines with 518 anti-cancer compounds including cytotoxic chemo- and targeted therapeutics. The prediction of sensitivity patterns is correlated with extensive genomic data to identify genetic features	>1000 cancer cell lines >1000 cancer cell lines 44 HNSCC lines	https://www.cancerrxgene.org	Iorio et al., *Cell*, 2016 [195]

Protein Atlas

Name	Institution	Description	Scale	URL	Reference
The Human Protein Atlas	Swedish-based program, funded by Knut and Alice Wallenberg Foundation	Mapping all the human proteins in cells, tissues, and organs using integration of various omics technologies, including antibody-based imaging, mass spectrometry-based proteomics, transcriptomics, and systems biology. It consists of six separate parts, including Tissue Atlas, Cell Atlas, Pathology Atlas, Blood Atlas, the Brain Atlas, and the Metabolic Atlas	>700 antibodies for protein expression >5 million IHC cancer tissue images	https://www.proteinatlas.org	Uhlén et al., *Science*, 2015 [196]

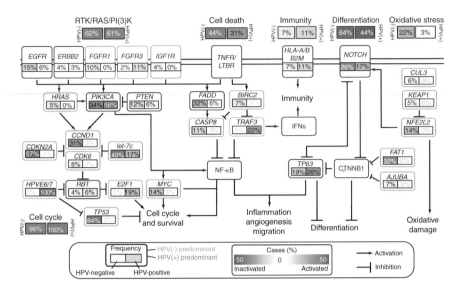

Fig. 7.5 Deregulation of signaling pathways and transcription factors. Key affected pathways, components, and inferred functions are summarized in the main text and Supplementary Information section 7 for $n = 279$ samples. The frequency (%) of genetic alterations for HPV(−) and HPV(+) tumors are shown separately within sub-panels and highlighted. Pathway alterations include homozygous deletions, focal amplifications, and somatic mutations. Activated and inactivated pathways/genes and activating or inhibitory symbols are based on predicted effects of genome alterations and/or pathway functions

Overview of TCGA Project and the Individual Biomarker Paper of HNSCC

TCGA project was initiated in 2006 and funded by the National Cancer Institute (NCI) and the National Human Genome Research Institute (NHGRI) of the National Institutes of Health (NIH) [191]. This was a landmark cancer genomics program that molecularly characterized 33 major cancer types, utilizing multiple platforms of high-throughput technologies and bioinformatics analyses. In 2018, TCGA Research Network completed the exciting journey, which generated over 2.5 petabytes of genomic, epigenomic, transcriptomic, and proteomic data, and published over 30 cancer type-specific "Marker" papers (Table 7.1). The "Marker" papers were defined as the unique papers published by TCGA cancer-specific consortium group of each cancer type, to distinguish with other papers using TCGA datasets [192].

Nature published the HNSCC TCGA "Marker" paper focusing on head and neck cancers in January 2015 [98]. This publication analyzed 279 patient samples, including 244 HPV(−) and 36 HPV(+) HNSCC, of which the final pathway summary figure illustrated the frequency of the most altered oncogene and tumor suppressor genes in HNSCC (Fig. 7.5, reproduced with permission from [98]). These critical molecules were organized into the major pathways, including growth receptor/cell cycle, cell death, immunity, cell differentiation, and oxidative stress. Several genomic alterations affected the tumor necrosis factor receptor (TNFR) components and inflammatory pathways that converge upon the NF-κB-mediated signaling. The gains in 11q13/22 encode *FADD*, *BIRC2/3*, and/or loss at 14q32 *TRAF3*, which regulates the classical and alternative NF-κB/REL family transcription factors and pathways important in cell death, migration, and inflammation in HNSCC. The loss of 3p and resulting duplication of isochromosome 3q in most HNSCC result in gains of mitogenic kinase *PIK3CA*, or alternatively, mutation of *PIK3CA*, especially in HPV(+) tumors, represents the most commonly altered oncogenes in HNSCC, also implicated in NF-κB activation. The loss of NOTCH or 3q gain of TP63 has been implicated in enhanced activation of ΔNTP63 oncogene that promotes stemness, oncogenesis, and the inflammatory phenotype of HNSCC.

A concurrent study of this cohort revealed 35 tumors (12.5%) showed detectable high-risk HPV types 16, 33, or 35, based on exome and transcriptome sequencing data. This study revealed that HPV viral genome integration promotes host tumorigenesis through oncogene amplification, disruption of tumor suppressors, driving chromosomal rearrangements, and altering gene expression and DNA methylation patterns [197]. So far, HNSCC TCGA project has completed the genomic analysis of ~530 tumor tissues, including ~81 HPV+ tumor tissues and more than 40 matched normal tissue samples. The technologies used six different "omic" platforms, including exome-seq, DNA copy-number array, DNA methylation array, mRNA-seq, miRNA-seq, and reverse phase protein array (RPPA, Table 7.1).

Three Major Themes of TCGA Pan-Cancer Atlas Project Include "Cell of Origin," "Oncogenic Process," and "Signaling Pathways"

We participated in the TCGA Pan-Cancer Atlas project, which conducted a multiplatform analysis of 3527 tumor samples from 12 cancer types, including HNSCC [198]. Through the multiplatform classification and integrated analysis of the datasets from five genomic platforms and RPPA, we revealed that SCCs from head and neck, lung, and a subset of bladder cancers merged into one subtype, including characteristic *TP53* alterations, copy gain of chromosome 3q with amplification and predominant expression of ΔN isoform of p63, and high expression of immune and proliferation pathway genes. This study correlated multiplatform classification and integrated analysis of genomic and expression signatures with tissue of origin and laid the foundation for the subsequent TCGA Pan-Cancer Atlas projects [198].

TCGA Pan-Cancer Atlas then collected and analyzed more than 11,000 samples across 33 different major cancer types, publishing 30 papers in the Cell Press journals, including three Flagship papers focusing on the three major themes of "Cell of Origin" [199], "Oncogenic Processes" [200], and "Signaling Pathways" [201]

(Table 7.1). Under the major theme of "Cell of Origin," which is based on organ systems or differentiation status, we chaired and led the pan-squamous project (PanSCC) to study tumor aggregation based on the histological subtypes of squamous cancers, including those from the head and neck, lung, esophagus, cervical, and bladder [190]. The pathogenesis of most SCCs is associated with smoking and/or HPV infection, and we observed that these tumors share and harbor 3q, 5p, and 11q recurrent chromosomal CNVs.

Another major theme is "Oncogenic Process" [200], which provided an overview of oncogenic molecular processes across 33 major cancer types. This project focused on the cancer mutation status and revealed (i) how germline genome affects somatic genomic landscape in a pathway-dependent fashion; (ii) how genomic mutations impact expression, signaling, and multi-omic profiles; and (iii) how mutation burdens and drivers influence immune cell composition in the microenvironment. Interestingly, driver mutations exhibited a high impact on the immune communication network in HNSCC TME, as among the top cancer types [202]. Most HNSCC samples exhibited high expression of IFNγ dominant and wound-healing gene signatures [203]. The third theme is "Signaling Pathways" [201], which generated the alteration map of ten signaling pathways. The authors developed a reusable, curated pathway template that includes a catalog of driver genes, which showed that 57% of tumors have at least one potentially actionable drug target alteration in these pathways.

Landscape Characterization of Human Cell Lines Using High-Throughput Technologies

The Cancer Cell Line Encyclopedia (CCLE) project was initiated in parallel to TCGA study to conduct a detailed genetic and pharmacologic characterization of a large panel of human cancer models [204]. So far, this project has collected >1700 cell lines from >30 major cancer types with integrated computational analyses that link distinct genomic patterns with pharmacologic drug sensitivities [205] (Table 7.1). For HNSCC, most of these cell lines analyzed are established from tumors in the oral cavity and other head and neck sites, without complete and detailed clinical and pathological information, such as HPV status. Another large collection of HNSCC cell lines by the University of Michigan has been established to fill in these gaps, designated as UM-SCC lines. This collection contains tumors from more than 100 HNSCC patients with detailed clinical and pathological information, including HPV status. Our laboratory has characterized 26 HNSCC lines using exome-seq and RNA-seq, which included 15 HPV− and 11 HPV+ lines, of which 18 are UM-SCC lines [158]. In this study, we found that the copy gains of chromosomes 3q, 5p, and 11q are linked to increased oncogene expression, including *TP63*, *PIK3CA*, and *ACTL6A* from 3q and *YAP1*, *CCND1*, and *FADD/BIRC2/3* from 11q loci, consistent with TCGA data. Thus, these cell lines recapitulated genomic alterations of more aggressive HNSCC tumor subtypes, wherein concurrent 3q26.3 amplification and *TP53* mutation are associated with worse survival. In addition, Ludwig et al. studied 14 UM-SCC cell lines from the oral cavity to denote the mutational profile, CNV, and gene and protein expression of each cell line [206]. They identified dominant genetic alterations of *PIK3CA* amplification, *CDKN2A* deletion, and a high prevalence of *TP53* and *CASP8* mutations. Furthermore, this group also investigated a panel of 16 cell lines derived from laryngeal squamous cell carcinoma [207]. The dominant genetic aberrations included *PIK3CA*, *EGFR*, *CDKN2A*, *TP53*, *NOTCH*, and *FAT1* genes. Moreover, van Harten et al. genetically characterized a panel of 24 HNSCC cell lines, including 9 UM-SCC lines, which represent HPV+, HPV−, and cell lines with a genetic predisposition, such as Fanconi anemia (FA) [208]. These FA-derived cell lines share comparable CNV and mutation patterns with sporadic HPV− HNSCC. In contrast, a subclass of CN-silent, HPV−, *TP53* wild-type, and *CASP8* mutation HNSCC lines were separated from the majority of HNSCC tumors and resembled 84 HNSCC cases from TCGA, which showed CN-silent and enriched for the female gender, *HRAS* and *CASP8* mutations. These genomic characterizations of HNSCC lines provide useful preclinical models for in-depth mechanistic studies of biomarkers and the identification of new therapeutic strategies.

Genome-Wide Gene Perturbation and Interrogation with Functional Analyses

To study the functional genomics of the cell lines, the DRIVE project, designated for "Deep RNAi Interrogation of Viability Effects in cancer" was conducted [209]. This assessed the knockdown effects of 7837 genes using ~20 shRNAs per gene in 398 cancer cell lines, including 10 HNSCC cell lines (Table 7.1). More recently, taking advantage of the CRISPR-Cas9 technology, 18,009 genes were knocked down in 324 human cancer cell lines from 30 cancer types, and a data-driven framework to prioritize candidates for cancer therapeutics was developed [210]. Among these cell lines, 34 HNSCC cell lines were screened, and the prioritized therapeutic targets were identified with approved drugs, such as *EGFR*, *TUBB4B*, *TYMS*, *CDK6*, and *HMGCR*. This dataset provides a rich resource of cancer driver genes and prioritized known and predicted cancer drug targets.

This project also generated RPPA data using 213 antibodies across 899 CCLE cell lines and studied protein expression with gene dependence or drug sensitivities [205]. These datasets are collected in DepMap, which stands for "Explore the Cancer Dependency Map" (https://depmap.org/portal/). This dataset provides open access to key cancer dependencies to empower the research community to make discoveries related to cancer vulnerabilities (Table 7.1). DepMap portal also incorporated drug screening data designated as PRISM, which stands for "Profiling Relative Inhibition Simultaneously in Mixtures" [211–213]. This integrated analysis added powerful tools to identify better predictive biomarkers and genetic dependencies to study cancer-related inflammation, develop new treatment strategies, and repurpose drugs for precision oncology and more effective therapeutics.

The HNSCC TCGA datasets provided a unique way to study inflammation gene expression regulated by the aberrant NF-κB activation in the tumor microenvironment. Concurrently, we analyzed the genome and transcriptome alterations of 279 HNSCC specimens from TCGA cohort and identified 61 genes involved in NF-κB and inflammatory pathways [214]. The most frequently altered 30 genes were distributed across 96% of HNSCC samples, and their expression was associated with genomic copy-number alterations. We compared the NF-κB and proinflammatory and related gene lists in TCGA data with the 26 HNSCC cell lines as discussed above and observed that most expression signatures studied are consistent between the data from TCGA and HNSCC cell lines. Using RNAi screening through an NF-κB reporter line, we observed that knockdown of *TNFR*, *LTBR*, or selected downstream signaling components revealed crosstalk between the classic and alternative NF-κB pathways. Improved survival was observed in HNSCC patients with elevated gene expression in T cell activation, immune checkpoints, and IFNγ and STAT pathways, which are modulated by NF-κB and proinflammatory genes. The gene signature of NF-κB activation and proinflammation could serve as potential biomarkers to identify therapeutic and prognostic targets in further preclinical and clinical investigations.

In summary, the high-throughput technologies of genomics, transcriptomics, and proteomics, combined with computation of large datasets, allowed us to achieve the comprehensive genome-wide characterization of each cancer type, which significantly accelerated cancer research. TCGA and Pan-Cancer Atlas projects cross-analyzed over 11,000 tumors from 33 major cancers, leading to the identification of previously unrecognized molecular biomarkers and a more accurate classification of new subgroups within each cancer type. In addition, the CCLE project provided a detailed catalog of a large panel of human cancer models, through integrated genome-wide gene perturbation with functional and pharmacologic drug sensitivity analyses. The altered NF-κB and proinflammatory signatures identified in these large-scaled investigations of HNSCC human tissues and cell lines are consistent with our previous laboratory observations. These large-scaled open source datasets provide unique information codes to specifically match the tumor genetic or expression defects with patient outcomes, which could lead to tailored precision medicine, including diagnosis and treatments.

Overall Conclusions and Future Directions

Inflammatory factors are deregulated in HNC, and aberrant activation of NF-κB underpins many of their effects on tumor cells and the TME. Pathways implicated in aberrant activation of NF-κB are frequently impinged by genomic alterations discovered by TCGA and present in the tumor cell lines used as models for mechanistic and preclinical studies to identify potential targets for prevention or therapy.

TNF is a key mediator of cytotoxic therapies and immune responses, to which HNSCCs become resistant via NF-κB-regulated prosurvival mediators. Integration of structural genomics from TCGA, these cell line models, and functional screens for molecules that inhibit TNF-induced NF-κB proinflammatory and prosurvival signaling using siRNA, CRISPR, or drug libraries could help identify key drivers, mediators, and druggable targets that have synthetic lethal activity with TNF and interrupt their deleterious effects on the malignant phenotype and immunity. We have developed an NF-κB reporter screening platform and completed a genome-wide siRNA screen that has identified unexpected candidates for which validation, mechanistic, and preclinical studies of potential therapeutics are underway.

Acknowledgments The authors thank Nyall London, Jr., MD, PhD (HNSB, NIDCD/NIH), and Georgia Z Chen, PhD, (Emory University, Atlanta, GA) for reading this review article and providing helpful comments and suggestions.

Authors' Contributions Jun Jeon wrote the cytokine section, Ramya Viswanathan wrote the NF-κB section, Ethan Morgan wrote the ubiquitination section, Zhong Chen wrote the genomics section, and Carter Van Waes wrote the introduction and overall conclusions. Zhong Chen, Ramya Viswanathan, and Ethan Morgan designed and drew the figures. Zhong Chen made the table. Ramya Viswanathan managed literature citations. All authors revised and approved the final version of the manuscript.

Funding Information This project is supported by NIDCD intramural projects Z01-DC-00016, 73, 74. This research was made possible through the NIH Medical Research Scholars Program, a public-private partnership supported jointly by the NIH and contributions to the Foundation for the NIH from the Doris Duke Charitable Foundation (DDCF Grant #2014194); the American Association for Dental Research; the Colgate-Palmolive Company, Genentech, Elsevier; and other private donors.

References

1. Elenbaas B, Weinberg RA. Heterotypic signaling between epithelial tumor cells and fibroblasts in carcinoma formation. Exp Cell Res. 2001;264(1):169–84.
2. Folkman J. Role of angiogenesis in tumor growth and metastasis. Semin Oncol. 2002;29(6, Supplement 16):15–8.
3. Peltanova B, Raudenska M, Masarik M. Effect of tumor microenvironment on pathogenesis of the head and neck squamous cell carcinoma: a systematic review. Mol Cancer. 2019;18:63.
4. Richmond A. Nf-kappa B, chemokine gene transcription and tumour growth. Nat Rev Immunol. 2002;2(9):664–74.
5. Setrerrahmane S, Xu H. Tumor-related interleukins: old validated targets for new anti-cancer drug development. Mol Cancer. 2017;16:153.
6. Baker KJ, Houston A, Brint E. IL-1 family members in cancer; two sides to every story. Front Immunol. 2019;10:1197.
7. Weber A, Wasiliew P, Kracht M. Interleukin-1 (IL-1) pathway. Sci Signal. 2010;3(105):cm1.
8. Zhu W, London NR, Gibson CC, Davis CT, Tong Z, Sorensen LK, et al. Interleukin receptor activates a MYD88-ARNO-ARF6 cascade to disrupt vascular stability. Nature. 2012;492(7428):252–5.

9. Dong G, Chen Z, Kato T, Van Waes C. The host environment promotes the constitutive acti-vation of nuclear factor-kappaB and proinflammatory cytokine expression during metastatic tumor progression of murine squamous cell carcinoma. Cancer Res. 1999;59(14):3495–504.

10. Loukinova E, Chen Z, Van Waes C, Dong G. Expression of proangiogenic chemokine Gro 1 in low and high metastatic variants of Pam murine squamous cell carcinoma is differentially regulated by IL-1alpha, EGF and TGF-beta1 through NF-kappaB dependent and independent mechanisms. Int J Cancer. 2001;94(5):637–44.

11. Smith CW, Chen Z, Dong G, Loukinova E, Pegram MY, Nicholas-Figueroa L, et al. The host environment promotes the development of primary and metastatic squamous cell carcinomas that constitutively express proinflammatory cytokines IL-1alpha, IL-6, GM-CSF, and KC. Clin Exp Metastasis. 1998;16(7):655–64.

12. Thomas GR, Chen Z, Leukinova E, Van Waes C, Wen J. Cytokines IL-1α, IL-6, and GM-CSF constitutively secreted by oral squamous carcinoma induce down-regulation of CD80 costim-ulatory molecule expression: restoration by interferon γ. Cancer Immunol Immunother. 2004;53(1):33–40.

13. Allen C, Duffy S, Teknos T, Islam M, Chen Z, Albert PS, et al. Nuclear factor-kappaB-related serum factors as longitudinal biomarkers of response and survival in advanced oropharyngeal carcinoma. Clin Cancer Res. 2007;13(11):3182–90.

14. Chen Z, Colon I, Ortiz N, Callister M, Dong G, Pegram MY, et al. Effects of interleukin-1alpha, interleukin-1 receptor antagonist, and neutralizing antibody on proinflammatory cytokine expression by human squamous cell carcinoma lines. Cancer Res. 1998;58(16):3668–76.

15. Chen Z, Malhotra PS, Thomas GR, Ondrey FG, Duffey DC, Smith CW, et al. Expression of proinflammatory and proangiogenic cytokines in patients with head and neck cancer. Clin Cancer Res. 1999;5(6):1369–79.

16. Duffey DC, Chen Z, Dong G, Ondrey FG, Wolf JS, Brown K, et al. Expression of a dominant-negative mutant inhibitor-kappaBalpha of nuclear factor-kappaB in human head and neck squamous cell carcinoma inhibits survival, proinflammatory cytokine expression, and tumor growth in vivo. Cancer Res. 1999;59(14):3468–74.

17. Wolf JS, Chen Z, Dong G, Sunwoo JB, Bancroft CC, Capo DE, et al. IL (interleukin)-1alpha promotes nuclear factor-kappaB and AP-1-induced IL-8 expression, cell survival, and prolif-eration in head and neck squamous cell carcinomas. Clin Cancer Res. 2001;7(6):1812–20.

18. Derakhshan A, Chen Z, Van Waes C. Therapeutic small molecules target inhibitor of apopto-sis proteins in cancers with deregulation of extrinsic and intrinsic cell death pathways. Clin Cancer Res. 2017;23(6):1379–87.

19. Choudhary MM, France TJ, Teknos TN, Kumar P. Interleukin-6 role in head and neck squa-mous cell carcinoma progression. World J Otorhinolaryngol Head Neck Surg. 2016;2(2):90–7.

20. Hong SH, Ondrey FG, Avis IM, Chen Z, Loukinova E, Cavanaugh PF, et al. Cyclooxygenase regulates human oropharyngeal carcinomas via the proinflammatory cytokine IL-6: a general role for inflammation? FASEB J. 2000;14(11):1499–507.

21. Lee TL, Yeh J, Van Waes C, Chen Z. Epigenetic modification of SOCS-1 differentially reg-ulates STAT3 activation in response to interleukin-6 receptor and epidermal growth factor receptor signaling through JAK and/or MEK in head and neck squamous cell carcinomas. Mol Cancer Ther. 2006;5(1):8–19.

22. da Silva JM, Soave DF, Moreira dos Santos TP, Batista AC, Russo RC, Teixeira MM, et al. Significance of chemokine and chemokine receptors in head and neck squamous cell carci-noma: a critical review. Oral Oncol. 2016;56:8–16.

23. Chan L-P, Wang L-F, Chiang F-Y, Lee K-W, Kuo P-L, Liang C-H. IL-8 promotes HNSCC progression on CXCR1/2-meidated NOD1/RIP2 signaling pathway. Oncotarget. 2016;7(38):61820–31.

24. Loukinova E, Dong G, Enamorado-Ayalya I, Thomas GR, Chen Z, Schreiber H, et al. Growth regulated oncogene-alpha expression by murine squamous cell carcinoma promotes tumor growth, metastasis, leukocyte infiltration and angiogenesis by a host CXC receptor-2 depen-dent mechanism. Oncogene. 2000;19(31):3477–86.

25. Bancroft CC, Chen Z, Dong G, Sunwoo JB, Yeh N, Park C, et al. Coexpression of proangio-genic factors IL-8 and VEGF by human head and neck squamous cell carcinoma involves coactivation by MEK-MAPK and IKK-NF-kappaB signal pathways. Clin Cancer Res. 2001;7(2):435–42.
26. Bancroft CC, Chen Z, Yeh J, Sunwoo JB, Yeh NT, Jackson S, et al. Effects of pharmacologic antagonists of epidermal growth factor receptor, PI3K and MEK signal kinases on NF-kappaB and AP-1 activation and IL-8 and VEGF expression in human head and neck squamous cell carcinoma lines. Int J Cancer. 2002;99(4):538–48.
27. Vandercappellen J, Van Damme J, Struyf S. The role of CXC chemokines and their receptors in cancer. Cancer Lett. 2008;267(2):226–44.
28. Dong G, Chen Z, Li ZY, Yeh NT, Bancroft CC, Van Waes C. Hepatocyte growth factor/scat-ter factor-induced activation of MEK and PI3K signal pathways contributes to expression of proangiogenic cytokines interleukin-8 and vascular endothelial growth factor in head and neck squamous cell carcinoma. Cancer Res. 2001;61(15):5911–8.
29. Dong G, Lee TL, Yeh NT, Geoghegan J, Van Waes C, Chen Z. Metastatic squamous cell carci-noma cells that overexpress c-Met exhibit enhanced angiogenesis factor expression, scattering and metastasis in response to hepatocyte growth factor. Oncogene. 2004;23(37):6199–208.
30. Worden B, Yang XP, Lee TL, Bagain L, Yeh NT, Cohen JG, et al. Hepatocyte growth fac-tor/scatter factor differentially regulates expression of proangiogenic factors through Egr-1 in head and neck squamous cell carcinoma. Cancer Res. 2005;65(16):7071–80.
31. Siemeister G, Martiny-Baron G, Marme D. The pivotal role of VEGF in tumor angiogenesis: molecular facts and therapeutic opportunities. Cancer Metastasis Rev. 1998;17(2):241–8.
32. Kowanetz M, Ferrara N. Vascular endothelial growth factor signaling pathways: therapeutic perspective. Clin Cancer Res. 2006;12(17):5018–22.
33. Lalla RV, Boisoneau DS, Spiro JD, Kreutzer DL. Expression of vascular endothelial growth factor receptors on tumor cells in head and neck squamous cell carcinoma. Arch Otolaryngol Head Neck Surg. 2003;129(8):882–8.
34. Arnold L, Enders J, Thomas SM. Activated HGF-c-Met axis in head and neck cancer. Cancers (Basel). 2017;9(12):169.
35. Aebersold DM, Landt O, Berthou S, Gruber G, Beer KT, Greiner RH, et al. Prevalence and clinical impact of Met Y1253D-activating point mutation in radiotherapy-treated squamous cell cancer of the oropharynx. Oncogene. 2003;22(52):8519–23.
36. Hong IS. Stimulatory versus suppressive effects of GM-CSF on tumor progression in multiple cancer types. Exp Mol Med. 2016;48(7):e242.
37. Hansen G, Hercus TR, McClure BJ, Stomski FC, Dottore M, Powell J, et al. The structure of the GM-CSF receptor complex reveals a distinct mode of cytokine receptor activation. Cell. 2008;134(3):496–507.
38. Suh HS, Kim MO, Lee SC. Inhibition of granulocyte-macrophage colony-stimulating factor signaling and microglial proliferation by anti-CD45RO: role of Hck tyrosine kinase and phos-phatidylinositol 3-kinase/Akt. J Immunol. 2005;174(5):2712–9.
39. Ninck S, Reisser C, Dyckhoff G, Helmke B, Bauer H, Herold-Mende C. Expression profiles of angiogenic growth factors in squamous cell carcinomas of the head and neck. Int J Cancer. 2003;106(1):34–44.
40. Gutschalk CM, Herold-Mende CC, Fusenig NE, Mueller MM. Granulocyte colony-stimulating factor and granulocyte-macrophage colony-stimulating factor promote malignant growth of cells from head and neck squamous cell carcinomas in vivo. Cancer Res. 2006;66(16):8026–36.
41. Cohen RF, Contrino J, Spiro JD, Mann EA, Chen LL, Kreutzer DL. Interleukin-8 expres-sion by head and neck squamous cell carcinoma. Arch Otolaryngol Head Neck Surg. 1995;121(2):202–9.
42. Mann EA, Spiro JD, Chen LL, Kreutzer DL. Cytokine expression by head and neck squamous cell carcinomas. Am J Surg. 1992;164(6):567–73.

43. Woods KV, El-Naggar A, Clayman GL, Grimm EA. Variable expression of cytokines in human head and neck squamous cell carcinoma cell lines and consistent expression in surgical specimens. Cancer Res. 1998;58(14):3132–41.
44. Yamamura M, Modlin RL, Ohmen JD, Moy RL. Local expression of antiinflammatory cytokines in cancer. J Clin Invest. 1993;91(3):1005–10.
45. Woodford D, Johnson SD, De Costa A-MA, Young MRI. An inflammatory cytokine milieu is prominent in premalignant oral lesions, but subsides when lesions progress to squamous cell carcinoma. J Clin Cell Immunol. 2014;5(3):230.
46. Johnson SD, De Costa A-MA, Young MRI. Effect of the premalignant and tumor microenvironment on immune cell cytokine production in head and neck cancer. Cancers (Basel). 2014;6(2):756–70.
47. Juretić M, Cerović R, Belušić-Gobić M, Brekalo Pršo I, Kqiku L, Špalj S, et al. Salivary levels of TNF-α and IL-6 in patients with oral premalignant and malignant lesions. Folia Biol (Praha). 2013;59(2):99–102.
48. Shkeir O, Athanassiou M, Lapadatescu M, Papagerakis P, Czerwinski MJ, Bradford CR, et al. In vitro cytokines release profile: predictive value for metastatic potential in head and neck squamous cell carcinomas. Head Neck. 2013;35(11):1542–50.
49. Duffey DC, Crowl-Bancroft CV, Chen Z, Ondrey FG, Nejad-Sattari M, Dong G, et al. Inhibition of transcription factor nuclear factor-kappaB by a mutant inhibitor-kappaBalpha attenuates resistance of human head and neck squamous cell carcinoma to TNF-alpha caspase-mediated cell death. Br J Cancer. 2000;83(10):1367–74.
50. Eytan DF, Snow GE, Carlson SG, Schiltz S, Chen Z, Van Waes C. Combination effects of SMAC mimetic birinapant with TNFalpha, TRAIL, and docetaxel in preclinical models of HNSCC. Laryngoscope. 2015;125(3):E118–24.
51. Lu H, Yan C, Quan XX, Yang X, Zhang J, Bian Y, et al. CK2 phosphorylates and inhibits TAp73 tumor suppressor function to promote expression of cancer stem cell genes and phenotype in head and neck cancer. Neoplasia. 2014;16(10):789–800.
52. Lu H, Yang X, Duggal P, Allen CT, Yan B, Cohen J, et al. TNF-alpha promotes c-REL/DeltaNp63alpha interaction and TAp73 dissociation from key genes that mediate growth arrest and apoptosis in head and neck cancer. Cancer Res. 2011;71(21):6867–77.
53. Druzgal CH, Chen Z, Yeh NT, Thomas GR, Ondrey FG, Duffey DC, et al. A pilot study of longitudinal serum cytokine and angiogenesis factor levels as markers of therapeutic response and survival in patients with head and neck squamous cell carcinoma. Head Neck. 2005;27(9):771–84.
54. Astradsson T, Sellberg F, Berglund D, Ehrsson YT, Laurell GFE. Systemic inflammatory reaction in patients with head and neck cancer—an explorative study. Front Oncol. 2019;9:1177.
55. Stanam A, Gibson-Corley KN, Love-Homan L, Ihejirika N, Simons AL. Interleukin-1 blockade overcomes erlotinib resistance in head and neck squamous cell carcinoma. Oncotarget. 2016;7(46):76087–100.
56. Braunschweiger PG, Basrur VS, Cameron D, Sharpe L, Santos O, Perras JP, et al. Modulation of cisPlatin cytotoxicity by interleukin-1 alpha and resident tumor macrophages. Biotherapy. 1997;10(2):129–37.
57. Freund-Brown J, Chirino L, Kambayashi T. Strategies to enhance NK cell function for the treatment of tumors and infections. Crit Rev Immunol. 2018;38(2):105–30.
58. Bier H, Hoffmann T, Haas I, van Lierop A. Anti-(epidermal growth factor) receptor monoclonal antibodies for the induction of antibody-dependent cell-mediated cytotoxicity against squamous cell carcinoma lines of the head and neck. Cancer Immunol Immunother. 1998;46(3):167–73.
59. Espinosa-Cotton M, Rodman Iii SN, Ross KA, Jensen IJ, Sangodeyi-Miller K, McLaren AJ, et al. Interleukin-1 alpha increases anti-tumor efficacy of cetuximab in head and neck squamous cell carcinoma. J Immunother Cancer. 2019;7(1):79.

60. Jinno T, Kawano S, Maruse Y, Matsubara R, Goto Y, Sakamoto T, et al. Increased expression of interleukin-6 predicts poor response to chemoradiotherapy and unfavorable prognosis in oral squamous cell carcinoma. Oncol Rep. 2015;33(5):2161–8.
61. Lee TL, Yeh J, Friedman J, Yan B, Yang X, Yeh NT, et al. A signal network involving coactivated NF-kappaB and STAT3 and altered p53 modulates BAX/BCL-XL expression and promotes cell survival of head and neck squamous cell carcinomas. Int J Cancer. 2008;122(9):1987–98.
62. Sriuranpong V, Park JI, Amornphimoltham P, Patel V, Nelkin BD, Gutkind JS. Epidermal growth factor receptor-independent constitutive activation of STAT3 in head and neck squamous cell carcinoma is mediated by the autocrine/paracrine stimulation of the interleukin 6/gp130 cytokine system. Cancer Res. 2003;63(11):2948–56.
63. Bu LL, Yu GT, Wu L, Mao L, Deng WW, Liu JF, et al. STAT3 induces immunosuppression by upregulating PD-1/PD-L1 in HNSCC. J Dent Res. 2017;96(9):1027–34.
64. Liu Q, Yu S, Li A, Xu H, Han X, Wu K. Targeting interleukin-6 to relieve immunosuppression in tumor microenvironment. Tumour Biol. 2017;39(6):1010428317712445.
65. Park SJ, Nakagawa T, Kitamura H, Atsumi T, Kamon H, Sawa S, et al. IL-6 regulates in vivo dendritic cell differentiation through STAT3 activation. J Immunol. 2004;173(6):3844–54.
66. Wang T, Niu G, Kortylewski M, Burdelya L, Shain K, Zhang S, et al. Regulation of the innate and adaptive immune responses by Stat-3 signaling in tumor cells. Nat Med. 2004;10(1):48–54.
67. Johnson DE, O'Keefe RA, Grandis JR. Targeting the IL-6/JAK/STAT3 signalling axis in cancer. Nat Rev Clin Oncol. 2018;15(4):234–48.
68. Leong PL, Andrews GA, Johnson DE, Dyer KF, Xi S, Mai JC, et al. Targeted inhibition of Stat3 with a decoy oligonucleotide abrogates head and neck cancer cell growth. Proc Natl Acad Sci U S A. 2003;100(7):4138–43.
69. Sen M, Thomas SM, Kim S, Yeh JI, Ferris RL, Johnson JT, et al. First-in-human trial of a STAT3 decoy oligonucleotide in head and neck tumors: implications for cancer therapy. Cancer Discov. 2012;2(8):694–705.
70. Liu H, Shen J, Lu K. IL-6 and PD-L1 blockade combination inhibits hepatocellular carcinoma cancer development in mouse model. Biochem Biophys Res Commun. 2017;486(2):239–44.
71. Lu C, Talukder A, Savage NM, Singh N, Liu K. JAK-STAT-mediated chronic inflammation impairs cytotoxic T lymphocyte activation to decrease anti-PD-1 immunotherapy efficacy in pancreatic cancer. Onco Targets Ther. 2017;6(3):e1291106.
72. Mace TA, Shakya R, Pitarresi JR, Swanson B, McQuinn CW, Loftus S, et al. IL-6 and PD-L1 antibody blockade combination therapy reduces tumour progression in murine models of pancreatic cancer. Gut. 2018;67(2):320–32.
73. Cohen EEW, Harrington KJ, Hong DS, Mesia R, Brana I, Perez Segura P, et al. A phase Ib/II study (SCORES) of durvalumab (D) plus danvatirsen (DAN; AZD9150) or AZD5069 (CX2i) in advanced solid malignancies and recurrent/metastatic head and neck squamous cell carcinoma (RM-HNSCC): updated results. Ann Oncol. 2018;29(Supplement 8):viii372–99.
74. Schalper KA, Carleton M, Zhou M, Chen T, Feng Y, Huang SP, et al. Elevated serum interleukin-8 is associated with enhanced intratumor neutrophils and reduced clinical benefit of immune-checkpoint inhibitors. Nat Med. 2020;26(5):688–92.
75. Yuen KC, Liu LF, Gupta V, Madireddi S, Keerthivasan S, Li C, et al. High systemic and tumor-associated IL-8 correlates with reduced clinical benefit of PD-L1 blockade. Nat Med. 2020;26(5):693–8.
76. Sanmamed MF, Perez-Gracia JL, Schalper KA, Fusco JP, Gonzalez A, Rodriguez-Ruiz ME, et al. Chavnges in serum interleukin-8 (IL-8) levels reflect and predict response to anti-PD-1 treatment in melanoma and non-small-cell lung cancer patients. Ann Oncol. 2017;28(8):1988–95.
77. Greene S, Robbins Y, Mydlarz WK, Huynh AP, Schmitt NC, Friedman J, et al. Inhibition of MDSC trafficking with SX-682, a CXCR1/2 inhibitor, enhances NK-cell immunotherapy in head and neck cancer models. Clin Cancer Res. 2020;26(6):1420–31.
78. Sun SC. The noncanonical NF-kappaB pathway. Immunol Rev. 2012;246(1):125–40.

79. Zhang Q, Lenardo MJ, Baltimore D. 30 years of NF-kappaB: a blossoming of relevance to human pathobiology. Cell. 2017;168(1–2):37–57.

80. House CD, Grajales V, Ozaki M, Jordan E, Wubneh H, Kimble DC, et al. IKappaKappaepsilon cooperates with either MEK or non-canonical NF-kB driving growth of triple-negative breast cancer cells in different contexts. BMC Cancer. 2018;18(1):595.

81. Khongthong P, Roseweir AK, Edwards J. The NF-KB pathway and endocrine therapy resistance in breast cancer. Endocr Relat Cancer. 2019;26(6):R369–R80.

82. Sakamoto K, Maeda S. Targeting NF-kappaB for colorectal cancer. Expert Opin Ther Targets. 2010;14(6):593–601.

83. Soleimani A, Rahmani F, Ferns GA, Ryzhikov M, Avan A, Hassanian SM. Role of the NF-kappaB signaling pathway in the pathogenesis of colorectal cancer. Gene. 2020;726: 144132.

84. Taniguchi K, Karin M. NF-kappaB, inflammation, immunity and cancer: coming of age. Nat Rev Immunol. 2018;18(5):309–24.

85. Van Waes C. Nuclear factor-kappaB in development, prevention, and therapy of cancer. Clin Cancer Res. 2007;13(4):1076–82.

86. Giuliani C, Bucci I, Napolitano G. The role of the transcription factor nuclear factor-kappa B in thyroid autoimmunity and cancer. Front Endocrinol (Lausanne). 2018;9:471.

87. Liu T, Zhang L, Joo D, Sun SC. NF-kappaB signaling in inflammation. Signal Transduct Target Ther. 2017;2:17023.

88. Cartwright T, Perkins ND, Wilson CL. NFKB1: a suppressor of inflammation, ageing and cancer. FEBS J. 2016;283(10):1812–22.

89. Kaltschmidt B, Greiner JFW, Kadhim HM, Kaltschmidt C. Subunit-specific role of NF-kappaB in cancer. Biomedicines. 2018;6(2):44.

90. Vander Broek R, Snow GE, Chen Z, Van Waes C. Chemoprevention of head and neck squamous cell carcinoma through inhibition of NF-kappaB signaling. Oral Oncol. 2014;50(10):930–41.

91. Ben-Neriah Y. Regulatory functions of ubiquitination in the immune system. Nat Immunol. 2002;3(1):20–6.

92. Christian F, Smith EL, Carmody RJ. The regulation of NF-kappaB subunits by phosphorylation. Cells. 2016;5(1):12.

93. Arun P, Brown MS, Ehsanian R, Chen Z, Van Waes C. Nuclear NF-kappaB p65 phosphorylation at serine 276 by protein kinase A contributes to the malignant phenotype of head and neck cancer. Clin Cancer Res. 2009;15(19):5974–84.

94. Sakurai H, Chiba H, Miyoshi H, Sugita T, Toriumi W. IkappaB kinases phosphorylate NF-kappaB p65 subunit on serine 536 in the transactivation domain. J Biol Chem. 1999;274(43):30353–6.

95. Ondrey FG, Dong G, Sunwoo J, Chen Z, Wolf JS, Crowl-Bancroft CV, et al. Constitutive activation of transcription factors NF-(kappa)B, AP-1, and NF-IL6 in human head and neck squamous cell carcinoma cell lines that express pro-inflammatory and pro-angiogenic cytokines. Mol Carcinog. 1999;26(2):119–29.

96. Dong G, Loukinova E, Chen Z, Gangi L, Chanturita TI, Liu ET, et al. Molecular profiling of transformed and metastatic murine squamous carcinoma cells by differential display and cDNA microarray reveals altered expression of multiple genes related to growth, apoptosis, angiogenesis, and the NF-kappaB signal pathway. Cancer Res. 2001;61(12):4797–808.

97. Loercher A, Lee TL, Ricker JL, Howard A, Geoghegen J, Chen Z, et al. Nuclear factor-kappaB is an important modulator of the altered gene expression profile and malignant phenotype in squamous cell carcinoma. Cancer Res. 2004;64(18):6511–23.

98. Cancer Genome Atlas Network. Comprehensive genomic characterization of head and neck squamous cell carcinomas. Nature. 2015;517(7536):576–82.

99. Zhang J, Chen T, Yang X, Cheng H, Spath SS, Clavijo PE, et al. Attenuated TRAF3 fosters activation of alternative NF-kappaB and reduced expression of antiviral interferon, TP53, and RB to promote HPV-positive head and neck cancers. Cancer Res. 2018;78(16):4613–26.

100. Chen T, Zhang J, Chen Z, Van Waes C. Genetic alterations in TRAF3 and CYLD that regulate nuclear factor kappaB and interferon signaling define head and neck cancer subsets harboring human papillomavirus. Cancer. 2017;123(10):1695–8.

101. Mishra A, Bharti AC, Varghese P, Saluja D, Das BC. Differential expression and activation of NF-kappaB family proteins during oral carcinogenesis: role of high risk human papillomavirus infection. Int J Cancer. 2006;119(12):2840–50.

102. Gupta S, Kumar P, Kaur H, Sharma N, Gupta S, Saluja D, et al. Constitutive activation and overexpression of NF-kappaB/c-Rel in conjunction with p50 contribute to aggressive tongue tumorigenesis. Oncotarget. 2018;9(68):33011–29.

103. Freudlsperger C, Burnett JR, Friedman JA, Kannabiran VR, Chen Z, Van Waes C. EGFR-PI3K-AKT-mTOR signaling in head and neck squamous cell carcinomas: attractive targets for molecular-oriented therapy. Expert Opin Ther Targets. 2011;15(1):63–74.

104. Vivanco I, Sawyers CL. The phosphatidylinositol 3-kinase AKT pathway in human cancer. Nat Rev Cancer. 2002;2(7):489–501.

105. Dan HC, Cooper MJ, Cogswell PC, Duncan JA, Ting JP, Baldwin AS. Akt-dependent regulation of NF-κB is controlled by mTOR and Raptor in association with IKK. Genes Dev. 2008;22(11):1490–500.

106. Dan HC, Ebbs A, Pasparakis M, Van Dyke T, Basseres DS, Baldwin AS. Akt-dependent activation of mTORC1 complex involves phosphorylation of mTOR (mammalian target of rapamycin) by IkappaB kinase alpha (IKKalpha). J Biol Chem. 2014;289(36):25227–40.

107. Tanaka K, Babic I, Nathanson D, Akhavan D, Guo D, Gini B, et al. Oncogenic EGFR signaling activates an mTORC2-NF-kappaB pathway that promotes chemotherapy resistance. Cancer Discov. 2011;1(6):524–38.

108. Wilson W 3rd, Baldwin AS. Maintenance of constitutive IkappaB kinase activity by glycogen synthase kinase-3alpha/beta in pancreatic cancer. Cancer Res. 2008;68(19):8156–63.

109. Nottingham LK, Yan CH, Yang X, Si H, Coupar J, Bian Y, et al. Aberrant IKKalpha and IKKbeta cooperatively activate NF-kappaB and induce EGFR/AP1 signaling to promote survival and migration of head and neck cancer. Oncogene. 2014;33(9):1135–47.

110. Freudlsperger C, Bian Y, Contag Wise S, Burnett J, Coupar J, Yang X, et al. TGF-beta and NF-kappaB signal pathway cross-talk is mediated through TAK1 and SMAD7 in a subset of head and neck cancers. Oncogene. 2013;32(12):1549–59.

111. Shaulian E, Karin M. AP-1 as a regulator of cell life and death. Nat Cell Biol. 2002;4(5):E131–6.

112. Atsaves V, Leventaki V, Rassidakis GZ, Claret FX. AP-1 transcription factors as regulators of immune responses in cancer. Cancers (Basel). 2019;11(7):1037.

113. Hussain S, Bharti AC, Salam I, Bhat MA, Mir MM, Hedau S, et al. Transcription factor AP-1 in esophageal squamous cell carcinoma: alterations in activity and expression during human papillomavirus infection. BMC Cancer. 2009;9:329.

114. Mishra A, Bharti AC, Saluja D, Das BC. Transactivation and expression patterns of Jun and Fos/AP-1 super-family proteins in human oral cancer. Int J Cancer. 2010;126(4):819–29.

115. Gupta S, Kumar P, Kaur H, Sharma N, Saluja D, Bharti AC, et al. Selective participation of c-Jun with Fra-2/c-Fos promotes aggressive tumor phenotypes and poor prognosis in tongue cancer. Sci Rep. 2015;5:16811.

116. Faust RA, Gapany M, Tristani P, Davis A, Adams GL, Ahmed K. Elevated protein kinase CK2 activity in chromatin of head and neck tumors: association with malignant transformation. Cancer Lett. 1996;101(1):31–5.

117. Gapany M, Faust RA, Tawfic S, Davis A, Adams GL, Ahmed K. Association of elevated protein kinase CK2 activity with aggressive behavior of squamous cell carcinoma of the head and neck. Mol Med. 1995;1(6):659–66.

118. Yu M, Yeh J, Van Waes C. Protein kinase casein kinase 2 mediates inhibitor-kappaB kinase and aberrant nuclear factor-kappaB activation by serum factor(s) in head and neck squamous carcinoma cells. Cancer Res. 2006;66(13):6722–31.

119. Brown MS, Diallo OT, Hu M, Ehsanian R, Yang X, Arun P, et al. CK2 modulation of NF-kappaB, TP53, and the malignant phenotype in head and neck cancer by anti-CK2 oligonucleotides in vitro or in vivo via sub-50-nm nanocapsules. Clin Cancer Res. 2010;16(8):2295–307.

120. Bian Y, Han J, Kannabiran V, Mohan S, Cheng H, Friedman J, et al. MEK inhibitor PD-0325901 overcomes resistance to CK2 inhibitor CX-4945 and exhibits anti-tumor activity in head and neck cancer. Int J Biol Sci. 2015;11(4):411–22.
121. Chen Z, Yan B, Van Waes C. The role of the NF-kappaB transcriptome and proteome as biomarkers in human head and neck squamous cell carcinomas. Biomark Med. 2008;2(4):409–26.
122. Allen CT, Conley B, Sunwoo JB, Van Waes C. CCR 20th anniversary commentary: preclinical study of proteasome inhibitor bortezomib in head and neck cancer. Clin Cancer Res. 2015;21(5):942–3.
123. Allen C, Saigal K, Nottingham L, Arun P, Chen Z, Van Waes C. Bortezomib-induced apoptosis with limited clinical response is accompanied by inhibition of canonical but not alternative nuclear factor-κB subunits in head and neck cancer. Clin Cancer Res. 2008;14(13):4175–85.
124. Gaykalova DA, Manola JB, Ozawa H, Zizkova V, Morton K, Bishop JA, et al. NF-kappaB and stat3 transcription factor signatures differentiate HPV-positive and HPV-negative head and neck squamous cell carcinoma. Int J Cancer. 2015;137(8):1879–89.
125. Liu Y, Denlinger CE, Rundall BK, Smith PW, Jones DR. Suberoylanilide hydroxamic acid induces Akt-mediated phosphorylation of p300, which promotes acetylation and transcriptional activation of RelA/p65. J Biol Chem. 2006;281(42):31359–68.
126. Webster GA, Perkins ND. Transcriptional cross talk between NF-kappaB and p53. Mol Cell Biol. 1999;19(5):3485–95.
127. Herzog A, Bian Y, Vander Broek R, Hall B, Coupar J, Cheng H, et al. PI3K/mTOR inhibitor PF-04691502 antitumor activity is enhanced with induction of wild-type TP53 in human xenograft and murine knockout models of head and neck cancer. Clin Cancer Res. 2013;19(14):3808–19.
128. Leiker AJ, DeGraff W, Choudhuri R, Sowers AL, Thetford A, Cook JA, et al. Radiation enhancement of head and neck squamous cell carcinoma by the dual PI3K/mTOR inhibitor PF-05212384. Clin Cancer Res. 2015;21(12):2792–801.
129. Mohan S, Vander Broek R, Shah S, Eytan DF, Pierce ML, Carlson SG, et al. MEK inhibitor PD-0325901 overcomes resistance to PI3K/mTOR inhibitor PF-5212384 and potentiates antitumor effects in human head and neck squamous cell carcinoma. Clin Cancer Res. 2015;21(17):3946–56.
130. Day TA, Shirai K, O'Brien PE, Matheus MG, Godwin K, Sood AJ, et al. Inhibition of mTOR signaling and clinical activity of rapamycin in head and neck cancer in a window of opportunity trial. Clin Cancer Res. 2019;25(4):1156–64.
131. Vermorken JB, Herbst RS, Leon X, Amellal N, Baselga J. Overview of the efficacy of cetuximab in recurrent and/or metastatic squamous cell carcinoma of the head and neck in patients who previously failed platinum-based therapies. Cancer. 2008;112(12):2710–9.
132. Van Waes C, Allen CT, Citrin D, Gius D, Colevas AD, Harold NA, et al. Molecular and clinical responses in a pilot study of gefitinib with paclitaxel and radiation in locally advanced head-and-neck cancer. Int J Radiat Oncol Biol Phys. 2010;77(2):447–54.
133. Pernas FG, Allen CT, Winters ME, Yan B, Friedman J, Dabir B, et al. Proteomic signatures of epidermal growth factor receptor and survival signal pathways correspond to gefitinib sensitivity in head and neck cancer. Clin Cancer Res. 2009;15(7):2361–72.
134. Kuriakose MA, Ramdas K, Dey B, Iyer S, Rajan G, Elango KK, et al. A randomized double-blind placebo-controlled phase IIB trial of curcumin in oral leukoplakia. Cancer Prev Res (Phila). 2016;9(8):683–91.
135. Hanahan D, Weinberg RA. Hallmarks of cancer: the next generation. Cell. 2011;144(5):646–74.
136. Corn JE, Vucic D. Ubiquitin in inflammation: the right linkage makes all the difference. Nat Struct Mol Biol. 2014;21(4):297–300.
137. Hu H, Sun S-C. Ubiquitin signaling in immune responses. Cell Res. 2016;26(4):457–83.
138. Komander D, Clague MJ, Urbé S. Breaking the chains: structure and function of the deubiquitinases. Nat Rev Mol Cell Biol. 2009;10(8):550–63.
139. Ji Z, He L, Regev A, Struhl K. Inflammatory regulatory network mediated by the joint action of NF-kB, STAT3, and AP-1 factors is involved in many human cancers. Proc Natl Acad Sci U S A. 2019;116(19):9453–62.

140. Wang G, Gao Y, Li L, Jin G, Cai Z, Chao J-I, et al. K63-linked ubiquitination in kinase activation and cancer. Front Oncol. 2012;2:5.
141. Ea C-K, Deng L, Xia Z-P, Pineda G, Chen ZJ. Activation of IKK by TNFalpha requires site-specific ubiquitination of RIP1 and polyubiquitin binding by NEMO. Mol Cell. 2006;22(2):245–57.
142. Wang C, Deng L, Hong M, Akkaraju GR, Inoue J, Chen ZJ. TAK1 is a ubiquitin-dependent kinase of MKK and IKK. Nature. 2001;412(6844):346–51.
143. Winston JT, Strack P, Beer-Romero P, Chu CY, Elledge SJ, Harper JW. The SCFbeta-TRCP-ubiquitin ligase complex associates specifically with phosphorylated destruction motifs in IkappaBalpha and beta-catenin and stimulates IkappaBalpha ubiquitination in vitro. Genes Dev. 1999;13(3):270–83.
144. Li X, Commane M, Jiang Z, Stark GR. IL-1-induced NFkappa B and c-Jun N-terminal kinase (JNK) activation diverge at IL-1 receptor-associated kinase (IRAK). Proc Natl Acad Sci U S A. 2001;98(8):4461–5.
145. Griesinger AM, Josephson RJ, Donson AM, Mulcahy Levy JM, Amani V, Birks DK, et al. Interleukin-6/STAT3 pathway signaling drives an inflammatory phenotype in Group A ependymoma. Cancer Immunol Res. 2015;3(10):1165–74.
146. Haas TL, Emmerich CH, Gerlach B, Schmukle AC, Cordier SM, Rieser E, et al. Recruitment of the linear ubiquitin chain assembly complex stabilizes the TNF-R1 signaling complex and is required for TNF-mediated gene induction. Mol Cell. 2009;36(5):831–44.
147. Tokunaga F, Sakata S-I, Saeki Y, Satomi Y, Kirisako T, Kamei K, et al. Involvement of linear polyubiquitylation of NEMO in NF-kappaB activation. Nat Cell Biol. 2009;11(2):123–32.
148. Harhaj EW, Dixit VM. Deubiquitinases in the regulation of NF-κB signaling. Cell Res. 2011;21(1):22–39.
149. Catrysse L, Vereecke L, Beyaert R, van Loo G. A20 in inflammation and autoimmunity. Trends Immunol. 2014;35(1):22–31.
150. Shembade N, Ma A, Harhaj EW. Inhibition of NF-kappaB signaling by A20 through disruption of ubiquitin enzyme complexes. Science. 2010;327(5969):1135–9.
151. Iliopoulos D, Jaeger SA, Hirsch HA, Bulyk ML, Struhl K. STAT3 activation of miR-21 and miR-181b-1 via PTEN and CYLD are part of the epigenetic switch linking inflammation to cancer. Mol Cell. 2010;39(4):493–506.
152. Hrdinka M, Fiil BK, Zucca M, Leske D, Bagola K, Yabal M, et al. CYLD limits Lys63- and Met1-linked ubiquitin at receptor complexes to regulate innate immune signaling. Cell Rep. 2016;14(12):2846–58.
153. Enesa K, Zakkar M, Chaudhury H, Luong LA, Rawlinson L, Mason JC, et al. NF-kappaB suppression by the deubiquitinating enzyme Cezanne: a novel negative feedback loop in proinflammatory signaling. J Biol Chem. 2008;283(11):7036–45.
154. Xu G, Tan X, Wang H, Sun W, Shi Y, Burlingame S, et al. Ubiquitin-specific peptidase 21 inhibits tumor necrosis factor alpha-induced nuclear factor kappaB activation via binding to and deubiquitinating receptor-interacting protein 1. J Biol Chem. 2010;285(2):969–78.
155. Goncharov T, Niessen K, de Almagro MC, Izrael-Tomasevic A, Fedorova AV, Varfolomeev E, et al. OTUB1 modulates c-IAP1 stability to regulate signalling pathways. EMBO J. 2013;32(8):1103–14.
156. Wiener R, Zhang X, Wang T, Wolberger C. The mechanism of OTUB1-mediated inhibition of ubiquitination. Nature. 2012;483(7391):618–22.
157. Sun W, Tan X, Shi Y, Xu G, Mao R, Gu X, et al. USP11 negatively regulates TNFalpha-induced NF-kappaB activation by targeting on IkappaBalpha. Cell Signal. 2010;22(3):386–94.
158. Cheng H, Yang X, Si H, Saleh AD, Xiao W, Coupar J, et al. Genomic and transcriptomic characterization links cell lines with aggressive head and neck cancers. Cell Rep. 2018;25(5):1332–45.e5.
159. Morgan EL, Chen Z, Van Waes C. Regulation of NFκB Signalling by Ubiquitination: A Potential Therapeutic Target in Head and Neck Squamous Cell Carcinoma?. Cancers (Basel). 2020;12(10):2877.

160. Hajek M, Sewell A, Kaech S, Burtness B, Yarbrough WG, Issaeva N. TRAF3/CYLD mutations identify a distinct subset of human papillomavirus-associated head and neck squamous cell carcinoma. Cancer. 2017;123(10):1778–90.

161. Ge Z, Leighton JS, Wang Y, Peng X, Chen Z, Chen H, et al. Integrated genomic analysis of the ubiquitin pathway across cancer types. Cell Rep. 2018;23(1):213–26.e3.

162. Arabi A, Ullah K, Branca RMM, Johansson J, Bandarra D, Haneklaus M, et al. Proteomic screen reveals Fbw7 as a modulator of the NF-κB pathway. Nat Commun. 2012;3(1):976–11.

163. Nateri AS, Riera-Sans L, Da Costa C, Behrens A. The ubiquitin ligase SCFFbw7 antagonizes apoptotic JNK signaling. Science. 2004;303(5662):1374–8.

164. Davis RJ, Welcker M, Clurman BE. Tumor suppression by the Fbw7 ubiquitin ligase: mechanisms and opportunities. Cancer Cell. 2014;26(4):455–64.

165. Lee D-F, Kuo H-P, Liu M, Chou C-K, Xia W, Du Y, et al. KEAP1 E3 ligase-mediated downregulation of NF-kappaB signaling by targeting IKKbeta. Mol Cell. 2009;36(1):131–40.

166. Drainas AP, Lambuta RA, Ivanova I, Serçin Ö, Sarropoulos I, Smith ML, et al. Genome-wide screens implicate loss of cullin ring ligase 3 in persistent proliferation and genome instability in TP53-deficient cells. Cell Rep. 2020;31(1):107465.

167. Liu J, Shaik S, Dai X, Wu Q, Zhou X, Wang Z, et al. Targeting the ubiquitin pathway for cancer treatment. Biochim Biophys Acta. 2015;1855(1):50–60.

168. Hideshima T, Richardson PG, Anderson KC. Mechanism of action of proteasome inhibitors and deacetylase inhibitors and the biological basis of synergy in multiple myeloma. Mol Cancer Ther. 2011;10(11):2034–42.

169. Oerlemans R, Franke NE, Assaraf YG, Cloos J, van Zantwijk I, Berkers CR, et al. Molecular basis of bortezomib resistance: proteasome subunit beta5 (PSMB5) gene mutation and overexpression of PSMB5 protein. Blood. 2008;112(6):2489–99.

170. Siegel DS, Martin T, Wang M, Vij R, Jakubowiak AJ, Lonial S, et al. A phase 2 study of single-agent carfilzomib (PX-171-003-A1) in patients with relapsed and refractory multiple myeloma. Blood. 2012;120(14):2817–25.

171. Chen Z, Ricker JL, Malhotra PS, Nottingham L, Bagain L, Lee TL, et al. Differential bortezomib sensitivity in head and neck cancer lines corresponds to proteasome, nuclear factorkappaB and activator protein-1 related mechanisms. Mol Cancer Ther. 2008;7(7):1949–60.

172. Sunwoo JB, Chen Z, Dong G, Yeh N, Crowl Bancroft C, Sausville E, et al. Novel proteasome inhibitor PS-341 inhibits activation of nuclear factor-kappa B, cell survival, tumor growth, and angiogenesis in squamous cell carcinoma. Clin Cancer Res. 2001;7(5):1419–28.

173. Kim J, Guan J, Chang I, Chen X, Han D, Wang C-Y. PS-341 and histone deacetylase inhibitor synergistically induce apoptosis in head and neck squamous cell carcinoma cells. Mol Cancer Ther. 2010;9(7):1977–84.

174. Fulda S, Vucic D. Targeting IAP proteins for therapeutic intervention in cancer. Nat Rev Drug Discov. 2012;11(2):109–24.

175. Varfolomeev E, Blankenship JW, Wayson SM, Fedorova AV, Kayagaki N, Garg P, et al. IAP antagonists induce autoubiquitination of c-IAPs, NF-kappaB activation, and TNFalphadependent apoptosis. Cell. 2007;131(4):669–81.

176. Shiozaki EN, Chai J, Rigotti DJ, Riedl SJ, Li P, Srinivasula SM, et al. Mechanism of XIAP-mediated inhibition of caspase-9. Mol Cell. 2003;11(2):519–27.

177. Eytan DF, Snow GE, Carlson S, Derakhshan A, Saleh A, Schiltz S, et al. SMAC mimetic birinapant plus radiation eradicates human head and neck cancers with genomic amplifications of cell death genes FADD and BIRC2. Cancer Res. 2016;76(18):5442–54.

178. Perimenis P, Galaris A, Voulgari A, Prassa M, Pintzas A. IAP antagonists Birinapant and AT-406 efficiently synergise with either TRAIL, BRAF, or BCL-2 inhibitors to sensitise BRAFV600E colorectal tumour cells to apoptosis. BMC Cancer. 2016;16(1):624–16.

179. Fulda S. Promises and challenges of Smac mimetics as cancer therapeutics. Clin Cancer Res. 2015;21(22):5030–6.

180. Tolcher AW, Bendell JC, Papadopoulos KP, Burris HA, Patnaik A, Fairbrother WJ, et al. A phase I dose-escalation study evaluating the safety tolerability and pharmacokinetics of

CUDC-427, a potent, oral, monovalent IAP antagonist, in patients with refractory solid tumors. Clin Cancer Res. 2016;22(18):4567–73.

181. Hurwitz HI, Smith DC, Pitot HC, Brill JM, Chugh R, Rouits E, et al. Safety, pharmacokinetics, and pharmacodynamic properties of oral DEBIO1143 (AT-406) in patients with advanced cancer: results of a first-in-man study. Cancer Chemother Pharmacol. 2015;75(4):851–9.

182. Zhao X-Y, Wang X-Y, Wei Q-Y, Xu Y-M, Lau ATY. Potency and selectivity of SMAC/DIABLO mimetics in solid tumor therapy. Cell. 2020;9(4):1012.

183. Matzinger O, Viertl D, Tsoutsou P, Kadi L, Rigotti S, Zanna C, et al. The radiosensitizing activity of the SMAC-mimetic, Debio 1143, is TNFα-mediated in head and neck squamous cell carcinoma. Radiother Oncol. 2015;116(3):495–503.

184. Pierce JW, Schoenleber R, Jesmok G, Best J, Moore SA, Collins T, et al. Novel inhibitors of cytokine-induced IkappaBalpha phosphorylation and endothelial cell adhesion molecule expression show anti-inflammatory effects in vivo. J Biol Chem. 1997;272(34):21096–103.

185. Yang L, Kumar B, Shen C, Zhao S, Blakaj D, Li T, et al. LCL161, a SMAC-mimetic, preferentially radiosensitizes human papillomavirus-negative head and neck squamous cell carcinoma. Mol Cancer Ther. 2019;18(6):1025–35.

186. Xiao R, An Y, Ye W, Derakhshan A, Cheng H, Yang X, et al. Dual antagonist of cIAP/XIAP ASTX660 sensitizes HPV− and HPV+ head and neck cancers to TNFα, TRAIL, and radiation therapy. Clin Cancer Res. 2019;25(21):6463–74.

187. Ye W, Gunti S, Allen CT, Hong Y, Clavijo PE, Van Waes C, et al. ASTX660, an antagonist of cIAP1/2 and XIAP, increases antigen processing machinery and can enhance radiation-induced immunogenic cell death in preclinical models of head and neck cancer. Onco Targets Ther. 2020;9(1):1710398.

188. Stratton MR, Campbell PJ, Futreal PA. The cancer genome. Nature. 2009;458(7239):719–24.

189. Lawrence MS, Stojanov P, Polak P, Kryukov GV, Cibulskis K, Sivachenko A, et al. Mutational heterogeneity in cancer and the search for new cancer-associated genes. Nature. 2013;499(7457):214–8.

190. Campbell JD, Yau C, Bowlby R, Liu Y, Brennan K, Fan H, et al. Genomic, pathway network, and immunologic features distinguishing squamous carcinomas. Cell Rep. 2018;23(1):194–212.e6.

191. Hutter C, Zenklusen JC. The Cancer Genome Atlas: creating lasting value beyond its data. Cell. 2018;173(2):283–5.

192. The TCGA Legacy. Cell. 2018;173(2):281–2.

193. Consortium GT, Laboratory DA, Coordinating Center -Analysis Working G, Statistical Methods groups-Analysis Working G, Enhancing Gg, Fund NIHC, et al. Genetic effects on gene expression across human tissues. Nature. 2017;550(7675):204-13.

194. Tsherniak A, Vazquez F, Montgomery PG, Weir BA, Kryukov G, Cowley GS, et al. Defining a Cancer Dependency Map. Cell. 2017;170(3):564–76 e16

195. Iorio F, Knijnenburg TA, Vis DJ, Bignell GR, Menden MP, Schubert M, et al. A Landscape of Pharmacogenomic Interactions in Cancer. Cell. 2016;166(3):740-54.

196. Uhlen M, Fagerberg L, Hallstrom BM, Lindskog C, Oksvold P, Mardinoglu A, et al. Proteomics. Tissue-based map of the human proteome. Science. 2015;347(6220):1260419.

197. Parfenov M, Pedamallu CS, Gehlenborg N, Freeman SS, Danilova L, Bristow CA, et al. Characterization of HPV and host genome interactions in primary head and neck cancers. Proc Natl Acad Sci U S A. 2014;111(43):15544–9.

198. Hoadley KA, Yau C, Wolf DM, Cherniack AD, Tamborero D, Ng S, et al. Multiplatform analysis of 12 cancer types reveals molecular classification within and across tissues of origin. Cell. 2014;158(4):929–44.

199. Hoadley KA, Yau C, Hinoue T, Wolf DM, Lazar AJ, Drill E, et al. Cell-of-origin patterns dominate the molecular classification of 10,000 tumors from 33 types of cancer. Cell. 2018;173(2):291–304.e6.

200. Ding L, Bailey MH, Porta-Pardo E, Thorsson V, Colaprico A, Bertrand D, et al. Perspective on oncogenic processes at the end of the beginning of cancer genomics. Cell. 2018;173(2):305–20.e10.
201. Sanchez-Vega F, Mina M, Armenia J, Chatila WK, Luna A, La KC, et al. Oncogenic signaling pathways in the Cancer Genome Atlas. Cell. 2018;173(2):321–37.e10.
202. Bailey MH, Tokheim C, Porta-Pardo E, Sengupta S, Bertrand D, Weerasinghe A, et al. Comprehensive characterization of cancer driver genes and mutations. Cell. 2018;174(4):1034–5.
203. Thorsson V, Gibbs DL, Brown SD, Wolf D, Bortone DS, Ou Yang TH, et al. The immune landscape of cancer. Immunity. 2018;48(4):812–30.e14.
204. Barretina J, Caponigro G, Stransky N, Venkatesan K, Margolin AA, Kim S, et al. The Cancer Cell Line Encyclopedia enables predictive modelling of anticancer drug sensitivity. Nature. 2012;483(7391):603–7.
205. Ghandi M, Huang FW, Jane-Valbuena J, Kryukov GV, Lo CC, McDonald ER 3rd, et al. Next-generation characterization of the Cancer Cell Line Encyclopedia. Nature. 2019;569(7757):503–8.
206. Ludwig ML, Kulkarni A, Birkeland AC, Michmerhuizen NL, Foltin SK, Mann JE, et al. The genomic landscape of UM-SCC oral cavity squamous cell carcinoma cell lines. Oral Oncol. 2018;87:144–51.
207. Mann JE, Kulkarni A, Birkeland AC, Kafelghazal J, Eisenberg J, Jewell BM, et al. The molecular landscape of the University of Michigan laryngeal squamous cell carcinoma cell line panel. Head Neck. 2019;41(9):3114–24.
208. van Harten AM, Poell JB, Buijze M, Brink A, Wells SI, Rene Leemans C, et al. Characterization of a head and neck cancer-derived cell line panel confirms the distinct TP53-proficient copy number-silent subclass. Oral Oncol. 2019;98:53–61.
209. McDonald ER 3rd, de Weck A, Schlabach MR, Billy E, Mavrakis KJ, Hoffman GR, et al. Project DRIVE: a compendium of cancer dependencies and synthetic lethal relationships uncovered by large-scale, deep RNAi screening. Cell. 2017;170(3):577–92.e10.
210. Behan FM, Iorio F, Picco G, Goncalves E, Beaver CM, Migliardi G, et al. Prioritization of cancer therapeutic targets using CRISPR-Cas9 screens. Nature. 2019;568(7753):511–6.
211. Corsello SM, Bittker JA, Liu Z, Gould J, McCarren P, Hirschman JE, et al. The Drug Repurposing Hub: a next-generation drug library and information resource. Nat Med. 2017;23(4):405–8.
212. Corsello SM, Nagari RT, Spangler RD, Rossen J, Kocak M, Bryan JG, et al. Discovering the anticancer potential of non-oncology drugs by systematic viability profiling. Nat Cancer. 2020;1(2):235–48.
213. Yu C, Mannan AM, Yvone GM, Ross KN, Zhang YL, Marton MA, et al. High-throughput identification of genotype-specific cancer vulnerabilities in mixtures of barcoded tumor cell lines. Nat Biotechnol. 2016;34(4):419–23.
214. Yang X, Cheng H, Chen J, Wang R, Saleh A, Si H, et al. Head and neck cancers promote an inflammatory transcriptome through coactivation of classic and alternative NF-kappaB pathways. Cancer Immunol Res. 2019;7(11):1760–74.

Chapter 8
Pain Associated with Head and Neck Cancers

Justin M. Young and Stephen Thaddeus Connelly

Introduction

Cancers of the head and neck are insidious and progressive entities that may present with a wide variety of symptoms depending on the location of the primary lesion. Lesions may be located in various anatomical structures including the sinuses, nasal cavity, salivary glands, tongue or lips, oral cavity, pharynx, or larynx. Depending on which of these sites are affected, there may be stereotypical symptoms that present or accompany the primary focus, but it is not necessarily a "one size fits all" presentation. Therefore, diagnosticians must realize there are no definitive patterns of pain that exist.

In general, a primary presenting lesion or mass or "sore" is detected first, commonly by the patient. In the head and neck region including oral cavity, the lips, gums, tongue, and cheeks are commonly affected structures. Contiguous structures such as the salivary glands, nasal cavity, and sinuses usually have initial masses or lesions that are more obscure and difficult to detect physically until they become quite advanced in size or begin to affect adjacent structures. Also, deeper structures, such as the nasopharynx or larynx, require special diagnostic modalities for detection, but usually these are not performed unless specific events encourage the consultation with a specialist. There is a high degree of variability among primary care physicians when synthesizing information that may ultimately lead to a timely

J. M. Young (✉)
Private Practice, San Francisco, CA, USA

Department of Oral & Maxillofacial Surgery, University of the Pacific, Arthur A. Dugoni School of Dentistry, San Francisco, CA, USA

S. T. Connelly
Department of Oral and Maxillofacial Surgery, University of California San Francisco (UCSF) School of Dentistry, San Francisco, CA, USA

San Francisco VA Health Care System, San Francisco, CA, USA

© Springer Nature Switzerland AG 2021
R. El Assal et al. (eds.), *Early Detection and Treatment of Head & Neck Cancers*, https://doi.org/10.1007/978-3-030-69852-2_8

185

referral to such specialist. Certainly, pain is one of the more straightforward presenting symptoms that helps lead to detection. Therefore, the symptoms of these more, "non-visible" primary lesions usually are indistinct until a later stage.

Within the easily visible structure of the oral cavity, hereafter understood to represent the mouth, lips, gums, tongue, and cheeks, usually a white or red sore is visible. This is commonly accompanied by pain or bleeding, a non-healing ulcer, and inflammation that affects regional structures. Symptoms are characteristically described as: (i) difficulty with swallowing, breathing, or speaking, (ii) pain with swallowing (dysphagia) or eating, (iii) chronic sore throat or neck pain (odynophagia), (iv) frequent headaches, (v) difficulty hearing or ringing in the ears (tinnitus), (vi) chronic nasal congestion with or without frequent nosebleeds (epistaxis), (vii) swelling around the eyes or double vision (diplopia), (viii) numbness or weakness of the facial muscles, and (ix) abnormal voice changes (hoarseness).

Certainly, the symptomatology indicates what the affected primary structure might be. For example, laryngeal primary lesions involve voice changes, difficulty with or painful swallowing, even a mass or lump in the throat, and enlarged lymph nodes even at a very early stage. In addition, coughing and choking with ingestion of foods and liquids, as well as unintentional aspiration of small volume of reflux materials (microaspiration), can be present. Therefore, constellations of symptoms may certainly point toward the area of the primary lesion, but not always.

In the oral cavity, there are several key common sites where lesions tend to develop more frequently, possibly due to static pooling of irritants, toxins, alcohol, or other carcinogens. These are in order of frequency, the sides of the tongue and floor of the mouth, the gum tissue behind the wisdom tooth or last molar (retromolar trigone), of the lateral and ventral surfaces of the tongue itself. Also, the gums, insides of cheeks and lips, and the roof of the mouth can develop irritation or lesions that can be detected at a very early stage.

In general, the evaluation of pain as a presenting symptom in head and neck cancers, leading to further diagnostic actions, is poorly understood. Most of the current understanding in this area comes from poorer-quality modalities such as self-reporting questionnaires as opposed to prospective or retrospective analyses [1]. Analysis shows that head and neck cancer (HNC) has prevalent reporting of pain, and certainly there are some factors that are associated with increased levels or pain appreciation [1–4]. However, the pain in HNC is overall poorly understood. We can all agree that changes in an area with dense innervation and presence of multiple overlapping critical anatomical structures in a confined area logically would have to be painful [1]. However, unique to oral cancers, the great majority of which are squamous cell carcinomas, is that they are accompanied by severe pain. Therefore, lesions that may be dysplastic or in situ typically do not produce pain [2–4]. Once conversion occurs, pain is a characteristic presenting symptom. This pain is usually associated with function, since the dynamic musculoskeletal components surrounding the oral cavity are constantly in motion with chewing, speaking, and swallowing [3]. Pain is not a common symptom associated with lesions outside the oral cavity, such as the base of the tongue, sinuses, larynx, and other areas previously mentioned.

Subsequently, we will further explore and elucidate the various modalities of pain associated with HNC by reviewing the contemporary state of knowledge in this area and then discuss modalities of treatment as well as avenues for further exploration.

Mechanisms of Head and Neck Cancer Pain

It is well established that the initial symptom leading to a diagnosis of most HNC and more commonly in oral squamous cell carcinoma (OSCC) in patients is lesion-specific pain [5]. The current theories explaining the overwhelming prevalence of pain in OSCC imply that the presence of a large number of soluble factors, generated by the cancer cells themselves, causes changes in the "microenvironment" of the lesion and allows a cascade of events that trigger, enhance, sensitize, and then perpetuate nociceptive pathways [2, 4]. Additionally, the experience of pain is subjective and is highly variable depending on the lesion and individual. Possible factors that correlate with oral cancer pain include (i) related to the primary lesion that include histological type (e.g., differentiation), (ii) presence of distant spread, and (iii) whether or not the lesion is situated near a site of musculoskeletal functioning, as many oral squamous cell lesions are. It has been demonstrated that oro-masticatory functions such as chewing, drinking, talking, and swallowing increase the perception of pain in patients with diagnosed OSCC [3]. This nociceptive activation is rare and not associated with other types of head and neck squamous cell carcinoma (HNSCC) such as nasopharyngeal or laryngeal [4]. As the initial lesion progresses, there are corresponding alterations in the surrounding microenvironment that may contribute to the development and perpetuation of oral cancer pain (summarized in Fig. 8.1). These changes occur in adjacent cells and tend to reflect the development of a tissue reparative versus a proinflammatory phenotype of the surrounding microenvironment. It is presumed that other HNSCC would also behave similarly, due to the common pathways of tumorigenesis. Thus, as in other cancers, such as breast cancer, more aggressive lesions tend to be associated with a tissue reparative phenotype where cells such as fibroblasts, macrophages, and other immune cells are influenced to participate in an environment geared toward repair. This is evident by the various cytokine profiles these cells emit and respond to; however, at this point it is not well understood how this might contribute to oral cancer pain [2, 4–9].

There are candidate mediators that may participate in the generation of pain, which include cancer- or microenvironment-secreted soluble factors such as endothelin-1, chemokines, integrins, and proteases or their activated receptors (PAR-2), as well as the nerve growth factor (NGF) and neurturin (NRTN) and others [2, 4, 6–10]. The complex signaling interplay between these mediators is just now becoming better understood. Focusing on what is now known, the major signaling pathways appear to be those summarized next.

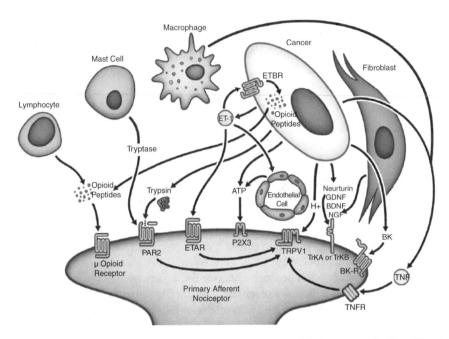

Fig. 8.1 Representation of various mediators that may be responsible for cancer pain. Key: *BDNF* brain-derived neurotrophic factor; *BK* bradykinin; *BK-R* bradykinin receptor; *ET-1* endothelin-1; *ETAR* endothelin A receptor; *ETBR* endothelin B receptor; *GDNF* glial-derived neurotrophic factor; *NGF* nerve growth factor; *PAR2* protease-activated receptor 2; *TrkA* tyrosine kinase receptor A; *TrkB* tyrosine kinase receptor B; *TRPV1* transient receptor potential vanilloid 1. (Reprinted by copyright permissions from Ref. [4])

Nerve Growth Factor

Typically secreted to promote local growth of afferent sensory neurons, a higher concentration of NGF in the cancer microenvironment, via activation of its sensitive high-affinity tyrosine kinase receptor, allows proliferation, activation, and invasion of many cancer types. In addition, thermal hyperalgesia, mechanical hyperalgesia, and sensitization may occur. NGF also may play a role in immunomodulation affecting lymphocytes and causing mast cell degranulation and an overall increase in substance P and CGRP from the spinal cord. Both of these substances are involved on the propagation of pain signals and ultimately sensitization. This may explain its role in the development of hyperalgesia. It is thought that NGF's involvement with "perineural" spread of many types of cancers can cause continued pain even after surgical resection [10, 11]. Angiogenesis and neurogenesis are thought to have interrelated pathways of activation. NGF alone may be key in angiogenesis in the tumor microenvironment and is well documented as a harbinger of pain (Fig. 8.2) [2, 4, 10–12].

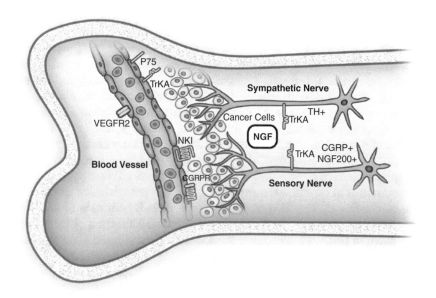

Fig. 8.2 NGF stimulates both angiogenesis and neurogenesis. NGF acts through TrkA to generate sensory and sympathetic nerve fibers that innervate the cancer microenvironment, and both fiber types contribute to cancer pain. Key: *CGRP* calcitonin gene-related protein; *CGRPR* calcitonin gene-related protein receptor; *NGF* nerve growth factor; *NK1* neurokinin-1 receptor; *SP* substance P; *TH* tyrosine hydroxylase; *TrkA* tyrosine kinase receptor A; *VEGF* vascular endothelial growth factor; *VEGFR* vascular endothelial growth factor receptor. (Reprinted by copyright permissions from Ref. [4])

Endothelin-1

Endothelin-1 mRNA and protein expression is elevated within the HNSCC cancer microenvironment and appears to be a potent vasoactive peptide producing nociception and is a main modulator of cancer pain [4, 6]. Its downstream targets are two G-protein-coupled receptors (classes A and B). Class A receptors are located primarily on peripheral sensory neurons, while class B targets are non-myelinated Schwann cells of the sciatic nerve and dorsal root ganglion satellite cells. These latter targets are implicated in inflammatory pain and vasodilation [4–7]. There seems to be a complex, poorly understood interplay between these two receptors that may control a complex cascade that leads to control over nociception in the cancer microenvironment. The testing of agonist and antagonists to these receptors in animal models has led to surprising results, but as of now, no clinically relevant treatment mechanism has emerged [8, 9]. Quite often, agonist attenuates pain, while antagonist elicits pain. Therefore, the effect appears multifactorial and counterintuitive and perhaps suggests a balance between the stimulation of these two targets.

Proteases and Protease-Activated Receptors

Proteolytic activity of HNC is a key mechanism in carcinogenesis, tissue invasion, metastasis, and the propagation of cancer pain [3]. Proteases and proteolytic peptides (trypsin, tryptase, and serine protease) have been identified in a wide range of cancers such as renal cell carcinoma, prostate carcinoma, and colorectal cancer [11]. Many of these peptides have been shown to directly increase nociceptive signaling, via intracellular pathways that begin with the activation of a protease-associated receptor (PAR) ultimately causing the release of substance P and CGRP from C-fibers. PAR-2, one of these specific receptors, has been well characterized. Located on sensory receptors, it is capable of mediating mechanical allodynia when experimentally injected into mice that are otherwise cancer-free [3, 13]. This leads one to speculate if activation of PAR-type mechanisms contributes to the characteristic pain under function or mechanical pain as noted in OSCC [3, 13]. There are a wide variety of proteolytic processes in the HNC environment. Other key actors are matrix metalloproteinases 8 and 9, neurotrypsin, complement factor B, and plasminogen. Especially with MMPs 8 and 9, the balance between normal and affected cancerous tissues indicates aggressiveness, biological behavior, and metastatic spread [3]. This is a well-known facet of any process that involves complement and it's activation or normal inflammatory cascades. In vivo targeting of proteolytic processing may be a future therapeutic target [14].

How Treatment Modalities Can Cause Pain?

It is well appreciated that HNC-related pain is resolved upon successful resection of the tumor. However, the sequelae of the various treatment regimens often entail significant amounts of pain. Surgery and radiotherapy that are the main treatment modalities often worsen normal biomechanics, oral masticatory function, and quality of life in the majority of patients [13, 15]. This is due, in part, to mucositis, epithelial atrophy, neuropathy, TMD, or myofascial pain [3, 15]. Mucositis alone has severe effects on oral and masticatory function, dental health, swallowing, and saliva secretion. This process also predisposes radiation therapy patients to fungal infection as normal mucosal immunity becomes impaired. These urgent procedures intended to remove the primary lesion are often life altering to the individual and require long recovery intervals. Radical excision in and of itself can destroy normal structures allowing sensitization, central pain phenomenon, and development of neuropathic pain [15]. Immediately after surgical treatment, other variables, such as speech intelligibility and mobility disorders in the head, neck, and shoulder regions, become more apparent [15].

Chronic Pain Pathophysiology

Here, we briefly review the pathophysiology of the development and perpetuation of pain, in general, to appreciate the why, how, when, and where interventions may benefit the patient. During normal function, nociception is carefully balanced via ascending and descending signals that are ultimately directed by the central nervous system (CNS). The incoming signals travel from the nociceptors in peripheral tissues to the brain via primary afferents of the dorsal root ganglia and the dorsal horn of the spinal cord. Secondary signals are relayed to the brain for processing and response. The responses are either for: modulation, fear, anxiety, enhancement, or withdrawal. Any perturbation in this balance between ascending signals and descending modulating responses will tip the scales toward several processes that perpetuate pain appreciation by the individual. Tissue injury, whether from surgery or radiation therapy, will normally cause acute pain that resolves during or prior to normal tissue healing. Most current pain control modalities are utilized during this step. By contrast, chronic pain develops when normal somatosensory function becomes prolonged and higher central mechanisms participate in perpetuation of the pain (Fig. 8.3) [16–19].

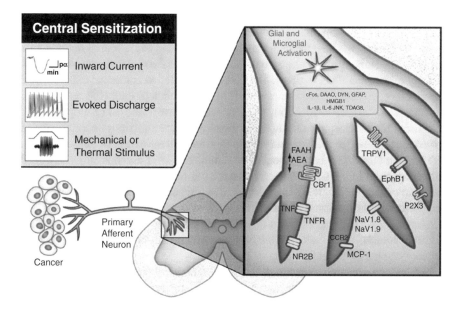

Fig. 8.3 Summarization of cancer related upregulation of pain signals. There are multiple pathways involved. Key: *AEA* anandamide; *CBr1* cannabinoid receptor 1; *CCR2* chemokine C-C motif receptor 2; *DAAO* d-amino acid oxidase; *DYN* = dynorphin; *EphB1* = ephrin B ligand receptor; *FAAH* fatty acid amide hydrolase; *GFAP* glial fibrillary acidic protein; *HMGB1* high-mobility group protein 1; *JNK* c-jun N-terminal kinase; *MCP-1* monocyte chemoattractant protein-1; *NR2B* NMDA (N-methyl-D-aspartate) receptor subunit; *TDAG8* T-cell death-associated gene 8; *TNF* tumor necrosis factor; *TNFR* tumor necrosis factor receptor; *TRPV1* transient receptor potential vanilloid 1. (Reprinted by copyright permissions from Ref. [4])

Modulation

Development of pathologic pain processing pathways is established upon prolonged and continued stimulation of the second-order neurons via release of synaptic release of excitatory amino acids and neuropeptides (e.g., substance P and glutamate), which bind and activate post-synaptic receptors of second-order neurons in the dorsal horn [20–22]. Excessive N-methyl-D-aspartate (NMDA)- and α-amino-3-hydroxy-5-methyl-4-isoxazolepropionic acid (AMPA)-mediated signaling reflects a hyperexcitability state that amplifies sensory responses and possibly contributes to the activation of higher-order brain regions that can lead to "central sensitization" [17, 20–22]. In this state, brainstem control of descending pain modulatory pathways becomes impaired, where the balance between descending inhibition and excitation is altered, and excitation dominates. Pain perception is continued and enhanced by ascending pain pathway sensitization and disinhibited by impaired descending inhibitory. The brain now receives altered, abnormal sensory messages.

Nociceptor activation does not, in and of itself, necessarily produce pain. Some persons with marked spinal pathology are asymptomatic, while others experience severe, chronic, disabling pain without apparent organic injury [15, 20]. Patient responses to analgesic therapy also vary substantially. Because of this, many treatments for pain control have to be tailored to the individual. Many typical treatments such as NSAIDs and opioids alone may be unsuccessful. A key factor in this pain response variability is how the pain message is modulated in the central nervous system [15, 20]. Tumor growth has been demonstrated to have direct effects on the morphology of peripheral nerve fibers. This has been studied in epidermal cells because many of these fibers here are nociceptors [23]. The squamous epithelial cells present in most head and neck mucosal surfaces would have these same impairments. Sensitization of nociceptors during tumor development results from a combination of nerve injury, release of inflammatory mediators, and release of algesic substances [2].

The pain signal can be augmented or diminished as it ascends from its dorsal horn entry point to the CNS and arrives in the cerebral cortex where it is processed and appreciated. Peripheral tissue injury or disease pathology and pain intensity are subject to modification and interference in the various pathways [17, 21, 22, 24]. Without treatment and prevention of enduring modification or sensitization from repeated stimuli, CNS pain modulation abnormalities persist and may become refractory to intervention [24, 25].

In HNC, neuropathic pain can develop when nerve fibers in any segment of the somatosensory system become dysfunctional or transmit signals inappropriately even without a lesion or disease such as in the case of regional lymph node spread or metastasis [26, 27]. This may occur before the cancer microenvironment has been established. Research has led to "altered nociception" as a proposed pain mechanism descriptor when chronic pain is neither nociceptive (e.g., tissue damage) nor neuropathic (e.g., nerve pathology) [21, 26, 28]. Maladaptive CNS neuroplasticity in chronic pain has been recognized since the early 2000s as a disease process of its own right, and translation into clinical practice of oncology and HNC surgery is long overdue [29].

New Frontiers

Next, we will explore some current treatment modalities, areas for future research, and novel proposed treatment methods. Some of these modalities show promise in other disciplines, but their use may be translated to management of pain in HNC. To date, the mainstays of pain management in HNC have been non-steroidal medication and opioid analgesics, as previously mentioned. These formulations fail in most instances, and clinical management of pain remains elusive and archaic. Also, as discussed, the multitude of elements eliciting pain in the cancer microenvironment and post-surgical pain require advanced modalities and continued research to provide HNC patients the best quality of life after surgery and concomitant therapies. Non surgical interventions are discussed.

Compounded Analgesic Formulations

Analgesic medications compounded for topical use are gaining popularity in chronic pain management. They may have application for HNSCC patients, especially in the realm of mucositis after potential radiation therapy, and treatment of site-related pain. Compounded analgesic formulations typically combine three or more analgesic drugs to achieve multiple complementary effects at the lowest doses possible rather than higher doses of the individual component medications. Topical formation of ketamine suspended in artificial saliva has been shown in a case series to offer significant relief for refractory oral mucositis [30]. Other commonly utilized combinations include flurbiprofen, tramadol, clonidine, cyclobenzaprine, bupivacaine, baclofen, phenytoin, gabapentin, and lidocaine [31].

Many small uncontrolled trials show compounded analgesic formulations' efficacy, but this approach must balance local penetration against systemic exposure and potential toxicity [32, 33]. Compounding is not FDA-regulated; vehicle formulation and active drug concentration should be standardized for greater confidence in compounded analgesic formulations for consistent safety and efficacy [32, 33]. Therefore, these compounded medications need additional studies to determine if they can be utilized in the dynamic musculoskeletal environment of HNSCC and OSCC.

Tapentadol

Tapentadol is a mu-opioid receptor agonist and norepinephrine reuptake inhibitor combined in a single molecule [34]. The extended release formulation is effective in diverse chronic pain, with or without a neuropathic pain component [35, 36]. Researchers found function, health status, and quality of life improved during long-term treatment [36]. The drug has a good safety profile with gastrointestinal (GI) tolerability more favorable than other opioids and a low risk of withdrawal after cessation [35, 36]. In studies, tapentadol was as effective as oxycodone in a nociceptive and neuropathic chronic low back pain model, with better GI tolerability and treatment adherence [37]. Importantly, mu-opioid receptor binding affinity of tapentadol is 18-fold lower than morphine, suggesting lower abuse potential than standard opioids [37].

Cebranopadol and NKTR-181

There are two novel opioid analgesics in development and testing that are designed to improve safety over standard opioids. Cebranopadol is a mu-opioid receptor agonist and nociceptin/orphanin FQ peptide opioid receptor agonist that may improve respiratory depression safety [38]. NKTR-181 is a long-acting mu-opioid receptor agonist with structural properties that alter its brain-entry kinetics and may limit abuse potential, and early studies show good long-term pain control [39].

Neurochemistry

Given the presence of a complex milieu of neurochemical modulators in any cancer microenvironment, especially in OSCC, it is safe to say that there may be a number of novel therapeutic targets that have yet to be discovered. Many of the soluble mediators in the microenvironment have been discovered by creating antagonists to their action [2, 4]. Not all antagonists have been explored. It appears that a delicate balance exists between some of the mediators in the OSCC environment. For example, the interplay between endothelin A and B receptors has had unpredictable outcomes when these receptors are agonized or antagonized respectively [2, 4, 9, 10]. Bradykinin has a direct effect on endothelin-1 expression, but agonism and antagonism of its receptors and its concomitant second-order effects remain unpredictable as well [4]. The milieu of mediators in the cancer microenvironment does not fit into the discrete categories of inflammatory, neuropathic, or dysfunctional (musculoskeletal) but rather have complex interplay that is still being explored. Post-translational modification of receptors and continued switching of intracellular signaling pathways as receptors are activated or deactivated, ligand effects, and changes in excitability make these therapeutic targets poorly suited toward enduring treatment [37, 38, 40].

Future Perspective

There are several other potential treatment targets on the horizon. For example, microRNA (miRNA), inhibitory segments of messenger RNA, may be able to prevent translational processing of proteins involved in the initiation and maintenance of pain signals [37, 40]. While some miRNAs have a role in maintenance of pain, over-expression of other miRNAs may have a role in promoting resolution most likely through modulation of chemokines. A considerable disadvantage of genetic therapies for pain is that we do not yet understand the consequences of long-term inhibition of these pathways; moreover, the route to market for genetic therapies is complex [37, 40]. Antibody or immunological therapies also hold promise in this arena. There are ongoing trials which target NGF, a soluble factor mentioned earlier that has an important role not only in pain but also propagation of cancers. NGF activity would be lessened as antibody neutralizes it's effect. The downside is that it may also block the proactive mechanism of pain appreciation at the CNS level.

Epigenetic therapies are also arising, which target abnormal genetic elements that prolong abnormal transcription of proteins that underlie chronic pain. For example, regulation of histone acetylation has been shown to play a role in the pathophysiology of pain [37, 38, 40]. Moreover, the modification of the epigenetic state of a specific locus may allow transcriptional silencing [40].

In summary, as research and trials continue, there are promising developments that may deliver further relief to our HNC patient population that is already compromised. With that, hopefully the struggle against the surgical and biomechanical implications of treatment, such as pain, will become easier for patients that have to endure these treatments and associated impairment of lifestyle and function.

References

1. Macfarlane TV, Wirth T, Ranasinghe S, et al. Head and neck cancer pain: systematic review of prevalence and associated factors. J Oral Maxillofac Res. 2012;3(1):e1.
2. Schmidt BL. The neurobiology of cancer pain. J Oral Maxillofac Surg. 2015;73(12 Suppl):S132–5.
3. Connelly ST, Schmidt BL. Evaluation of pain in patients with oral squamous cell carcinoma. J Pain. 2004;5(9):505–10.
4. Schmidt BL. The neurobiology of cancer pain. Neuroscientist. 2014;20(5):546–62.
5. Marshall JA, Mahanna GK. Cancer in the differential diagnosis of orofacial pain. Dent Clin North Am. 1997;41(2):355–65.
6. Lam DK, Dang D, Zhang J, Dolan JC, Schmidt BL. Novel animal models of acute and chronic cancer pain: a pivotal role for PAR2. J Neurosci. 2012;32:14178.
7. Nelson J, Bagnato A, Battistini B, Nisen P. The endothelin axis: emerging role in cancer. Nat Rev Cancer. 2003;3:110–6.
8. Pickering V, Jay Gupta R, Quang P, et al. Effect of peripheral endothelin-1 concentration on carcinoma-induced pain in mice. Eur J Pain. 2008;12:293.
9. Quang PN, Schmidt BL. Endothelin-A receptor antagonism attenuates carcinoma-induced pain through opioids in mice. J Pain. 2010;11(7):663–71.
10. Levi-Montalcini R, Skaper SD, Dal Toso R, Petrelli L, Leon A. Nerve growth factor: from neurotrophin to neurokine. Trends Neurosci. 1996;19(11):514–20.
11. Schmidt BL, Hamamoto DT, Simone DA, Wilcox GL. Mechanism of cancer pain. Mol Interv. 2010;10(3):164–78.
12. Nico B, Mangieri D, Benagiano V, Crivellato E, Ribatti D. Nerve growth factor as an angiogenic factor. Microvasc Res. 2008;75:135–41.
13. Yang Y, Zhang P, Li W. Comparison of orofacial pain of patients with different stages of precancer and oral cancer. Sci Rep. 2017;7(1):203.

14. Hardt M, Lam DK, Dolan JC, Schmidt BL. Surveying proteolytic processes in human cancer microenvironments by microdialysis and activity-based mass spectrometry. Proteomics Clin Appl. 2011;5(11–12):636–43.

15. Gellrich NC, Schimming R, Schramm A, Schmalohr D, Bremerich A, Kugler J. Pain, function, and psychologic outcome before, during, and after intraoral tumor resection. J Oral Maxillofac Surg. 2002;60(7):772–7.

16. Fornasari D. Pharmacotherapy for neuropathic pain: a review. Pain Ther. 2017;6(1):25–33.

17. Colloca L, Ludman T, Bouhassira D, et al. Neuropathic pain. Nat Rev Dis Primers. 2017;3:17002.

18. Finnerup NB, Attal N, Haroutounian S, et al. Pharmacotherapy for neuropathic pain in adults: systematic review, meta-analysis and updated NeuPSIG recommendations. Lancet Neurol. 2015;14(2):162–73.

19. Binder A, Baron R. The pharmacological therapy of chronic neuropathic pain. Dtsch Arztebl Int. 2016;113(37):616–25.

20. Rose M. Neck pain in adults. NetCE course reference material #94130.

21. Baron R, Hans G, Dickenson AH. Peripheral input and its importance for central sensitization. Ann Neurol. 2013;74(5):630–6.

22. Bannister K, Dickenson AH. What the brain tells the spinal cord. Pain. 2016;157(10):2148–51.

23. Simone DA, Nolano M, Johnson T, Wendelschafer-Crabb G, Kennedy WR. Intradermal injection of capsaicin in humans produces degeneration and subsequent reinnervation of epidermal nerve fibers: correlation with sensory function. J Neurosci. 1998;18(21):8947–59.

24. Yarnitsky D. Role of endogenous pain modulation in chronic pain mechanisms and treatment. Pain. 2015;156(Suppl 1):S24–31. Fornasari D. Pain mechanisms in patients with chronic pain. Clin Drug Investig. 2012;32(1):45–52.

25. Worley SL. New directions in the treatment of chronic pain. PT. 2016;41(2):107–14.

26. Spahr N, Hodkinson D, Jolly K, Williams S, Howard M, Thacker M. Distinguishing between nociceptive and neuropathic components in chronic low back pain using behavioral evaluation and sensory examination. Musculoskelet Sci Pract. 2017;27:40–8.

27. Fornasari D. Pain mechanisms in patients with chronic pain. Clin Drug Investig. 2012;32(1):45–52.

28. Förster M, Mahn F, Gockel U, et al. Axial low back pain: one painful area—many perceptions and mechanisms. PLoS One. 2013;8(7):e68273.

29. Woolf CJ, American College of Physicians, American Physiological Society. Pain: moving from symptom control toward mechanism-specific pharmacologic management. Ann Intern Med. 2004;140(6):441–51.

30. Slatkin NE, Rhiner M. Topical ketamine in the treatment of mucositis pain. Pain Med. 2003;4(3):298–303.

31. Knezevic NN, Tverdohleb T, Nikibin F, Knezevic I, Candido KD. Management of chronic neuropathic pain with single and compounded topical analgesics. Pain Manag. 2017;7(6):537–58.

32. Derry S, Conaghan P, Da Silva JA, et al. Topical NSAIDs for chronic musculoskeletal pain in adults. Cochrane Database Syst Rev. 2016;4:CD007400.

33. Hesselink JMK. Topical analgesics: critical issues related to formulation and concentration. J Pain Relief. 2016;5:274.

34. Manion J, Waller MA, Clark T, Massingham JN, Gregory Neely G. Developing modern pain therapies. Front Neurosci. 2019;13:1370.

35. Baron R, Eberhart L, Kern KU, et al. Tapentadol prolonged release for chronic pain: a review of clinical trials and 5 years of routine clinical practice data. Pain Pract. 2017;17(5):678–700.

36. Sánchez Del Águila MJ, Schenk M, Kern KU, Drost T, Steigerwald I. Practical considerations for the use of tapentadol prolonged release for the management of severe chronic pain. Clin Ther. 2015;37(1):94–113.

37. Tramullas M, Francés R, de la Fuente R, Velategui S, Carcelén M, García R, Llorca J, Hurlé MA. MicroRNA-30c-5p modulates neuropathic pain in rodents. Sci Transl Med. 2018;10(453):eaao6299.

38. Christoph A, Eerdekens MH, Kok M, Volkers G, Freynhagen R. Cebranopadol, a novel first-in-class analgesic drug candidate: first experience in patients with chronic low back pain in a randomized clinical trial. Pain. 2017;158(9):1813–24.
39. Miyazaki T, Choi IY, Rubas W, et al. NKTR-181: a novel mu-opioid analgesic with inherently low abuse potential. J Pharmacol Exp Ther. 2017;363(1):104–13.
40. Stover JD, Farhang N, Berrett KC, Gertz J, Lawrence B, Bowles RD. CRISPR epigenome editing of AKAP150 in DRG neurons abolishes degenerative IVD-induced neuronal activation. Mol Ther. 2017;25:2014–27.

Chapter 9
Emerging Trends in Oral Mucoadhesive Drug Delivery for Head and Neck Cancer

Solange Massa, Ayman Fouad, Mehdi Ebrahimi, and Peter Luke Santa Maria

Introduction

Oral mucoadhesive drug delivery systems are pharmaceutical formulations designed to interact with the mucus layer to augment the efficiency and resident time of the active compound at the site of absorption. The oral mucosa provides an ideal surface for local or systemic drug delivery. For local drug delivery, mucoadhesive systems can allow for on-site delivery, reduce systemic side effects, and augment the drugs' resident time in the oral cavity. For systemic drug delivery, mucoadhesive systems can be used to avoid the first-pass metabolism and provide direct and painless administration. Saliva facilitates the water-based dissolution of the active ingredient and interacts with the mucosal mucins providing a surface anchor for the drug delivery system. However, creating a mucoadhesive system for local or systemic delivery can be a challenging endeavor. The challenges and limitations of the oral mucosa include local enzymatic degradation, variable pH in the oral cavity, unpleasant taste or odors of drugs, drug delivery dosage limits, and being limited to drugs undergoing passive diffusion. Considerations must be made for the possibility of swallowing the tablet where it is absorbed by the conventional oral route. The oral mucosa

S. Massa · P. L. S. Maria (✉)
Department of Otolaryngology, Head & Neck Surgery, Stanford University,
Stanford, CA, USA
e-mail: psm01@stanford.edu

A. Fouad
Department of Otolaryngology, Head & Neck Surgery, Stanford University,
Stanford, CA, USA

Department of Otolaryngology, Head & Neck Surgery, Tanta University, Tanta, Egypt

M. Ebrahimi
Department of Oral Rehabilitation, Prince Philip Dental Hospital,
The University of Hong Kong, Pok Fu Lam, Hong Kong, China

© Springer Nature Switzerland AG 2021
R. El Assal et al. (eds.), *Early Detection and Treatment of Head & Neck Cancers*, https://doi.org/10.1007/978-3-030-69852-2_9

is also less permeable compared to other sections of the gastrointestinal tract like the small intestine.

When a mucoadhesive compound attaches to the mucosa, it goes through stages of mucoadhesion: first the contact stage and then the consolidation stage. Mucosal adhesion is explained by several theories which include diffusion, adsorption, electronic, fracture, and wetting theories. Using varied dosage forms that go from liquid to solid, and utilizing the appropriate components, oral mucoadhesive drug delivery systems can be used to obtain the desired outcome locally and systemically. Mucoadhesive materials can be formulated in a way to further improve drug bioavailability, absorption, and transport while minimizing undesirable systemic effects. This chapter provides a basic overview of the histological structure of oral mucosa allowing for a better understanding of the mechanism of action of oral mucoadhesive agents. This is followed by a discussion of the available and emerging oral mucoadhesive drug delivery formulations for management of head and neck cancer and related conditions.

Histological Structure of the Oral Mucosa and Saliva Components

The oral mucosa comprises a complex set of layers interacting with each other through cellular adhesions [1]. Histological examination of the oral mucosa reveals that there are three distinctive functional layers: the epithelial lining, the basement membrane, and the connective tissue layer [2, 3]. The oral cavity has varied epithelial thickness depending on the anatomical location observed. In humans, the mouth floor thickness is aproximately 100 μm, 220 μm in the lateral tongue, 250 μm in the hard palate, and 300 μm in the inner cheek [4], and is the primary site for the development of most oral pathologies, including ulcers and malignancies. The connective tissue layer below supports the basement membrane, which in turn supports the epithelium [5] (Fig. 9.1).

The Epithelial Layer

The main function of the epithelial layer is to act as a barrier to protect the underlying structures [6]. In general, the permeability of the oral mucosa varies depending on the physical and chemical nature of a substance administered [3]. The basal layer is the source of progenitor cells that gives rise to the more superficial layers. Keratinocytes from the basal layer to the top layer differ in shape, size, and maturation [7]. The epithelial lining has two distinct functional zones in the oral cavity: (i) a non-keratinized epithelium and (ii) a keratinized epithelium. The non-keratinized epithelium is the mucus-secreting zone as it has membrane coating cholesterol sulfate and glucosylceramide granules [8]. It entails the floor of the mouth, tongue undersurface, and soft palatal mucosa, as well as buccal and labial mucosa. The

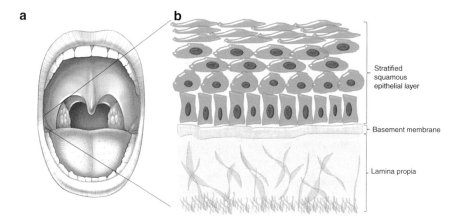

Fig. 9.1 (**a**) Anatomical and (**b**) histological schematics of the oral cavity. (Reproduced with copyright permission from Chris Gralapp, MA, CMI)

keratinized epithelium is the masticatory and barrier zone, as it has neutral lipids composed of ceramide and acyl ceramide [9]. It includes the dorsal tongue, hard palate mucosa, and the gingival mucosa.

The Basement Membrane

The main functions of the basement membrane are to provide support to the epithelium and anchor it to the underlying connective tissue [10]. The basement membrane has two distinctive layers: the basal lamina and the reticular connective tissue [11]. The basal lamina can be subdivided into the lamina lucida, a thin clear layer adjacent to the surface epithelium, and a lamina densa, a thick dense layer close to the reticular connective tissue. The lamina lucida is composed mainly of dystroglycan, entactins, laminin, and integrins, and there is some debate as to whether this is simply an artifact of tissue preparation [12]. The lamina densa contains heparan sulfate-rich proteoglycan perlecan coated collagen IV [13]. The basement membrane is attached to the underlying connective tissue layer by collagen VII [13, 14].

The Connective Tissue

The main function of the connecting tissue is to provide scaffolding for the whole of the mucosa and to be the main nutrition source for the lamina propria, a connective tissue-based structure that sits below the basement membrane [14]. There are three main constituents of the connective tissue: fibers from collagen and elastin [15]; cells that include fibroblasts, adipocytes, macrophages, mast cells, and leukocytes; and a system of glycosaminoglycans and proteoglycans to hold water and collagen fibers in the intercellular spaces [16, 17].

Saliva, Mucus, and Mucins

The saliva is the main lubricant of the oral cavity. Its daily secretion ranges between 0.5 and 2 liters with a pH ranging from 5.5 to 7 [18]. Saliva is more than 95% water, and the water-rich environment it creates is the fundamental idea behind using a hydrophilic polymeric material for transmucosal drug delivery. This thin, translucent, and viscid secretion adheres to the epithelium with a mean layer thickness of 50–450 μm in humans. It is originally secreted by goblet cells, but it can also be produced by specialized mucous cells in exocrine glands. It is composed of lipids (1–2%), mineral salts (1%), immunoglobulins, mucins, and other free proteins (0.5–1%). The viscosity of saliva is due to the presence of mucus linked to mucin fibers with a high capacity to bind water and affect drug delivery [19]. Mucins are glycoproteins composed of 25% amino acids and 75% carbohydrates [20] and are present in the oral epithelium as either membrane-bound (MUC1, 3, and 4) [21] or freely in saliva (MUC2 and 5AC). MUC7 and MUC5B form a mucus network attached to MUC1 [22] (Fig. 9.2) that is connected to the epithelium. Although mucus has a negative charge promoted by sialic acid and sulfate residues, drug delivery systems can be designed to leverage this property, but this also provides a challenging environment for drug attachment and delivery [23, 24].

Mucoadhesive Theories

The exact mechanisms of how the coupling between drug delivery systems and mucosal surfaces occurs are not well understood. It is believed to occur in two

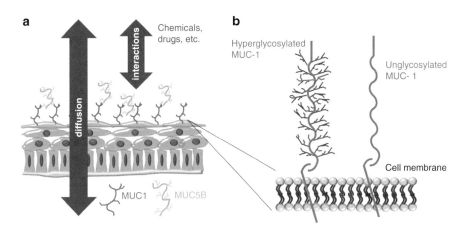

Fig. 9.2 (**a**) MUC1 expressed in the oral mucosa attached to salivary mucin MUC5B. (**b**) MUC1 showned as a transmembrane protein in the mucosal surface

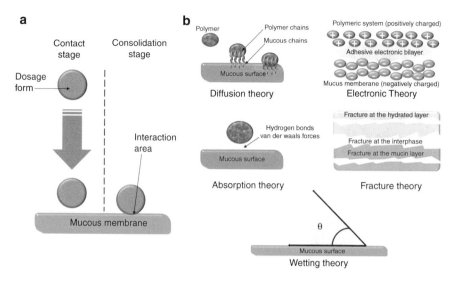

Fig. 9.3 Mucoadhesive theories. (**a**) Two phases, contact and consolidation, describe the interaction of the mucoadhesive compound with the mucosal surface. (**b**) Five mucoadhesive theories that explain the relationship between mucoadhesive surfaces and delivery systems: diffusion, electronic, absorption, fracture, and wetting

stages: (i) the contact stage and (ii) the consolidation stage. In the contact stage, the material contacts the mucosa in a swelling and spreading mechanism. The consolidation stage is initiated by moisture when the mucoadhesive compound links to the surface by van der Waals and hydrogen bonds [25]. From a physical and chemical perspective, several bonding theories have been suggested to explain how a material behaves like a mucoadhesive (Fig. 9.3).

Diffusion Theory

The main concept for the diffusion theory is the semipermanent adhesive bond production through the entanglement between the mucus glycoproteins and the mucoadhesive polymer chains [26]. Many factors impact the inter-diffusion of the macromolecules such as adequate flexibility of the polymer chain, good solubility of one element in the other, adequate polymer exposure, a sufficient match between both chemical structures, and the bioadhesive polymer diffusion coefficient. The materials with solubility parameters close to the mucus glycoproteins have the strongest bioadhesive bonds [27, 28].

Electronic Theory

At the center of the electronic theory is the electron transfer that occurs upon contact between two electrically different structures. Assuming that both the bioadhesive and the target biological surface have a different electronic formulation, when these two surfaces come in contact with each other, electron transfer occurs resulting in the development of a charged double electrical layer. When this electrical double layer is formed between the mucus and the polymer, there is a resultant attraction force that keeps the two together [29, 30].

Absorption Theory

The absorption theory describes atomic surface forces that occur after initial contact. In this theory, two types of chemical bonds occur: (a) a primary unfavorable covalent bond as it may produce a permanent bond and (b) a secondary bond with attraction forces such as van der Waals, hydrogen bonds, electrostatic forces, and hydrophobic bonds [31]. In the case of polymers, hydrogen bonds are the main interfacial forces given that these systems contain carboxyl groups.

Fracture Theory

The main concept behind the fracture theory is that the fracture force S_m required to separate two surfaces is equivalent to the adhesive power. The fracture force S_m is the result of $S_m = F_m/A_\Theta$ where F_m is the ratio of the maximal detachment force and A_Θ is the surface area [32].

Wetting Theory

The wetting theory describes the relationship between a liquid and a mucoadhesive surface mainly defined by the contact angle of the substance with the surface. The interfacial tension predicts the spreading of the bioadhesive polymer on a biological surface. The spreading coefficient (S) is measured by Young's equation $\gamma_{SG} = \gamma_{SL} + \gamma_{LG} \, COS\Theta$ where γ is the interfacial tension between two components, γ_{SG} is solid-gas surface tension, γ_{SL} is solid-liquid surface tension, γ_{LG} is liquid-gas surface tension, and Θ is the contact angle and can be easily measured [33, 34]. Ideally, the contact angle should be as close to zero as possible, defining good spreadability.

Oral Mucoadhesive Drug Delivery System Formulations for Head and Neck Cancer

There are numerous commercially available oral mucoadhesive systems; however, few are specifically for head and neck conditions. In particular, the applications for head and neck oncology are limited to pain control as well as the management of radiation-induced oral mucositis and xerostomia. Table 9.1 summarizes the available oral mucoadhesive agents for head and neck cancer and other head and neck conditions. Even though there have been many clinical trials on the oral mucoadhesive system, few systems have successfully passed clinical trials to enter the market [35, 36] (Table 9.2).

In general, available oral mucoadhesive drug delivery formulations entail solids, semisolids, and liquid formulations. The first-generation mucoadhesive agents were natural or synthetic hydrophilic polymers of cationic, anionic, or non-ionic nature. The second-generation mucoadhesive agents involve the use of multifunctional biomaterials with the ability to incorporate both hydrophilic and lipophilic drugs with a more intelligent mechanism of mucoadhesion. Recently, the advent of nanoparticle drug delivery systems for mucoadhesive administration demonstrated an improved drug permeability and release kinetics as well as higher resistance to enzymatic degradation and reduced undesirable systemic effects [36–38]. For more information regarding recent developments in nanoparticle drug delivery systems, the interested reader can refer to the related chapter in volume I in this book series.

Solids

The outcome when utilizing solid oral formulations is dependent on the manufacturing process, design, and solid phase type [39]. These formulations are ideal for localized, stable, and longer delivery times.

Tablets

Tablets represent the solid form of the mucoadhesive drug system, which can be prepared by powder mix compression. These tablets can be used for both local and systemic therapy. For local therapy, they can be used by direct application to the desired location. For systemic therapy, they protect the drug from enzymatic degradation and avoid the first-pass metabolism by holding the drug in close relation with the mucosal absorptive surface. In order for the tablet to be effective in the buccal environment, it should ideally dissolve at a faster rate compared to the orally swallowed tablets. The main drawbacks include being with bad taste and irritation which

Table 9.1 Commercial oral mucoadhesive formulations for head and neck conditions

No.	Application	Drug	Formulation	Commercial name
1	Xerostomia in radiation-induced head and neck cancer and Sjogren's syndrome	Pilocarpine HCl	Tablet, hydrogel buccal insert	*Piolobuc, Salegen*
2	Narcotic for opioid-dependent patient	Buprenorphine HCl and naloxone HCl	Tablet	*Subutex*
3	Pain	Sufentanil	Tablet	*Dsuvia, Zalviso*
4	Pain	Fentanyl citrate	Tablet, spray, film, lozenge	*Abstral, Actiq, Subsys, Fentora, Onsolis*
5	Pain	Buprenorphine	Tablet, film	*Temgesic, Belbuca*
6	Narcotic for opioid dependence	Buprenorphine + naloxone	Film	*Suboxone*
7	Sedation	Lorazepam	Tablet	*Ativan, Temesta Expidet Buccal*
8	Sedation	Oxazepam	Tablet	*Seresta Expidet Buccal*
9	Allergic rhinitis	Allergen extract	Tablet	*Grastek, Oralair, Odactra, Ragwitek*
10	Oral candidiasis	Nystatin	Oral liquid	*Nilstat, Mycostatin*
11	Oral candidiasis	Miconazole	Gel	*Daktarin, Decozol*
12	Oro-pharyngeal candidiasis	Miconazole	Tablet	*Loramyc, Lauriad*
13	Oral ulceration	Triamcinolone acetonide	Paste	*Kenalog in Orabase, Aftach*
14	Antimicrobial mouthwash	Chlorhexidine digluconate	Oromucosal gel	*Corsodyl gel*
15	Steroid	Hydrocortisone sodium succinate	Oromucosal pallets	*Corlan pellets*
16	Nausea/emesis	Prochlorperazine buccal	Tablet	*Buccastem*
17	Nausea/emesis	Prochlorperazine buccal	Tablet	*Tementil*
18	Migraines	Rizatriptan	Wafer	*Maxalt Wafers*
19	Epilepsy	Midazolam	Oral liquid	*Buccolam, Epistatus*

Table 9.2 Recent past and present clinical trials on oral mucoadhesive formulations related to head and neck oncology

No.	Title/year	Conditions	Interventions	Enrolment	Study phase/references
1	Dexamethasone to Treat Oral Lichen Planus (2005–2008)	Oral lichen planus	Drug: dexamethasone solution	70	Phase 2 [48]
2	Study of the safety of BEMA™ Fentanyl use for breakthrough pain in cancer subjects on chronic opioid therapy (2006–2008)	Cancer pain	Drug: BEMA fentanyl disc	244	Phase 3 [49]
3	Efficacy and safety study of Clonidine Lauriad® to treat oral mucositis (2010–2014)	Chemoradiotherapy-induced severe oral mucositis in patients with head and neck cancer	Drug: clonidine Lauriad® buccal tablet Drug: placebo Lauriad®	183	Phase 2 [50, 51]
4	A study to evaluate the efficacy of MuGard for the amelioration of oral mucositis in head and neck cancer patients (MuGard) (2011–2013)	Oral mucositis	Device: MuGard oral wound rinse Device: aqueous control rinse	120	Phase 4 [52, 53]
5	Clinical effect of phenytoin mucoadhesive paste on wound healing after oral biopsy (2012–2013)	Pain Wound healing	Drug: phenytoin paste Drug: placebo	40	Phase 1 [54]
6	Comparing triamcinolone acetonide mucoadhesive films with licorice mucoadhesive films (2013–2014)	Mucositis	Drug: triamcinolone acetonide film and licorice films (Aftogel Patch)	60	Phase 1 and phase 2 [55, 56]
7	Comparison of triamcinolone acetonide mucoadhesive film and Licorice mucoadhesive film effect on lichen planus (2014–2015)	Oral lichen planus	Drug: licorice film (Aftogel Patch) and triamcinolone acetonide film	60	Phase 2 [57]
8	Efficacy and safety of Forrad® for the management of radiation-induced mucositis in patients with nasopharyngeal carcinoma receiving IMRT (2016–2017)	Nasopharyngeal neoplasms Stomatitis	Drug: oral ulcer gargle (Forrad®) hydrogel and quadruple mixture (composed of dexamethasone, gentamicin, vitamin B12, and procaine)	90	Phase 2 [58]
9	Efficacy of curcumin in oral submucous fibrosis (ECOSMF) (2014–2018)	Oral submucous fibrosis	Drug: curcumin mucoadhesive gel, curcumin capsules, and curcumin mucoadhesive gel + curcumin capsules Drug: placebo capsule	200	Phase 2 [59, 60]

(continued)

Table 9.2 (continued)

No.	Title/year	Conditions	Interventions	Enrolment	Study phase/references
10	Efficacy of a dietary supplement (Aqualief®) in xerostomic patients (Aqualief) (2016–2017)	Xerostomia due to hyposecretion of salivary gland	Dietary supplement: Aqualief dietary tablet Supplement: placebo	60	Not applicable [61]
11	Dexamethasone solution for the treatment of oral lichen planus (2017–2019)	Oral lichen planus	Drug: MucoLox™ dexamethasone solution (Decadron Elixir)	24	Phase 2 [62]
12	Intra-oral treatment of OLP with Rivelin®-CLO Patches (2018–2019)	Oral lichen planus	Drug: clobetasol propionate (Rivelin®-CLO patches)	140	Phase 2 [63]
13	Effects of Aqualief® in patients with xerostomia as consequence of radiotherapy for head and neck cancer (2017–2020)	Xerostomia Asialia Hyposalivation Mouth dryness	Dietary supplement: Aqualief® tablet (a food supplement based on carnosine and hibiscus) Other: placebo	100	Not applicable [64]
14	Topical chamomile in preventing chemotherapy-induced oral mucositis (2019–2020)	Oral mucositis due to chemotherapy	Drug: chamomile topical oral gel (Carbopol® 970), Miconazole topical gel, BBC oral spray (anesthetics and anti-inflammatory agent), and Oracure gel (analgesic gel)	45	Phase 2 [65, 66]
15	Carnosine supplementation on quantity/quality of oral salivae. (PHoral) (2020–2020)	Oral diseases	Dietary supplement: Aqualief tablet Dietary supplement: placebo tablet	60	Not applicable [67, 68]
16	MucoLox formulation to mitigate mucositis symptoms in head/neck cancer (2018–2021)	Oral mucositis in head and neck cancer	Drug: MucoLox® polymer hydrogel and sodium bicarbonate	27	Phase 2 [69]
17	Clinical and biochemical assessment of the effect of topical use of Coenzyme Q10 versus topical corticosteroid in management of symptomatic oral lichen planus: randomized controlled clinical trial (2019–2021)	Oral lichen planus	Drug: co-enzyme Q10 mucoadhesive tablets (ubiquinol)	34	Phase 1 [70, 71]

Abbreviations: *BEMA* BioErodible MucoAdhesive, *IMRT* intensity-modulated radiotherapy

may affect patient acceptability, and the drug can be distributed with the saliva decreasing the effectiveness of local therapy. Tablets can be prepared by using a bioadhesive polymer alone or in combination and then incorporated with an active ingredient to form a matrix [40, 41].

Wafers

Wafers are excellent systems for multi-faceted delivery intentions. Bilayered wafers can provide a mucoadhesive layer while having a drug-loaded side for a prolonged and stable drug release. If ideal mechanical and chemical properties are achieved, wafers could be the system of choice for the treatment of oral cavity infections [42].

Bioadhesive Microspheres

Bioadhesive microspheres can be delivered in aqueous suspension, aerosol, paste, gel, or ointment. The main advantage of this system is that it has increased swelling ratios and has longer half-times than other formulations [43]. They are usually more accepted by the patients due to their small size and convenient administration. If desired, these systems can be designed to be retained inside the buccal cavity with fewer systemic adverse effects.

Semisolids

The structure of semisolids is similar to tablets with the difference in the excipient, which is usually dissolved or suspended in an aqueous or no aqueous base as a fine powder. Advantages over the tablet are being of acceptable mouth feeling and the possibility to be applied to the target region by using a syringe or finger. However, the amount of drug delivered may be variable and less localized [44].

Films and Patches

The patch is commonly prepared semisolid by forming a cast of the polymer, drug, and any excipients then allowing it to dry. The size of the patches is variable; however, the commonest size ranges from 1 to 3 cm with an elliptical shape to be used in the buccal mucosa effectively. They share the pros and cons of the tablets. Being more flexible and thinner than tablets, they appear to get more patient acceptance. However, their relative thin size makes them susceptible to overhydration and loss of bioadhesive characters [45].

Chewing Gum

Chewing gum formulations are usually a mixture of a gum core with plasticizers, fillers, and coloring agents in addition to the active compound. This system has good storage capabilities but low drug absorption and bioavailability given that the active drug is released upon mastication [46]. Several experimental works have been developed to assess this type of therapy to bypass the hepatic first-pass effect.

Ointment or Gel

Regarded as having some benefits over other formulations, gels or ointments can decrease the risk for allergies or irritability. They have an easy manufacturing process and the active compound is easy to incorporate into the delivery system. Additionally, gels can provide a faster release compared to solid systems [47].

Liquids or Suspensions

The main advantage of the liquid form is that it can be distributed throughout the buccal cavity. However, the main disadvantage is that it cannot be targeted to a certain region and the amount of the drug delivered is uncontrolled. Last, if the active compound is liable to enzymatic destruction from saliva, this system provides no or very small protection against degradation.

Components of Oral Mucoadhesive Drug Delivery Systems

When designing a buccal mucoadhesive drug delivery system, the primary goal is to deliver a desired active compound through the oral mucosal membrane for local or systemic effects. To achieve this, several formulation characteristics must be achieved. This includes (i) choosing the right drug substance, (ii) designing a good bioadhesive polymer system, and (iii) considering adding a backing membrane, plasticizers, and/or permeation enhancers.

Drug Substance

The mucoadhesive drug delivery system is based upon the desired pharmacokinetic properties of each drug. The ideal drug criteria must include (a) a small conventional single dose, (b) a molecular size ideally between 75 and 100 daltons, (c) biological half-life between 2 and 8 h, (d) exhibiting first-pass effect or pre-systemic drug elimination, (e) having passive drug absorption if possible [72, 73], and (f) stability at buccal pH.

Bioadhesive Polymers

Bioadhesive polymer selection and characterization are crucial for oral drug delivery system design. The ideal mucoadhesive polymer must (a) be of high molecular weight to promote mucus-polymer interaction, (b) have good swelling properties as a result of high crosslinking to avoid disintegration and protect the active compound, (c) promote the adhering of the active compound to the mucosa through flexible polymer chains, (d) have an optimum pH, (e) be environmentally inert, (f) be compatible with the biological membrane, (g) have a durable shelf life to be stored without decomposition, (h) be economically viable, and (i) be easily incorporated in the drug formula [74]. Another desirable characteristic is being able to control the release of the drug into the buccal cavity by embedding the drug into the polymer matrix [75].

Polymers can be classified by source (natural/synthetic) or by their solubility or charge among other classifications. If separated by charge, polymers can be anionic, cationic, and non-ionic polymers. The most commonly used anionic polymers are xanthan gum sodium alginate, sodium, pectin, and chitosan-EDTA PAA. The cationic polymers include compounds like chitosan, dextran, amino dextran, chitosan and DEAE-dextran, among others. The non-ionic polymers include Eudragit® analogs and polyacrylamides.

Backing Membrane

The main function of the backing membrane is to attach the bioadhesive material to the mucosa. This membrane should prevent drug loss outside of the mucosa and improve patient compliance; hence, it must be inert and impermeable to the drug and enhance penetration. Carbopol, magnesium stearate, hydroxypropyl methylcellulose (HPMC), hydroxypropyl cellulose (HPC), carboxymethylcellulose (CMC), and polycarbophil are the most commonly used materials for the formation of the backing membrane [76].

Plasticizers

A plasticizer is a substance used to increase plasticity and flexibility of a formulation. Plasticizers can be used to make a mucoadhesive buccal drug delivery system softer and can be added in large quantities to the formulations. Polymers, in particular, can be internally plasticized by modifying the polymer per se – or its monomers – or can be externally plasticized to increase flexibility upon formulation completion. The most commonly used plasticizers are sorbitol, propylene glycol, and glycerine [77].

Permeation Enhancers

Permeation enhancers are compounds designed to increase the mucosal permeation rate of the desired drug. When selecting a certain enhancer, there are several factors to consider including the drug physicochemical properties and administration site, as well as the nature of the vehicle and other excipients. All of these enhancers must be safe, reversible, non-irritant, and chemically inert.

They act through several mechanisms of action: (a) they change mucus rheology by reducing the viscosity of the mucus and saliva, (b) increase lipid bilayer membrane fluidity by disturbing the intracellular lipid packing in interaction with either lipid or protein components, (c) alter tight junctions to increase absorption, and (d) modify the drug's partition coefficient to enhance drug solubility [78].

Among the most common permeation enhancers we can find: (a) steroidal detergents including bile salts, saponins, sodium glycocholate, sodium taurocholate, and sodium glycol dihydro fusidate; (b) surfactants including ionic-cationic (cetyltrimethylammonium bromide), anionic (sodium lauryl sulfate), and non-ionic (sucrose esters); (c) fatty acids including lauric acid, caproic acid, and oleic acid; and (d) others like chelating agents such as salicylates and sulfoxides [79].

Conclusion

Mucoadhesive drug delivery formulation is a promising alternative to conventional drug administration. In the area of head and neck cancer, these systems are already in use for management of oral mucositis, xerostomia, and pain control. The advantages include large bioavailability because of their capacity to bypass the first-pass metabolism and enzymatic degradation of gastrointestinal tract; various dosage forms that include patches, films, spray, and others; and the possibility to be given to unresponsive or traumatized patients. Active drugs can also be released in a controlled or slow-release manner with the possibility to modify the absorption pattern. Currently, new delivery formulations are under investigation for management of oral potentially premalignant disorders. It is expected that more innovative formulations including nanoparticulate forms will finally reach clinical trials following comprehensive preclinical study and optimization that will result in a more efficient local and systemic drug delivery.

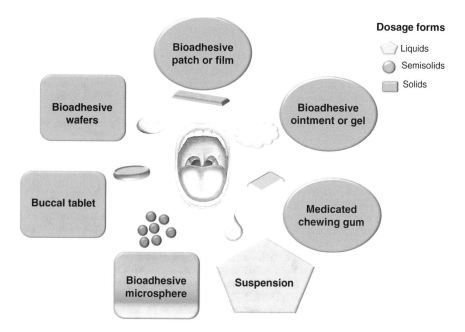

Fig. 9.4 Oral mucoadhesive formulations including solid, semisolid, and liquid drug delivery systems. (Reproduced with copyright permission from Chris Gralapp, MA, CMI)

Acknowledgments We would like to thank Chris Gralapp, certified medical illustrator, who provided the human mouth images for Figs. 9.1a and 9.4.

References

1. Chen J, Ahmad R, Li W, Swain M, Li Q. Biomechanics of oral mucosa. J R Soc Interface. 2015;12:20150325. https://doi.org/10.1098/rsif.2015.0325.
2. Harris D, Robinson JR. Drug delivery via the mucous membranes of the oral cavity. J Pharm Sci. 1992;81:1–10. https://doi.org/10.1002/jps.2600810102.
3. Squier CA. The permeability of oral mucosa. Crit Rev Oral Biol Med. 1991;2:13–32. https://doi.org/10.1177/10454411910020010301.
4. Prestin S, Rothschild SI, Betz CS, Kraft M. Measurement of epithelial thickness within the oral cavity using optical coherence tomography. Head Neck. 2012;34:1777–81. https://doi.org/10.1002/hed.22007.
5. Redler P, Lustig ES. Control of epithelial development in normal and pathological connective tissue from oral mucosa. Dev Biol. 1970;22:84–95. https://doi.org/10.1016/0012-1606(70)90007-2.
6. Luke DA. Cell proliferation in epithelium of murine oral mucosa in vivo and in vitro. An autoradiographic study using tritiated thymidine. Virchows Arch B Cell Pathol. 1979;29:343–9. https://doi.org/10.1007/BF02899365.

7. Jonek T, Gruszeczka B. Histological study of changes in the epithelium of the oral mucosa caused by estrogens in castrated mice. Czas Stomatol. 1976;29:767–72. http://www.ncbi.nlm. nih.gov/pubmed/1067954.
8. Adams D. The mucus barrier and absorption through the oral mucosa. J Dent Res. 1975;54 Spec No:B19–26. https://doi.org/10.1177/00220345750540021601.
9. Dale BA, Stern IB, Clagett JA. Initial characterization of the proteins of keratinized epithelium of rat oral mucosa. Arch Oral Biol. 1977;22:75–82. https://doi. org/10.1016/0003-9969(77)90081-4.
10. Watanabe I. Ultrastructure of the basal membrane of the mucosa of the hard palate of rats. Quintessencia. 1981;8:57–65. http://www.ncbi.nlm.nih.gov/pubmed/6954560.
11. Ricci V, Gasparini G. The structure of the basal membrane of the nasal mucosa in man, under the electron microscope. Boll Soc Ital Biol Sper. 1960;36:932–4. http://www.ncbi.nlm.nih. gov/pubmed/13741218.
12. Chan FL, Inoue S. Lamina lucida of basement membrane: an artefact. Microsc Res Tech. 1994;28:48–59. https://doi.org/10.1002/jemt.1070280106.
13. Adachi E, Hopkinson I, Hayashi T. Basement-membrane stromal relationships: interactions between collagen fibrils and the lamina densa. Int Rev Cytol. 1997;173:73–156. https://doi. org/10.1016/s0074-7696(08)62476-6.
14. Weijs TJ, Goense L, van Rossum PSN, Meijer GJ, van Lier ALHMW, Wessels FJ, Braat MNG, Lips IM, Ruurda JP, Cuesta MA, van Hillegersberg R, Bleys RLAW. The peri-esophageal connective tissue layers and related compartments: visualization by histology and magnetic resonance imaging. J Anat. 2017;230:262–71. https://doi.org/10.1111/joa.12552.
15. Sauer F, Oswald L, Ariza de Schellenberger A, Tzschätzsch H, Schrank F, Fischer T, Braun J, Mierke CT, Valiullin R, Sack I, Käs JA. Collagen networks determine viscoelastic properties of connective tissues yet do not hinder diffusion of the aqueous solvent. Soft Matter. 2019;15:3055–64. https://doi.org/10.1039/c8sm02264j.
16. Mourão PA. Proteoglycans, glycosaminoglycans and sulfated polysaccharides from connective tissues. Mem Inst Oswaldo Cruz. 1991;86(Suppl 3):13–22. https://doi. org/10.1590/s0074-02761991000700003.
17. Muir H. Chemistry and metabolism of connective tissue glycosaminoglycans (mucopolysaccharides). Int Rev Connect Tissue Res. 1964;2:101–54. https://doi.org/10.1016/ B978-1-4831-6751-0.50009-4.
18. Roblegg E, Coughran A, Sirjani D. Saliva: an all-rounder of our body. Eur J Pharm Biopharm. 2019;142:133–41. https://doi.org/10.1016/j.ejpb.2019.06.016.
19. Teubl BJ, Stojkovic B, Docter D, Pritz E, Leitinger G, Poberaj I, Prassl R, Stauber RH, Fröhlich E, Khinast JG, Roblegg E. The effect of saliva on the fate of nanoparticles. Clin Oral Investig. 2018;22:929–40. https://doi.org/10.1007/s00784-017-2172-5.
20. Bansil R, Stanley E, LaMont JT. Mucin biophysics. Annu Rev Physiol. 1995;57:635–57. https://doi.org/10.1146/annurev.ph.57.030195.003223.
21. Kho H-S. Oral epithelial MUC1 and oral health. Oral Dis. 2018;24:19–21. https://doi. org/10.1111/odi.12713.
22. Frenkel ES, Ribbeck K. Salivary mucins in host defense and disease prevention. J Oral Microbiol. 2015;7:29759. https://doi.org/10.3402/jom.v7.29759.
23. Agarwal S, Aggarwal S. Mucoadhesive polymeric platform for drug delivery; a comprehensive review. Curr Drug Deliv. 2015;12:139–56. https://doi.org/10.217 4/1567201811666140924124722.
24. Fröhlich E, Roblegg E. Mucus as barrier for drug delivery by nanoparticles. J Nanosci Nanotechnol. 2014;14:126–36. https://doi.org/10.1166/jnn.2014.9015.
25. Smart JD. The basics and underlying mechanisms of mucoadhesion. Adv Drug Deliv Rev. 2005;57:1556–68. https://doi.org/10.1016/j.addr.2005.07.001.
26. Andrews GP, Laverty TP, Jones DS. Mucoadhesive polymeric platforms for controlled drug delivery. Eur J Pharm Biopharm. 2009;71:505–18. https://doi.org/10.1016/j.ejpb.2008.09.028.
27. Fu Y, Kao WJ. Drug release kinetics and transport mechanisms of non-degradable and degradable polymeric delivery systems. Expert Opin Drug Deliv. 2010;7:429–44. https://doi. org/10.1517/17425241003602259.

28. Lee JW, Park JH, Robinson JR. Bioadhesive-based dosage forms: the next generation. J Pharm Sci. 2000;89:850–66. https://doi.org/10.1002/1520-6017(200007)89:7<850:: AID-JPS2>3.0.CO;2-G.

29. Guardado-Alvarez TM, Devi LS, Vabre J-M, Pecorelli TA, Schwartz BJ, Durand J-O, Mongin O, Blanchard-Desce M, Zink JI. Photo-redox activated drug delivery systems operating under two photon excitation in the near-IR. Nanoscale. 2014;6:4652–8. https://doi.org/10.1039/c3nr06155h.

30. Dodou D, Breedveld P, Wieringa PA. Mucoadhesives in the gastrointestinal tract: revisiting the literature for novel applications. Eur J Pharm Biopharm. 2005;60:1–16. https://doi.org/10.1016/j.ejpb.2005.01.007.

31. McGinty S, Pontrelli G. A general model of coupled drug release and tissue absorption for drug delivery devices. J Control Release. 2015;217:327–36. https://doi.org/10.1016/j.jconrel.2015.09.025.

32. Smart JD. Theories of mucoadhesion. In: Mucoadhesive mater drug delivery systems. Chichester: Wiley; 2014. p. 159–74. https://doi.org/10.1002/9781118794203.ch07.

33. Ugwoke MI, Agu RU, Verbeke N, Kinget R. Nasal mucoadhesive drug delivery: background, applications, trends and future perspectives. Adv Drug Deliv Rev. 2005;57:1640–65. https://doi.org/10.1016/j.addr.2005.07.009.

34. Cheng Y, Jiao X, Zhao L, Liu Y, Wang F, Wen Y, Zhang X. Wetting transition in nanochannels for biomimetic free-blocking on-demand drug transport. J Mater Chem B. 2018;6:6269–77. https://doi.org/10.1039/C8TB01838C.

35. Ebrahimi M. Standardization and regulation of biomaterials. In: Handbook biomater. biocompat.: Elsevier; United Kingdom 2020. p. 251–65. https://dokumen.pub/handbook-of-biomaterials-biocompatibility-woodhead-publishing-series-in-biomaterials-1nbsped-0081029675-9780081029671.html.

36. Hua S. Advances in nanoparticulate drug delivery approaches for sublingual and buccal administration. Front Pharmacol. 2019;10:1328. https://doi.org/10.3389/fphar.2019.01328.

37. Morales JO, Brayden DJ. Buccal delivery of small molecules and biologics: of mucoadhesive polymers, films, and nanoparticles. Curr Opin Pharmacol. 2017;36:22–8. https://doi.org/10.1016/j.coph.2017.07.011.

38. Hua S, de Matos MBC, Metselaar JM, Storm G. Current trends and challenges in the clinical translation of nanoparticulate nanomedicines: pathways for translational development and commercialization. Front Pharmacol. 2018;9:790. https://doi.org/10.3389/fphar.2018.00790.

39. Zhang GGZ, Law D, Schmitt EA, Qiu Y. Phase transformation considerations during process development and manufacture of solid oral dosage forms. Adv Drug Deliv Rev. 2004;56:371–90. https://doi.org/10.1016/j.addr.2003.10.009.

40. Nokhodchi A, Raja S, Patel P, Asare-Addo K. The role of oral controlled release matrix tablets in drug delivery systems. Bioimpacts. 2012;2:175–87. https://doi.org/10.5681/bi.2012.027.

41. Vivien-Castioni N, Gurny R, Baehni P, Kaltsatos V. Salivary fluoride concentrations following applications of bioadhesive tablets and mouthrinses. Eur J Pharm Biopharm. 2000;49:27–33. https://doi.org/10.1016/s0939-6411(99)00041-7.

42. Timur SS, Yüksel S, Akca G, Şenel S. Localized drug delivery with mono and bilayered mucoadhesive films and wafers for oral mucosal infections. Int J Pharm. 2019;559:102–12. https://doi.org/10.1016/j.ijpharm.2019.01.029.

43. Kockisch S, Rees GD, Young SA, Tsibouklis J, Smart JD. Polymeric microspheres for drug delivery to the oral cavity: an in vitro evaluation of mucoadhesive potential. J Pharm Sci. 2003;92:1614–23. https://doi.org/10.1002/jps.10423.

44. Boddupalli BM, Mohammed ZNK, Nath RA, Banji D. Mucoadhesive drug delivery system: an overview. J Adv Pharm Technol Res. 2010;1:381–7. https://doi.org/10.4103/0110-5558.76436.

45. Karki S, Kim H, Na S-J, Shin D, Jo K, Lee J. Thin films as an emerging platform for drug delivery. Asian J Pharm Sci. 2016;11:559–74. https://doi.org/10.1016/j.ajps.2016.05.004.

46. Aslani A, Rostami F. Medicated chewing gum, a novel drug delivery system. J Res Med Sci. 2015;20:403–11. http://www.ncbi.nlm.nih.gov/pubmed/26109999.

47. Fini A, Bergamante V, Ceschel GC. Mucoadhesive gels designed for the controlled release of chlorhexidine in the oral cavity. Pharmaceutics. 2011;3:665–79. https://doi.org/10.3390/pharmaceutics3040665.

48. ClinicalTrials.gov U.S. National Library of Medicine, dexamethasone to treat oral lichen planus, 2008. https://clinicaltrials.gov/ct2/show/NCT00111072.

49. ClinicalTrials.gov U.S. National Library of Medicine, study of the safety of BEMA™ fentanyl use for breakthrough pain in cancer subjects on chronic opioid therapy, 2012. https://clinicaltrials.gov/ct2/show/NCT00293020.

50. Giralt J, Tao Y, Kortmann R-D, Zasadny X, Contreras-Martinez J, Ceruse P, de la Vega FA, Lalla RV, Ozsahin EM, Pajkos G, Mazar A, Attali P, Bossi P, Vasseur B, Sonis S, Henke M, Bensadoun R-J. Randomized phase 2 trial of a novel clonidine mucoadhesive buccal tablet for the amelioration of oral mucositis in patients treated with concomitant chemoradiation therapy for head and neck cancer. Int J Radiat Oncol Biol Phys. 2020;106:320–8. https://doi.org/10.1016/j.ijrobp.2019.10.023.

51. ClinicalTrials.gov U.S. National Library of Medicine, efficacy and safety study of clonidine Lauriad® to treat oral mucositis, 2017. https://clinicaltrials.gov/ct2/show/NCT01385748.

52. ClinicalTrials.gov U.S. National Library of Medicine, a study to evaluate the efficacy of MuGard for the amelioration of oral mucositis in head and neck cancer patients (MuGard), 2013. https://clinicaltrials.gov/ct2/show/NCT01283906.

53. Allison RR, Ambrad AA, Arshoun Y, Carmel RJ, Ciuba DF, Feldman E, Finkelstein SE, Gandhavadi R, Heron DE, Lane SC, Longo JM, Meakin C, Papadopoulos D, Pruitt DE, Steinbrenner LM, Taylor MA, Wisbeck WM, Yuh GE, Nowotnik DP, Sonis ST. Multi-institutional, randomized, double-blind, placebo-controlled trial to assess the efficacy of a mucoadhesive hydrogel (MuGard) in mitigating oral mucositis symptoms in patients being treated with chemoradiation therapy for cancers of the head and neck. Cancer. 2014;120:1433–40. https://doi.org/10.1002/cncr.28553.

54. ClinicalTrials.gov U.S. National Library of Medicine, clinical effect of phenytoin mucoadhesive paste on wound healing after oral biopsy, 2012. https://clinicaltrials.gov/ct2/show/NCT01680042.

55. Ghalayani P, Emami H, Pakravan F, Nasr Isfahani M. Comparison of triamcinolone acetonide mucoadhesive film with licorice mucoadhesive film on radiotherapy-induced oral mucositis: a randomized double-blinded clinical trial. Asia Pac J Clin Oncol. 2017;13:e48–56. https://doi.org/10.1111/ajco.12295.

56. ClinicalTrials.gov U.S. National Library of Medicine, comparing triamcinolone acetonide mucoadhesive films with licorice mucoadhesive films, 2014. https://clinicaltrials.gov/ct2/show/NCT02075749.

57. ClinicalTrials.gov U.S. National Library of Medicine, comparison of triamcinolone acetonide mucoadhesive film and licorice mucoadhesive film effect on lichen planus, 2015. https://www.clinicaltrials.gov/ct2/show/NCT02453503.

58. ClinicalTrials.gov U.S. National Library of Medicine, efficacy and safety of forrad® for the management of radiation-induced mucositis in patients with nasopharyngeal carcinoma receiving IMRT, (2016). https://clinicaltrials.gov/ct2/show/NCT02735317.

59. ClinicalTrials.gov U.S. National Library of Medicine, efficacy of curcumin in oral submucous fibrosis (ECOSMF), 2018. https://clinicaltrials.gov/ct2/show/NCT03511261.

60. Hazarey VK, Sakrikar AR, Ganvir SM. Efficacy of curcumin in the treatment for oral submucous fibrosis – a randomized clinical trial. J Oral Maxillofac Pathol. 2015;19:145–52. https://doi.org/10.4103/0973-029X.164524.

61. ClinicalTrials.gov U.S. National Library of Medicine, efficacy of a dietary supplement (Aqualief®) in xerostomic patients (Aqualief), 2018. https://clinicaltrials.gov/ct2/show/NCT03612414.

62. ClinicalTrials.gov U.S. National Library of Medicine, dexamethasone solution for the treatment of oral lichen planus, 2018. https://clinicaltrials.gov/ct2/show/NCT02850601.

63. ClinicalTrials.gov U.S. National Library of Medicine, Intra-oral treatment of OLP with Rivelin®-CLO patches, 2020. https://clinicaltrials.gov/ct2/show/NCT03592342.

64. ClinicalTrials.gov U.S. National Library of Medicine, effects of Aqualief® in patients with xerostomia as consequence of radiotherapy for head and neck cancer, 2020. https://clinicaltrials.gov/ct2/show/NCT03601962.
65. Braga FTMM, Santos ACF, Bueno PCP, Silveira RCCP, Santos CB, Bastos JK, Carvalho EC. Use of Chamomilla recutita in the prevention and treatment of oral mucositis in patients undergoing hematopoietic stem cell transplantation: a randomized, controlled, phase II clinical trial. Cancer Nurs. 2015;38:322–9. https://doi.org/10.1097/NCC.0000000000000194.
66. ClinicalTrials.gov U.S. National Library of Medicine, Topical chamomile in preventing chemotherapy-induced oral mucositis, 2020. https://clinicaltrials.gov/ct2/show/NCT04317183.
67. ClinicalTrials.gov U.S. National Library of Medicine, Carnosine supplementation on quantity/ quality of oral salivae (PHoral), 2020. https://www.clinicaltrials.gov/ct2/show/NCT04295525.
68. Menon K, Mousa A, de Courten B. Effects of supplementation with carnosine and other histidine-containing dipeptides on chronic disease risk factors and outcomes: protocol for a systematic review of randomised controlled trials. BMJ Open. 2018;8:e020623. https://doi.org/10.1136/bmjopen-2017-020623.
69. ClinicalTrials.gov U.S. National Library of Medicine, MucoLox formulation to mitigate mucositis symptoms in head/neck cancer, 2020. https://clinicaltrials.gov/ct2/show/NCT03461354.
70. Bhagavan HN, Chopra RK. Plasma coenzyme Q10 response to oral ingestion of coenzyme Q10 formulations. Mitochondrion. 2007;7(Suppl):S78–88. https://doi.org/10.1016/j.mito.2007.03.003.
71. ClinicalTrials.gov U.S. National Library of Medicine, Clinical and biochemical assessment of the effect of topical use of coenzyme Q10 versus topical corticosteroid in management of symptomatic oral lichen planus: randomized controlled clinical trial, 2019. https://clinicaltrials.gov/ct2/show/NCT04091698.
72. Wen H, Jung H, Li X. Drug delivery approaches in addressing clinical pharmacology-related issues: opportunities and challenges. AAPS J. 2015;17:1327–40. https://doi.org/10.1208/s12248-015-9814-9.
73. Edsman K, Hägerström H. Pharmaceutical applications of mucoadhesion for the non-oral routes. J Pharm Pharmacol. 2005;57:3–22. https://doi.org/10.1211/0022357055227.
74. Sudhakar Y, Kuotsu K, Bandyopadhyay AK. Buccal bioadhesive drug delivery–a promising option for orally less efficient drugs. J Control Release. 2006;114:15–40. https://doi.org/10.1016/j.jconrel.2006.04.012.
75. Steward A, Bayley DL, Howes C. The effect of enhancers on the buccal absorption of hybrid (BDBB) α-interferon. Int J Pharm. 1994;104:145–9. https://doi.org/10.1016/0378-5173(94)90189-9.
76. Himanshi T, Sachdeva R. Transdermal drug delivery system: a review. Int J Pharm Sci Res. 2016; https://doi.org/10.13040/IJPSR.0975-8232.7(6).2274-90.
77. Das NG, Das SK. Development of mucoadhesive dosage forms of buprenorphine for sublingual drug delivery. Drug Deliv. 2004;11:89–95. https://doi.org/10.1080/10717540490280688.
78. Kováčik A, Kopečná M, Vávrová K. Permeation enhancers in transdermal drug delivery: benefits and limitations. Expert Opin Drug Deliv. 2020;17:145–55. https://doi.org/10.1080/17425247.2020.1713087.
79. Maher S, Brayden D, Casettari L, Illum L. Application of permeation enhancers in oral delivery of macromolecules: an update. Pharmaceutics. 2019;11:41. https://doi.org/10.3390/pharmaceutics11010041.

Index

© Springer Nature Switzerland AG 2021
R. El Assal et al. (eds.), *Early Detection and Treatment of Head & Neck
Cancers*, https://doi.org/10.1007/978-3-030-69852-2

Printed in the United States
by Baker & Taylor Publisher Services